GAMES
DOCTORS
PLAY

GAMES
DOCTORS
PLAY

Edited by

CLAUDE A. FRAZIER, M.D.

Asheville, North Carolina

With Forewords by

Gladys M. Heldman

Editor, World Tennis

James D. Telfer, M.D.

Publisher, Rx Sports and Travel

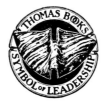

CHARLES C THOMAS • PUBLISHER

Springfield • Illinois • U.S.A.

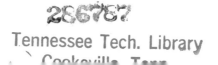

Published and Distributed Throughout the World by
CHARLES C THOMAS • PUBLISHER
Bannerstone House
301-327 East Lawrence Avenue, Springfield, Illinois, U.S.A.

© *1973, by* CHARLES C THOMAS • PUBLISHER

ISBN 0–398–02586–X

Library of Congress Catalog Card Number: 72–87000

With THOMAS BOOKS *careful attention is given to all details of manufacturing and design. It is the Publisher's desire to present books that are satisfactory as to their physical qualities and artistic possibilities and appropriate for their particular use.* THOMAS BOOKS *will be true to those laws of quality that assure a good name and good will.*

Printed in the United States of America

BB-14

I dedicate this book to the people with whom I have so often enjoyed playing tennis.

To Kay Frazier, my wife, David Henderson, my nephew, Calvin Frazier, my brother and my friend, Jim Woollcott—all challenging opponents.

To Jim Hamilton, Ronald C. Wilson, Norman Schellenger, Bretney Smith, Jr., Spaff Taylor, David Morgan, George Russell, Dell Sylvia, Hal Burrows, Jordan L. Maynard, Howard Hunt, Norman Jarrard, Dick Covington, Frank Fishburne, Bill Powell, Bobby Moore, Dick Frankel and Fred Farzanegan—all excellent, high-ranking tournament players.

CONTRIBUTORS

ARNOLD R. BEISSER, M.D.
Los Angeles, California

JOSEPH H. BELLINA, M.D.
New Orleans, Louisiana

JOHNNY A. BLUE, M.D.
Oklahoma City, Oklahoma

JACK BRAINARD, M.D.
Rochester, Minnesota

RICHARD L. BUTLER, M.D.
M.L.O.B.
Syracuse, New York

ARCHIE T. COFFEE, JR., M.D.
Charlotte, North Carolina

H. ROYER COLLINS, M.D.
Cleveland, Ohio

ROBERT P. CROUCH, M.D.
Asheville, North Carolina

AUGUST F. DARO, M.D.
Chicago, Illinois

PAUL DAVIDSON, M.D.
Morgantown, West Virginia

THOMAS N. DAVIS, III, M.D.
Lake Zurick, Illinois

DONALD B. FRANKEL, M.D.
Chicago, Illinois

KAY FRAZIER
Asheville, North Carolina

WILLIAM C. GRABB, M.D.
Ann Arbor, Michigan

JOHN B. GRAMLICH, M.D.
Cheyenne, Wyoming

TRAVIS C. GREEN, M.D.
Austin, Texas

JAMES P. HARNSBERGER, M.D.
Hot Springs, Virginia

WALDO E. HARRIS, M.D.
Portland, Oregon

ADRIAN C. KANAAR, M.D.
Poughkeepsie, New York

RUSSELL M. LANE, M.D.
Orono, Maine

DELANO MERIWETHER, M.D.
Boston, Massachusetts

GEORGE E. MOORE, M.D.
Buffalo, New York

WYLIE H. MULLEN, JR., M.D.
Joliet, Illinois

TIBOR NYILAS, M.D.
Elmhurst, New York

ALEXIUS RACHUN, M.D.
Ithaca, New York

EDWARD A. SHARPLESS, M.D.
Greensboro, North Carolina

ROBERT J. SPENCER, M.D.
Rochester, Minnesota

W. W. WALKER, M.D.
Gastonia, North Carolina

FOREWORD

Claude A. Frazier is a doctor, tennis player and humorist with whom I have been corresponding for a decade. Ten years ago he submitted a humorous article for publication in *World Tennis*. I wrote back to say we were holding it for possible future use, and the article was then put in the "hold" file. Numerous letters were exchanged as to the date when the article would first see print, and after several years of "holding," I regretfully informed Dr. Frazier that we would be unable to use it.

But Claude Frazier is more than just doctor, tennis player and humorist. He is also tenacious. After a quiescent period of two years, he resubmitted the article. Once again numerous letters on the subject were exchanged, with the article passing from my hands to his and back again. Again there was a lull of several years and again the article was resubmitted. By this time the file under "Frazier, Claude A." had become so bulky that I almost broke down and printed it.

After twenty-five years of experience with tennis playing doctors, I have discovered that many of them have the same attributes as Claude Frazier. They are witty, dedicated and tenacious. The following story illustrates not only their medical interest but their unlimited competitive instinct. The time was twenty-five years ago and the place was Rip's Tennis Courts in New York City (now the site of a tall Sutton Place apartment building). Court charges were very high at Rip's, and those of us who played there were either "on scholarship," stockbrokers, or doctors. It was an extremely hot day in midsummer, and I had been playing singles with a friend. I had managed to win the first set but was too exhausted to continue. We came into the little clubhouse and I fell into a chair, my face purple and my breath coming in short gasps.

A doctor friend came over to me, felt my forehead, took my pulse and remarked, "Gladys, you have sunstroke. Stay out of the sun for the rest of the day and for heaven's sake don't play any more tennis."

Fifteen minutes went by while I sat in the chair, still beet red but puffing less. Then the doctor stuck his head in the club-house door and said professionally,

"Hey, Gladys, we need a fourth."

GLADYS M. HELDMAN

FOREWORD

It doesn't seem too long ago that I remember reading the words of Francis Bacon that "Every man is a debtor to his profession." As a young rebel I felt that, while I owed my profession integrity and responsibility, I also did not desire to be indentured.

In relation to the Bacon dictum, I preferred to believe, in the words of the renowned Scottish poet Robert Burns, that something had gang a-gley. Musing on the title of Dr. Claude A. Frazier's book, "Games Doctors Play", I am reassured that I have followed the appropriate prescription.

My philosophy, accordingly, has been to establish a compatible mixture of business and recreational activities that blend into the 'toto homo'. Over the past six years, through the pleasant channel of Rx SPORTS and TRAVEL Magazine, I have had the welcome opportunity of meeting thousands of physicians and becoming acquainted with their varied leisure time pursuits.

There is an emphatic distinction between leisure and laziness. Leisure time, for a doctor, is simply the disposition of his hours and days when he is not ministering to the demands and responsibilities of his profession. Doctors are dedicated and responsive professionals whose vocation requires they devote long, concentrated hours to healing their fellow men.

To balance this intense humane application of the healing arts, doctors, like other citizens, need to relax and unwind or the overworked taut springs will deteriorate and break. To prevent this tragic occurrence, doctors should have a hobby, sports or recreational diversion which revives the mind, spirit and body after massing their energies and skills toward a healthy human race.

In sports, this expression of leisure time application is not to infer that doctors should become candidates for the Olympics or reach the summit of their sports accomplishments. Some have, and still do perform as champions—and I applaud them. But for the average doctor, sports or recreational participation means enjoyment on an amateur basis. And the key word here is enjoyment. The sports may differ, but if the result is enjoyment or competitive satisfaction, then the game has contributed its equivalent value.

As doctors' personalities and tastes differ, so also does their selection of games. Editor-Doctor Claude A. Frazier, whom I have known and appreciated for many years, has tackled and conquered a prodigious task in assembling the various categories of sports that doctors play. The range is extraordinary and every doctor who peruses this volume will attain the objective of the book's title—enjoyment, relaxation and pleasure.

JAMES D. TELFER, M.D.
Publisher
Rx SPORTS and TRAVEL Magazine

PREFACE

I was amazed and astounded at the variety of sports in which physicians not only participate but are outstanding. Many of them are more than outstanding—they are champions. This should not discourage the physician from joining in a sport, but rather entice him to find recreation and enjoyment in pursuing one.

Payne Thomas of Charles C Thomas, Publisher, has been enthusiastic about this book from the beginning. As I have received and read various chapters, I, too, have become very enthusiastic. I knew little about some of the sports, so I found these chapters informative as well as interesting.

At the request of Mr. Payne Thomas, my wife has consented to write a chapter. Kay is a champion in her own right. She is ranked in tennis in North Carolina, having won several tournaments. She ranks first with me.

The reader should know a little about the qualifications of the editor. Is he a champion in several different sports? The answer is no. Is he a great tennis player and a champion in tennis? In all humility, I must answer in the negative. (I gave this Preface to my wife to peruse and correct. In her haste she must have overlooked the preceding sentence.) I do enjoy various sports and have won a few trophies, but to be perfectly honest, I am not outstanding in any one particular sport. I enjoy tennis most of all and do play in tournaments when time and circumstance permit.

While attending college at West Virginia Institute of Technology, I won the table tennis tournament and played on the tennis team. The tennis trophies on my desk show that I have won some tournaments, but not against very stiff competition. When pitted against tough competition, I am slaughtered!

This brings to mind the places where I have played in tennis tournaments. The largest was in Lakeland, Florida, in the fall of 1970, where I finished in the finals of the senior doubles.

Some people like to go to a different place for each vacation. I have done this but always return to one favorite place in particular for a wonderful time—the *Homestead* in Hot Springs, Virginia. My wife and I have gone there to tennis tournaments more often than to any other place.

To my mind, it is the ideal place to go for a vacation, not only because tennis tournaments are held there, but because it is a great place to relax. There are so many activities available, i.e. fishing, swimming in the indoor or outdoor pool, bowling, horseback riding, skeet shooting, three fine golf courses, playground for children, indoor theatre and much more. One may wish to relax while reading on the spacious veranda, soaking in the hot springs after a tough tennis match, or listening to the music of the orchestra during dinner or afterwards in the lounge. More than all this, there is the warmth and friendliness

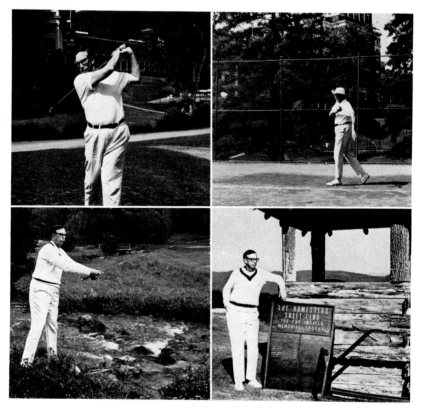

of the staff. Mr. Tom Lennon, President, Virginia Hot Springs, Inc., goes out of his way to make the guests feel at home. The *Homestead* has outstanding instructors in the various sports. Because of my interest in tennis I have come to know the tennis pro, Mr. Hal Burrows, an outstanding tennis player.

When I am there for a tennis tournament, I participate in other activities, too. I enjoy fishing in their well-stocked trout stream, swinging a golf club, shooting on the skeet range, and after a tennis match, soaking in the same warm springs that Thomas Jefferson used. One of my tennis partners once asked the attendant if the stones at the bottom of the pool were the same ones that Thomas Jefferson had stepped on. The attendant replied, "They are just a little smaller."

I feel that participation in a sport has been a blessing to me and allowed me to practice medicine more effectively. It has helped me to concentrate more fully on my writing. It has also fostered a closer family unity. A family that plays together, stays together.

I want to acknowledge the efficient help of my secretaries, Rosemarie Duda and Vivian Brotherton, who aided in the preparation of this manuscript.

CLAUDE A. FRAZIER

CONTENTS

GAMES
DOCTORS
PLAY

1

THE LOVE GAME

KAY FRAZIER

I have been asking myself for several weeks, as I considered how to write this chapter, Why me. Just why I have the privilege of contributing to this book, I am not exactly sure. Most editors' wives do not ordinarily contribute a chapter to a book. Since all of the other contributors are men, women's liberation crossed my mind, but since I am not wholeheartedly for this movement, I quickly discarded this thought. Recently, however, I found out that I am in fact writing because the publisher suggested it. He knows that I play tennis and he convinced my husband that a woman's point of view might add another dimension to the book. I am very flattered to be included.

Girls, do *you* feel included? I mean included in the sport which your husband enjoys. Do you participate together in a sport? If not, it is not too late to begin. If lack of time is your excuse, it likely is not a valid one, as one can usually find time to do what she really wishes to do.

I work full time in my husband's office as office manager, manage our busy household, and still have time for my favorite sport.

It has been said that there is more leisure time in America today than ever before in history. Man's lifespan is longer and his workspan shorter. So is woman's for that matter! The ability to play becomes vitally important under these conditions. The child who learns how to play, presumably becomes the adult

NOTE: Thank you Verna, Kathleen, Sicka, Kitty, Elma, Sarah, Ginny, and my many other tennis-playing friends for the many hours of fun and pleasure on the courts.

who knows how to play. He can move into old age more calmly and more confidently than the untrained. He can keep his interest alive until the very end, living fully all the days of his life in contrast to those who sit empty-handed, empty-minded, filled with a loneliness they have no means to combat. Has not each of use seen retired persons who fall into this latter category?

I play women's doubles regularly with a woman in her seventies. She is active, alert and an excellent tennis player. She is one of my favorite partners but also can be one of my most formidable opponents.

Creative play is not a sin, nor is it a luxury as some would have us believe. It is a companion and helpmate of work, and just as necessary a part of everyday living.

Balance is always a valuable component of any program. Even nature is continually engaged in a struggle to maintain a proper balance, and when the balance is disturbed, disaster results. Man as a child of nature must regulate his life and keep all the elements in balance, or disaster, in one form or another, may result.

It was no dull-witted, inexperienced fool who first made the statement, "All work and no play makes Jack a dull boy." But even in his play Jack must maintain a balance to assure a sturdy and vigorous growth—mentally, socially, physically and spiritually. No one would argue the point that to derive the full benefits from our food we must participate in the business of eating. To sit at a laden table and watch others eat while we sit by neither satisfies our physical hunger nor does it nourish us. Yet in our leisure time, we delude ourselves into thinking that by watching others at play, whether in the ball field or in the concert hall, we find nourishment and satisfaction for our needs. It is true that there is a place in our lives for passive forms of recreation, but our major emphasis must be on participation. The most important type of participation to my mind is the type that requires physical exercise.

I have read that psychiatrists throughout the country are disturbed by an odd upsurge of troubled people. These people have no serious marital or monetary problems. Their health is good, their children reasonably obedient. They complain of feeling depressed; often they become violently irritated with others without reason. They lie awake at night, plagued by feelings of anxiety. What's wrong? One Boston psychiatrist said that these people are bored.

What causes boredom? If the laboratory psychologists are correct, it is deprivation of stimuli. In extreme experiments where persons are allowed to lie for days in a dark room, cut off from all stimuli including light and sound, near-psychotic reactions occurred. Absolute boredom can literally drive one crazy. But the boredom from which most of us suffer is much more moderate. It creeps up slowly, when routine becomes so familiar that it no longer stimulates our minds and imaginations.

It cannot be denied that there is a direct relationship between the emotional, spiritual and physical health of man. Boredom can contribute to mental deterioration of any or all of these three aspects of man's makeup.

The more complex our lives become—the higher our civilization, the more numerous our inventions—and the more we complicate our lives with labor-saving devices, the greater the need becomes to escape boredom. More than ever in social history, man must be prepared to meet the challenge of leisure.

What are we to do? There are numerous possibilities, but I will attempt to discuss only one aspect: *develop a hobby!*

The word "hobby" has been used too often only for that type of activity in which people make something with their hands or gather things together in collection. Often the activities so termed have been of such low quality that the word has acquired an almost unfavorable reputation and many turn up their noses at the mention of it and snort, "Bah, hobbies, they're for children."

Webster defines a hobby as a favored pursuit, which would make the choice of activities practically limitless. Hobbies actually cover more than the categories of making and collecting things. They include doing things and learning things as well. Seldom does any hobbyist begin in one category and remain there.

Whether the hobbyist pursues a doing, making, learning or collecting hobby is not so important as whether the individual has put his time to creative use. Leisure is one of our most precious assets. How we use this time can contribute to the development of our personal well-being.

The primary purpose of my writing this chapter is not to tell you that we have more leisure time than ever before or to convince you of the importance of escaping boredom or developing a hobby. The purpose is to tell you about my hobby and its place in my life.

There are a number of hobbies which I enjoy. I like to play table tennis, bridge and the piano as well as sew, oil paint and swim. I also like to talk: this summer I won first place at the International Toastmistress Speech Contest in Phoenix, Arizona, competing against sixteen other contestants. I became a member of the Asheville Toastmistress Club a few years ago, because I was shy of public speaking. It was a handicap which I have learned to overcome.

When referring to a hobby in this chapter, I wish to consider one which is more of a sport and which involves physical activity—this is my chief hobby, tennis. This game itself is not a new one but one which has been played for a long time.

Tennis has its origin in the ancient game of handball, played in Greece long before the Christian era. During the Middle Ages it developed into a game of batting the ball between two opponents rather than against a wall. At first there were no boundary lines but gradually a court was developed, first in the shape of an hourglass and later into the rectangular shape we now have.

The early ball was made of leather and stuffed with hair. For protection in hitting the ball, a glove was worn. Then for greater protection, the cords were wrapped around the glove. Later an elongated paddle was used. With the need for a longer reach, the idea of a racket evolved from the combination of paddle and cords.

In the Middle Ages, the game was carried to England where it was played by the nobility. Not until the late 19th century, when the scoring and rules became simplified, did the common people become interested in the game. It soon became a more universal game in England and France, spreading rapidly to the colonies. Tennis was brought to the U.S. in 1875, by Mary Outerbridge, after a visit to Bermuda where the game was very popular. She brought racquets, net and balls and introduced the game to her friends on Staten Island. The game spread like wildfire over the East.

In 1881, the U.S. Lawn Tennis Association was formed in New York and Boston. Through this organization, the popularity of tennis spread even more.

How does one learn to play tennis? The chief factors are these—first, practice, second, practice, third, practice. One cannot learn by just going out occasionally to play for fun. He should first take lessons and learn the correct strokes from the very beginning—otherwise, many bad habits can soon be acquired which can take many extra hours to correct. Concentration is very important. One should keep his thoughts on the game and try to outsmart his opponent. Good footwork is important. In tennis the ball never comes in the same direction, at the same height, nor does it bounce in the same spot twice in succession. A tennis player is constantly busy moving all over the court during the entire game and mobility is essential.

Tennis is a game not only of skill but of stamina. Being in good physical condition is essential. A tournament match can last as long as two to four hours or longer in the heat of the day.

The game of tennis is most easily learned by a youngster, beginning preferably around the age of eight or nine years. Apparently, this is true in the learning of most sports. I was not so young when I began to play tennis. In fact, on our honeymoon I sat contentedly on the sideline of the tennis court and watched my husband play in a mixed doubles match: I had not yet become an active participant.

I have since learned to participate in this sport—not through self-motivation, but because of the encouragement and prodding of my husband, Claude. It was his idea in the early years of our marriage that we participate in a sport together. Since tennis had been for many years his preference, there was no question in his mind that this would be the game I would learn.

He began instructing me by standing at the net and throwing the ball to me to return. At first, I would either miss the ball entirely, or when I hit it, send it into the net or over the fence. Rarely would it go into the proper court, but when it did, Claude encouraged my confidence with praise. The next step he took was to hit the ball to me with his tennis racket instead of throwing it to me. One small step followed another in my learning process.

What a demonstration of patience Claude has exhibited. Any husband who has tried to instruct his wife in anything will immediately know what I mean. I was not always the "willing" pupil—in fact I was very obstinate and uncooperative at times. It was my position of wife, I suppose, that made me take out my frustrations on my husband.

I give Claude 90 percent of the credit for my learning to play tennis to the extent that it has become fun and not just work. When we went on vacations, he always encouraged me to take lessons from the tennis professionals, if one was anywhere nearby.

When I lacked confidence to ask another woman for a tennis match, my husband would arrange a game for me. In order to give me practice, he many times made me volley with his opponent to "warm him up" for their match.

After about two summers of intense encouragement and instruction from my husband, the "tennis bug" finally bit me. My husband wrote a textbook entitled, *Insect Allergy,* the first and only one of its kind. If I were to be technical, he no doubt would tell me there is no such insect as a "tennis bug." But it did bite me and I am not allergic to it. After this, I did not have to be asked twice to play. I was always ready and if no one was available to face me across the net, I would hit against the backboard. My best and most profitable competition during my early training stage were the young high school boys at a public park. They were eager to make the tennis team and the more practice they had, the better was their chance. They were always eager for a game even if their opposition was a female. Of course, games with other women, tennis clinics and reading many books on the subject of tennis were also helpful.

It was not until I began to enter tournaments and have a few wins behind me that I began to develop confidence. Confidence is a *must* in tennis if one wishes to be on the winning side.

I have not yet become good enough to beat my husband in a game, and furthermore I never will. Oh, I have tried and have even gone so far as to distract him enough to break his concentration. I can get a few points and perhaps a game or two, but never can I win a set. If I ever reached the point at which I *could* do so (no danger of this), I *would* not. I have had enough psychology courses in my college career to know that this is one situation I wish to avoid.

Tennis is not a game about which one learns everything in a few lessons. It is a game in which the person continues to learn for as long as he participates. Perfecting basic strokes, learning new strokes and tactics and keeping in good physical condition are the keys to making it truly a fun game. Even though I now have been playing for a number of years, I still need professional lessons to smooth out my game. Claude has continued to be my best and most severe critic. I constantly need encouragement from him to improve my court play.

In regard to keeping in good physical condition, I have found that jumping rope each day for a certain period of time is the best training away from the court. This helps to increase my stamina and aids me in covering the tennis court with more speed and alertness.

The rewards of my learning the game of tennis have been many. Foremost is physical well-being. A good tennis match is exhilarating. This is strictly a selfish reward, but it should be pointed out. Those with whom I come in contact will also benefit from this. My husband and I are appreciative of the fact that it makes it easier for us to get along with each other (unless of course we lost in a tournament).

After completing a busy day at the office, many times I am mentally and physically exhausted. After a quick trip from the office to the tennis courts for a couple of sets of vigorous tennis, I can return home completely refreshed; I am physically tired, but yet I feel relaxed, because mentally, I feel great!

The game of tennis has contributed to Claude's and my

marital happiness. It is something we can enjoy together. I often come in contact with tennis or golf "widows" whose husbands participate in a sport with which the wives are not involved. Perhaps most would say that this is by choice, but I am not so sure. For example, I could very easily have become a tennis "widow." It is undeniable that this similar interest of ours has strengthened our relationship.

Our most exciting vacations are those centered around a tennis tournament. We seldom leave home without packing our tennis gear; a tennis court at the hotel is a *must*, even when we go away on a business trip.

Naturally a tennis tournament is at times tense, but this setting can greatly improve one's game. At no other time on the courts do I concentrate so intently. These tournaments have been rewarding in other ways. With a great deal of work and a little luck, both my husband and I have added a number of trophies to our collection.

This leads to another important reward—meeting and becoming acquainted with other enthusiastic tennis players. I have made friends all over the world because of this mutual interest. One of our most exciting mixed doubles matches was a few years ago in Paris against a French couple who could not speak English. The game was arranged by the tennis professional at the tennis club. The *only* barrier which existed was the language one.

We so often hear today of the generation gap. Tennis can be a way for parents to bridge this gap with their children through mutual interest and respect for each other. It can work in any adult-youngster relationship. For example, I recently was in a finals match against a ranked junior tennis player. We have practiced against each other on several occasions and have become good friends. This has also occurred with other junior players.

There is little doubt in my mind that the game of tennis represents the ultimate in individual sports. You golf, swimming, boxing or bowling enthusiasts might consider these following facts. Tennis is international and can be played by both sexes the world over. It is a game the entire family can enjoy. It is relatively inexpensive. It requires skill and speed. It requires tremendous and undivided powers of concentration. It requires courage and the will to win. It offers a sufficient amount of exercise. It breeds sportsmanship, because the game calls for courtesy, a minimum of temperament and no alibis.

To add the new zest to life, I challenge you to wait no longer than today to begin tennis lessons. Better still, get your husband to join you. It can be a game of love.

2

TENNIS

EDWARD A. SHARPLESS

Tennis is for you. If you are old enough to read, but young enough to enjoy watching a pretty girl, if you are reasonably sound of mind and body and your arches have not completely collapsed in a heap of bone and cartilage, you ought to give it a try. It is an excellent sport for a young doctor. It is relatively inexpensive and can be enjoyed equally at the country club or in the city park. It keeps you trim, and it is a good way to meet girls. It is also an excellent sport for the busy doctor in his middle years. It provides relief from the tensions of a busy practice, and can provide just the right amount of exercise with only sixty to ninety minutes out of a busy schedule. In many cases it can be played year-round, indoors or outdoors, at night as well as during the day. For the older doctor approaching or even past retirement age it is still the sport. It provides good exercise for those stiff joints and sore bones, and it can help to keep that expanding waistline in check. They now have tournaments for those who are interested, starting with the ten year olds and under, all the way up to the 65 and over group.

The game has grown enormously in popularity in the past few years. Part of this is no doubt due to the increased coverage on TV. Also, thankfully, the sport is breaking some of its ties with the country club, which it must do to become a great national sport. Courts are springing up all over towns and cities, and the game is becoming more popular with the young people of both sexes and all races. The realization that it is one of the few sports which can be enjoyed by both both young and old has helped. Finally, the growing emphasis on exercise and weight control for maintaining good health has stimulated the interest in a universal sport, and many have latched onto tennis as the answer.

The game has been played on many different surfaces over the years. It all started on grass (lawn tennis), and since has been played on various types of clay or composition surfaces, on a variety of hardtop surfaces such as concrete, plastic, asphalt and Lay-kold®; and on carpet and canvas, especially indoors. Of these, the most serviceable and popular have been composition-clay courts and hard courts, and most courts today represent one of these types. Composition surfaces are probably the most popular, especially among the older players. The court is easy on the legs and feet, the bounce of the ball is relatively slow, and the game itself is slower paced with more emphasis on a well-rounded game utilizing all of the shots. Court maintenance is more of a problem though, and often the court cannot be used through the winter. Also, the court can really only be used for tennis. Many younger players, and some older ones, too, prefer hard courts. These surfaces are gaining in popularity and there are probably more new hard courts being constructed than any other kind. Because of a variety of new types of court construction material these can be installed quickly, easily and relatively inexpensively. They are practically maintenance free and they can be made to have a slower or faster bounce within certain limits depending on the smoothness or roughness of the surface. Lines merely need to be painted on. Furthermore, the game is generally a hard, fast type of play with few bad bounces. Those who prefer the power game usually prefer courts of this type.

The game can be played in three different ways, sometimes for quite different reasons. The three types of play are singles, doubles and mixed doubles. Each has its own personality and its own set of strategies. Try each and decide for yourself which you prefer.

SINGLES

Singles play is the backbone of the game. Everyone must play singles at some time if he is to be much of a player. Singles has the most interest for young people because it is the most vigorous way to play the game. It is also the simplest and purest form of tennis competition. Unquestionably, from a spectator's point of view singles *is* the game of tennis. Here most clearly is the drama of competition, the one-against-one spectacle of antagonist and protagonist. It most clearly portrays the competitive instinct that is in us all, the instinct which compels us to watch bullfighting, boxing, and even tournament golf. Singles play has another facet which should not be overlooked. It is a physically demanding sport that requires a significant amount of conditioning. Dr. Kenneth Cooper, in his book *Aerobics,* states that tennis is a relatively poor way of achieving and maintaining real physical conditioning (compared to jogging, cycling, swimming and so on). The health benefits from a program of physical activity are agreed on by most medical authorities. Dr. Cooper, for the first time, has scientifically calibrated various forms of exercise with physical conditioning. If one is able to adhere to one of Dr. Cooper's training schedules, one should indeed benefit from it. The rub is that few of us have the determination to adhere to one of his schedules. Aside from the handball/squash/basketball schedule, there is little enjoyment in his programs, unless you happen to enjoy running two to five miles, cycling 12 to 30 miles, or swimming some 3500 yards per week. If, however, one can play four to five hours of tennis mixed in with some running or cycling or even walking in a week, one can achieve an equivalent effect. Or if you can get the time, about seven to eight hours of singles tennis per week will achieve the same thing with no extra running, swimming, etc. I play tennis first and foremost because I love it, but I do not consider the health benefits to be negligible. I play singles because it is an excellent exercise, and it keeps me in good shape. My singles game is comparable to that of Little Orphan Annie, so it is certain that I am not in it for the money or trophies.

Singles does offer the player more. Since it is the purest form of tennis, it requires the highest degree of proficiency in all shots. True championship tennis on grass or hard courts is largely a game of serve, volley and smash. Some of our best players have risen to the top of the tennis heap on these three shots plus a modicum of service-return ability. The late John F. Kenfield, for many years the coach of the University of North Carolina tennis team, used to say that Victor Sexais, America's best singles player in 1951 and 1954, had a "sorry lot" of ground strokes (backhand and forehand strokes). Mr. Kenfield loved to talk about Vic, his most famous pupil, and I suspect that there was an element of tongue-in-cheek in his remarks. I remember thinking at the time that if Vic's ground strokes were "sorry," mine must have been unmentionable. It is true, though, that Vic was the best in his day largely because he played a superb power game of serve and volley tennis, and this type of game best fit the predominately grass surfaces of that day. When the average player plays singles, however, it becomes a game of serve and service return, of backhand and forehand, of drop shot and lob, and to a lesser extent volley and overhead smash. The good singles player must be well-rounded. Once on the singles court, he has no place to hide. If he has a weakness, his opponent will surely exploit it. Singles forces one to sharpen-up his game. Even when we arrive at the age when we feel that singles is too strenuous for a regular diet, we must play some singles just to stay in tune.

Let me add a word of caution. Singles can be an extremely taxing form of exercise, and especially as one grows older, one should not play strenuous singles on an infrequent basis. Nor should one go out on the first day of spring and play five tough sets after a long winter lay-off. Aside from the obvious stresses and strains placed on muscles and joints which are not in condition, the danger of a heart attack or fatal arrhythmia is probably considerable when the sport is approached on these terms. Thankfully in many areas tennis can now be played on a year-round basis, or at least the winter lay-off can be minimized. Also, if possible, the game of tennis should be combined with some other form of exercise such as calisthenics, weight lifting and running or cycling so that one can maintain a year-round training effect. Let us hope that the winter lay-off is a thing of the past. We should not forget the yearly physical examination either, which hopefully will include an exercise electrocardiogram. This may be the only simple test for a potentially dangerous degree of atherosclerosis of the coronary arteries of the heart. There have been a number of recorded examples of fatal "heart attacks" (probably mostly arrhythmias) which have occurred during or just after jogging or other types of physical exercise. Presumably many of these could have been avoided by a physical examination which included an exercise electrocardiogram.

Tactics for singles play vary considerably according to the sex, age and ability of the players, and to the type of court surface and sometimes other external conditions of play (such as night play, windy conditions and so on). Ideally the younger player who is in good shape and who is reasonably proficient in his stroke production will attempt to storm the net where it is easier to win the point. This is the basic tactic of the championship serve and volley game. The server follows his serve into the net, parrying the service return into the corners of the court. Once at the net he is in position to volley or smash away the opponent's returns. On a slower court surface, such as clay-composition, most players are not able to follow their serves in to the net every time. They must play a more cautious game, waiting for a weak return shot to gain the net behind a hard, well-placed approach shot. Always, though, the strokes of both players are oriented toward an eventual net rush. The one who gains the net position first feels an advantage, and provided his strokes are going properly, he will win the point. In this type of game the basic forehand and backhand ground strokes are less important. The forehand and backhand strokes can never be ignored, however; for one thing the service must be returned. If one's backhand is weak, he will find most of the opponent's shots, including the services, coming to his backhand. On slow courts, at night and with both older and very young players, the basic forehand and backhand strokes are the important part of the game. There are long exchanges of ground strokes from the back court, and the net is approached only when a good forcing shot is made. Some players with a weakness in their serve, volley or overhead, hardly ever come to the net. The defensive player who spurns net play may go far in the game, and he may win many matches, but there is usually an aggressive net rusher somewhere who can beat him. The power game should be the ideal for all boys learning the game and some of the girls, too. Few girls, though, seem to develop the power serve and volley game the way men do. Perhaps the strenuous rushes to the net and the requirement for a good overhead smash and volley are too taxing for the average woman. Perhaps the female philosophy of caution and control is responsible. Whatever the reason, women usually prefer basic back court tennis to the power game.

DOUBLES

Doubles play is somewhat different. Some players consider doubles important only after they have been put out of the singles event in a tournament. Some characters, myself among them, prefer doubles from the very beginning. By the very nature of the game it is a team effort, and for some this makes it attractive. For others the team aspect makes it repellent. Some excellent singles players cannot cut it in doubles and some will not even play. Other players who can hardly beat a well-coordinated chimpanzee in singles find themselves winning at doubles. There is no one explanation for this seeming paradox. Some who prefer doubles just do not like to be all alone out there on the court. Some who choose singles cannot put up with a partner's mistakes, and so prefer to make it or lose on their own. There are others who can hit one, two, or even three or more good shots in succession, but as the returns keep coming back, their efforts become more frantic. They start to think about the likelihood of an error, and naturally they themselves make the errors. This type of person does better in doubles, because, first of all, he has a partner with whom to share shots. In fact, this type of player may complement his partner by forcing setups that his partner can put away, shots that he himself might miss.

Also, it is easier to hide a weakness on the doubles court. If your backhand is weak, for example, it is easier to run around it in doubles play since the court you patrol is smaller. Another trick is to put your weak backhand in the middle of the court where your partner can take the shots coming into this area. Eventually a shot will come to your weakness. When it does, fake it one time with a hard purposeful swing. If the fates are on your side, it may go for a winner, and your opponents may never hit you that shot again all day.

While singles is the ideal of young boys, men and women are usually more turned on by doubles. For one thing, the "He can run, but he can't hide" philosophy is less applicable to doubles. One runs and hides and lobs and bloops and connives, and tries all sorts of unconventional shots and techniques. It seems that the natural gamesmanship that adults seem to possess is more applicable to doubles play; call it subtlety or experience if you prefer. The harmless looking but devilish dink shot aimed at the opponent's feet; the tantalizing touch lob just out of reach of the net man; the well-aimed volley right at the net man's genitals—these are typical weapons of the thoughtful doubles player. The power singles player designs to use these crafty shots, at least until he is past 35 years old. Do not be misled, however; the doubles team with the Arthur Ashe serves, the Marty Reissen volleys, and the John Newcomb overhead smashes, is in good shape. All the craft, cunning and *Stephan Potter tactics* in existence will come to no avail, because when the chips are down, the power team will carry the day in doubles as surely as it will in singles. Perhaps it is the fact that the kids with the lethal strokes do not set foot on the doubles court as often. Maybe it is because the average 35-and-over doubles player has given up the impossible dream of Davis Cup play, and has let his game slide into the more devious approaches of doubles play. Whatever the reasons, facts are facts. For most more "mature adults" (dirty old men), singles is the game to keep his body and strokes in shape, doubles is the game to *play*.

The vocabulary for singles is relatively simple: forehand, backhand, serve, volley, smash and sometimes lob and drop shot. All of these strokes are also applicable to doubles play, but additionally such terms as poach, volley lob and dink shot may creep in. Formations are used to facilitate the netward rush, and frequently signals are used between partners to counteract certain effective shots of the opposition, and to break up their rhythm of play. There is more obvious intent in doubles play to upset the other team's balance, to break up their concentration. Because of this, the final outcome of a close match seems less predictable in doubles than in singles. You may find that after your team has won the first set relatively easily, the tide may turn. Whereas you may have felt like John Henry the steel driving man in the first set, you may now find yourself chasing lobs all over the place, and swinging at them with the grace of a pregnant goonie bird in a windstorm.

Many people underrate doubles. By the time the doubles play is ready to start on TV, coverage has shifted to putt-putt golf or Lassie or something equally salubrious to the Neilson ratings. Also, doubles matches traditionally follow singles matches, and the purses are a fraction of the singles winnings in professional matches. If a player is only able to play one match, and is scheduled to play both doubles and singles, nine times out of ten he will default in doubles and play singles. Then, too, singles trophies are bigger than doubles trophies. Those of us who play doubles seriously do not mind the slight. These are the facts of life. For us victory is still as sweet, and defeat is just as agonizing. It was pointed out to my nine-year-old daughter in the following way. She had only been playing the game for a year and a half, and was entered in her first doubles match. Her partner had won the singles, but they were beaten in the doubles by two girls the partner had demolished in singles. After the doubles match the conversation between my daughter and partner was as follows:

Partner: How long have you been playing tennis?
Daughter: (eagerly) Oh, about a year and a half.
Partner: No wonder you're so bad.

There it is. The agony of defeat and the difficulties of partnership summed up in a few words. Difficult though the stresses may be in doubles, they are 100 times worse in mixed doubles.

MIXED DOUBLES

Mixed doubles is really quite a bizarre affair. *Mixed-up* doubles is what some people call it. The majority of serious males who will sweat and strain for hours on the singles court will play doubles, sometimes only when nothing better is at hand. However, play mixed doubles? Nevermore. They would rather play a glockenspiel duet with Tiny Tim than get into one set of mixed doubles. To some it is like playing with a built-in handicap, like playing on roller skates, for example. Mixed doubles is like bringing your wives along to your Friday night poker game. It is unreal, and should never be approached as a serious sport. However, when viewed in its proper, somewhat psychotic perspective, it can be enormous fun for all.

The tactics in singles are straightforward and forceful, like a John Wayne movie. In doubles they are sometimes devious, like a Hitchcock thriller. In mixed doubles they are as logical and organized as the Keystone Cops. In the first place power tennis, which is exaulted in singles and is quite useful in doubles, has no place at all in mixed doubles. The Women's Liberation movement which is shaking the roots of our society has not yet made its way to the mixed doubles court. Accordingly it is considered extremely bad form to attempt to drill a new belly button in your female opponent who is standing primly at the net facing you on your service return. I once watched a mixed doubles match at Forest Hills between the Graebners and the Susmans where anything went. The men appeared positively homocidal as they bounced overheads and volleys off the female opposition. The girls did survive and, in fact, got in a few licks of their own. There are few players around who are the likes of Carole Graebner and Karen Susman, so for most of us the mixed doubles court is no place for an overt show of hostility. *Underhanded* and *backstabbing* tactics are quite all right, and in fact that's the game, but nothing *overt*. The best mixed doubles player in town is a scholarly looking college professor who hits devilish dipping soft forehands, and puny overheads which plop at the opposing women's feet. Whenever he gets a setup, he makes a big show of hitting a hard one at the opposing man, but the bread and butter points come via Machiavellian bloopers which the ladies cannot quite come up with.

But for most men, the mixed doubles court is a most confusing place. Some of their best shots—the jaw-jarring serve, the chest-crunching volley, and the skull-splitting overhead—are strictly forbidden. If the man forgets himself for a second and drives a service return through the net man (or rather the net girl) he must quickly follow with rounds of diplomatic apology for his "bad aim," lest he be burdened with guilt feelings, or worse, crowd disfavor. If he charges to the net behind a well placed serve like the book says to do in doubles, he will probably find himself chasing a better placed lob over his partner's head, and feeling like the idiot of the year while his partner looks on helplessly. Her look is a model of benign pity and seems to say, "You know I would chase that mean shot if I could dear, but since those three Caesarian sections I just cannot run like a young thing anymore."

In doubles the standard play is for both members of the team to be either at the net or in the backcourt. Never play with one man up and one man back. That formation went out with striped knickers. In mixed doubles, though, you can hardly be successful any other way. If you both play back, you allow the other team to charge to the net, take the offensive and pound the ball through you, over you or by you, or to drop shot you. If you both come up, you face the inevitable risk of chasing lobs over your partner's head until your knees wobble and your vision grows dim.

Also, in mixed doubles the women seem to have all the advantages. It would be similar to Notre Dame playing Slippery Rock in basketball. If Notre Dame won, who would notice, but if Slippery Rock were to luck out, the whole world would seem to have eyes glued on that event. In mixed doubles the man versus woman exchanges can be most embarrassing. If the innocent-appearing sweet thing with larceny in her heart makes you look bad a few times, you can rapidly blow your cool. Then you lose and are humiliated in the process. No wonder so many men are afraid of mixed doubles. It is really not all bad, though, and it *can* be lots of fun. Women always seem to enjoy mixed doubles, no problem. Men can too, if they can apply these simple ground rules:

1. Do not expect artistic tennis. Mixed doubles is more like pop art tennis.

2. Place the majority of your shots and all of your real zingers at the opposing man. Let your partner do the hatchet work on the other girl.

3. When you do hit a shot at the other female, hit softly with spin and aim for her feet whenever possible.

4. Serve hard to the opposing male and purposely much softer to the girl, but with spin. This makes you look like a good guy and still makes it difficult for her.

5. Stay in the back court most of the time and hit easy looping shots to both players much of the time. Let them hit the hard ones and make the errors, you had best play it cool.

6. Place your partner at the net whenever possible and let her hit anything she can reach, but you will have to do most of the real leg work. High loopers and lobs help you from getting out of position if the opposition persists in lobbing your partner.

7. If your male opponent stands at the net while his partner is serving, hit frequent lobs over his head. If you can hit touch lobs, they are almost sure points.

8. If you really need a point badly, drop shot the girl if she is back, or hit a "wild" medium speed zinger at her if she is at the net. Then apologize for your bad aim, provided you win the point.

9. Finally above all remember that it is only a game and that there is no substitute for good sportsmanship. If you lose, shake hands with your opponents and tell your partner you enjoyed playing with her and accept the blame for the defeat, secure in the knowledge that it was really her fault.

This then, I hope, explains why tennis is one of the "games doctors play." I think it is an ideal sport for practically everyone. I realize that in many really large cities, adequate facilities may not be available to everyone, especially in ghetto areas where play facilities tend to be inadequate and space is often not available. In some of these cases, basketball, baseball or touch football may be more realistic sports activities than tennis. Some cities though, like Philadelphia, apparently have programs to get ghetto children involved in tennis, and we should all hope that more of this will become available in the future.

For the busy doctor there is no problem. All he needs is a tennis court, dressing and shower facilities, and an opponent. He has the time to play at least five hours per week, or, if not he is working too hard, the lunch hour is a particularly good time since it both provides the needed exercise and it cuts down on food intake, two conditions which would benefit most Americans.

3

SNOW WHITE AND THE TENNIS DWARFS

RICHARD L. BUTLER

Tennis to the doctor is like chess to the soldier, and similarly it may save his sanity, perhaps his life, certainly his liberty, and will delightfully abet his pursuit of happiness.

To be specific, knowing ourselves to be without fault or fallacy, tennis diverts and divests those frustrations and hostilities of life caused by the ever present "witches and warlocks." It substitutes "Snow White"—an elastic hirsute varicolored sphere—to be pummelled, cut, smashed, and driven over an obstacle within reasonable bounds against an imaginary "witch-lock" apparition. She is then unceremoniously discarded without loss of dignity, life, limb, or temper.

Why should a doctor faced with many time demands and perhaps other avocations and social obligations choose tennis as his princess? The answer is rather simple: tennis is bad exercise*, good fun, takes little time, demands concentration away from "evil spells," allows frustrations to fly to the winds, and is tiring.

The rules, skills, practice requirements, and so forth, I leave to the professional books, but there are some facets that every doctor should know in order to get his most out of the "Snow White" game.

TENNIS COMMANDMENTS

1. Thou shalt play in the heat (older joints and tendons).
2. Thou shalt drink an electrolyte solution between sets. (1 pkg. limeade, ¼ cup sugar, ¾ tbsp. Ca^{++} Sucaryl, ⅜ tsp. salt mix— 6.00 gm NaCl, 2.00 gm $NaHCO_3$, 2.00 gm $KHCO_3$; H_2O q.s.a.d. 2 qts.)
3. Thou shalt wear loose clothes (avoid a bellyache).
4. Thou shalt get the lightest shoes thou canst find (tired legs).

---

* Perhaps the fact that tennis is rather bad exercise may seem surprising, but a look at aerobics and how far down the list tennis ranks as a conditioner leaves little room for doubt about this.

24

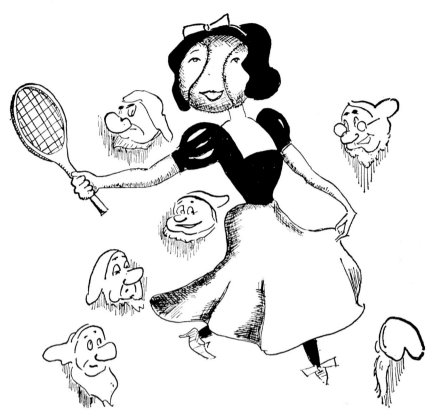

5. Thou shalt use the lightest, smallest gripped racquet thou canst find (only Charles Atlas uses a big, heavy one).
6. Thou shalt place a half-wet towel at the post for wiping and drying a slipping hand or bald pate (skin oil, not sweat, causes the racquet to move in your ungloved hand).
7. Thou shalt wear a golf glove to hold the racquet (particularly if a surgeon).
8. Thou shalt cover the balls of thy feet with benzoin and mole skin (no blisters).
9. Thou shalt find who thou canst beat and who thou canst not beat and play them alternately (no depression or false elation).
10. Thou shalt avoid tennis pecking orders and postmortems (artificial statures can be enervating).

The doctor/"Snow White" relationship is clearly abetted and compounded by dwarf opponents and partners. These being caricatures of mankind and perhaps providing a basic reason why tennis is so pleasantly necessary to the doctor. He can see, relate, understand, but in the game setting—the play if you will—need only transiently and amusingly burden himself with the following dwarfs:

> DOPEY—Wears high-top tennis shoes, trips over the tapes, hits the ball over the fences, and smiles vacuously about everything.
>
> GRUMPY—The net is never quite the right height and tapes not clean enough. He sticks absolutely to the rules (never leaves the court even under exhaustion), calls the balls a little close, and growls at your calls.
>
> HAPPY—Nothing bothers him, always says "good show," with a bad play; makes his opponent "take two," on an obviously bad serve; laughs hebephrenically when he misstrokes.
>
> SLEEPY—Delays the game for muscle strains or pulls; walks to receive each serve with his back towards his opponent turning around and holding up the game for the loose tape or twig on the court.
>
> DOC—Another physician who hates you for not sending him patients, always diagnosing your faulty play. He is to be avoided if at all possible.
>
> BASHFUL—Generously allows you to cover the whole court, is hesitant about stroking the ball and frequently double faults. He changes calls if looked at crossly, and he fears to perspire.
>
> SNEEZEY—Disconcerts his opponent and partner by sly, agitating motions; frequently throws serves up not striking them with the sun in his eyes; holds up a game with a cough, a little skip, tying his shoelace, or drops the ball on the court at an inappropriate moment.

No game a doctor plays would be complete without a brief perspective of its past and present. The origin of tennis, or more correctly lawn tennis, derived from the medieval sport, royal or court tennis. The original game combined qualities of both lawn tennis and squash. Field tennis was played as early as the 18th century and a game more nearly like lawn tennis by Lord Arthur Hervey later on. However, it was not until 1874 that Major Wingfield patented a game called Sphairistike which with only slight modifications developed into the game we know as lawn tennis and now abbreviate to tennis.

4

THE WORLD OF TABLE TENNIS

ROBERT P. CROUCH

My own interest in table tennis dates back to the end of World War II and the purchase of a secondhand table from a USO club that was closing. It became a basement relic but provided many hours of fun during high school days. During college and especially in medical school a table was always available. Even though crowded between rows of lockers, it was always in use at lunch and after school. Winners were always challenged so one was always under threat of losing his place at the table. After completion of medical school, my old sandpaper paddle was put up on a shelf never to be used again.

For Christmas, 1969, my number two son received a new tennis table. We put it on our large front porch which is walled on three sides. The fourth side is screened and has a southern exposure. Thus we developed a perfect spot for playing table tennis. Each day as I came home from work, regardless of how cold or hot or wet the weather or how exhausted I might be or how late it was in the evening, I was met by an eager, enthusiastic thirteen-year-old opponent who never seemed to tire. We managed to play three or four times a week. My son improved rapidly. Two months later, at the time of his fourteenth birthday, I remarked to my wife that in just another month or so I would no longer be able to beat my son. That year at fourteen he won the junior city championship, the district championship and placed fourth in the state tournament. I lost in the quarter finals in our city tournament.

Suddenly the thrill of competition and tournament play kindled a new interest that made us take a second look at the game of table tennis. We obtained and read all the books we

27

could find. Next we joined the United States Table Tennis Association and put new and adequate lights on our porch. We brought new sandwich paddles and most important of all we played as often as possible. We even purchased a training machine for Mike's practice.° Mike is now a good table tennis player and out of my class. He shows promise in developing into a great player. Even though his playing is far better than mine, I share with him the interest and devotion to the game. The thrill of competitive play is always present around our house. My hope is that I can arouse in the readers of this book some of this same interest and motivate you to take a second look at the sport of table tennis.

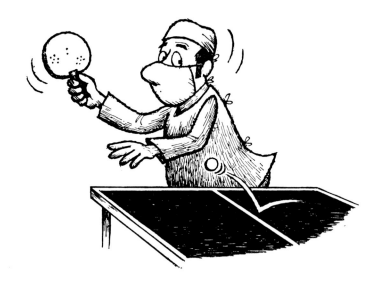

THE ROMANCE OF TABLE TENNIS

The weather was perfect. Exams were finished. Basketball season was over. Baseball was not in full swing. A perfect weekend with no commitments had finally arrived. Mike enthusiastically approached Cindy and asked, "How about spending the weekend playing table tennis at the lodge?" Can you imagine the entire family making plans for a table tennis week-

° The Robot © by Stiga.

end? Preparation might include getting all the homework done, the yard in good shape, the proper clothes, the car gassed and ready for the trip, the equipment ready, lunch packed and ready to leave before dark on a cold day. Something is strange. Families, and especially young people, simply do not plan a weekend for table tennis. The romantic appeal of skiing at the lodge, wearing the new beautiful clothes and warming by the fire simply does not exist for table tennis. Remember the mass hysteria of the crowds cheering at the football or basketball game? Can you imagine homecoming weekend or parents day celebrating table tennis competition between schools? Would you be surprised to see the newspapers announcing that the

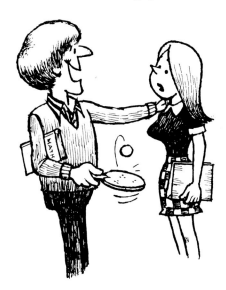

legislature of your state had proclaimed a Table Tennis Week? The surprising fact is that thousands of people in this country and multiple thousands of people over the world enjoy the game of table tennis.

In this chapter I shall introduce you to this exciting game of table tennis, a sport that offers more fun and more exercise to more people than does any other sport in existence. To call the sport "ping-pong" is akin to saying Bayer® instead of aspirin. Ping-Pong® is a trademark name that creates a false image of this fascinating game. Table tennis is a very popular tournament sport in the Orient and Europe, and there appears to be an increasing interest in tournament competition in the United States. Tables and equipment are available in many schools, recreational facilities, summer camps and in many private clubs. Almost every adult in the United States has played a game or two at some time in his life. Few, however, have played seriously enough or with adequate coaching and competition to learn to play the game well. While the game is fun and exciting even to the novice, the real thrill of the game comes with active competition in tournaments. What the game really

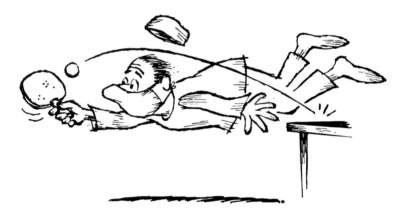

needs perhaps is an Arnold Palmer of table tennis. Arnie was a classmate of mine in college (any similarity unfortunately ends there), and even then his magnetism as well as his golfing ability was evident. He can be credited with the rise in popularity and the increased participation in the sport of golf. Unfortunately, so far no such advocate of table tennis has appeared, and so the game continues to occupy a minor interest in the minds and hearts of most athletes in this country.

ADVANTAGES ARE DISADVANTAGES

As I started to prepare a list of the many good points about table tennis, it suddenly dawned on me that these advantages actually help produce the lack of interest in the sport. Our society for some unknown reason seems to believe that a game or sport is more appealing of fascinating if it is an expensive sport or if an entire weekend or week is required to participate in the sport. The sport is even greater if one must go to great effort or travel great distances in order to play. The requirement of expensive or special clothing and highly specialized equipment seems to make the sport more desirable.

Table tennis can be played for fifteen minutes or for three or four hours. The proper equipment is available already in many places and can be purchased at a very minimum cost. The game can be played by two or more persons by both sexes and at almost any age regardless of the weather. It is an excellent game for the family, the summer camp, the school fraternity or the church recreation room. The real enthusiast will seek a table tennis club because this is the only satisfactory way a player can find good competition, adequate coaching and most of all the motivation for self-improvement. Table tennis clubs are available in most large cities in the United States. To my knowledge the Triangle Table Tennis Club of the Raleigh-Durham area is the only organized table tennis club in the state of North Carolina.

Probably no sport offers better exercise for young and old alike. The game, properly played, is extremely fast and provides a continuous sustained type of activity that provides fun and excitement to participants and spectators. It provides not only a means of getting exercise and having fun, it can serve as a method of families sharing precious moments together.

As with most sports, there are a few disadvantages such as the lack of body contact, the lack of glamor, the lack of available coaching, and most of all the lack of knowledge of how much fun and exercise can be obtained in the sport.

TRY IT—YOU'LL LIKE IT

The game has been called the pee-wee relative of lawn tennis by Dick Miles in an article in *Sports Illustrated*, November, 1970. This description, though accurate, needs some amplification. The game is played by striking with a paddle a hollow

spherical celluloid ball over a net fixed across a dark nonre-
flecting table top. The server's paddle hits the ball behind his
end of the table so that it bounces first on his side of the table,
then over the net onto his opponent's side. The ball is then
struck back directly across the net to the server's side, and to
and fro directly across the net after bouncing, until a point
is scored by failure of a player to make a good return. Service
alternates every five points and the winner is the player that

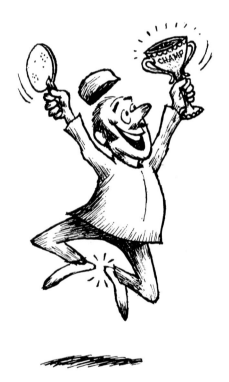

first scores twenty-one points. The game must be won by two
points and the service alternates if the score reaches twenty-all.
In doubles, the ball must first touch the server's right half-court
and after passing over the net must touch the receiver's right
court. Once in play after the serve, the ball may be placed
anywhere on the table as in singles except that partners must
alternate in returning the ball. A pamphlet, *Laws of Table Ten-*

nis, contains the rules and regulations about equipment and playing conditions for competition. This pamphlet is included in most table tennis sets purchased in this country and can be obtained directly from the United States Table Tennis Association.

The United States Table Tennis Association is a nonprofit organization functioning through state, district and local associations. Most table tennis clubs are affiliated with the United States Table Tennis Association. The members are people like me, and hopefully eventually you, who are interested in and enjoy table tennis. Membership in the United States Table Tennis Association is available to any person interested in table tennis, both champions and beginners. The membership dues are small and are used to support the activities of the association. Membership allows members to participate in sanctioned tournaments and receive the national publication *Table Tennis Topics.* There are many other advantages of belonging to the association. This author would urge all persons who have any interest to write to the United States Table Tennis Association, P.O. Box 815, Orange, Connecticut 06477.

In March, 1971, I competed in the 1971 United States Open Table Tennis Tournament in Atlanta, Georgia. In what other sport could an amateur like myself participate in a United States Open? The very good players from over the United States were present, and I learned a great deal. Most of all I enjoyed seeing the fastest indoor sport in the world played by the best players from all over the country. Undoubtedly this tournament has furthered my interest and hopefully my ability. They even had a division for senior players, and I found that this was my class. It was even more interesting and exciting to follow the progress of my son, Mike.

Some years ago when I finally completed my Specialty Boards, I thought I was through with all examinations. Now, much to my surprise, I recently found myself preparing to take an examination so I could become a qualified referee or umpire. I passed both the written and the practical examination and now I am a qualified umpire for the U.S.T.T.A.

THE NECESSARY EQUIPMENT

The enjoyment of any game is not dependent upon equipment. As one progresses from novice to intermediate player, equipment becomes more important. For the serious tournament player, proper equipment, lighting, clothing and adequate space are essential to the full enjoyment of the sport. A brief chapter does not permit a complete discussion of all of the proper equipment. The first essential is a racket. The majority of tournament players now use a racket covered with sponge rubber usually about one to two millimeters thick. This sponge is covered by a playing surface of rubber. The rubber surface has rubber pips that either face the playing surface or face the sponge. The flat surfaced sponge rubber bat is called an inverted bat because the layer of pips faces the sponge. When the pips face the playing surface, the racket is called a sandwich racket. Many international experts still use the old type of rubber racket without the sponge rubber.

Table tennis is a game of spin and the inverted sponge racket imparts a lot of spin to the ball with enormous speed. In contrast, the sandwich sponge racket sends the ball with less speed but more control. Sandpaper paddles are not acceptable in tournament competition. The playing surface of the paddle must be dark. Since I am not an expert, I can with a clear conscience recommend the inverted sandwich paddle to the beginning table tennis players.

The table must be nine feet by five feet and the playing surface thirty inches from the floor. The paint should be dark and never polished with wax. There should be as much light as possible over the table and the back court. Glare should be avoided. Three hundred watt bulbs with silver bowl bottoms and reflectors should be hung about eight feet over the playing surface. Remember to provide lighting for the back court.

Allow as much room as possible to permit adequate movement around the table. A tournament player often travels thirty feet behind the table to return the ball that has been slammed by his opponent. Even for intermediate players a minimum of seven to ten feet is needed behind the table.

Tournament rules prohibit wearing light-colored clothing. Dark-colored short-sleeved polo shirts and dark-colored tennis shorts are combined with tennis shoes to complete the customary clothing. It is better to wear the proper clothing each time you play or practice. The psychological effect and freedom of movement will improve your game.

Paddles and tables may be purchased in all good sporting stores and often in large department stores. There are many stores that specialize in table tennis equipment. The equipment

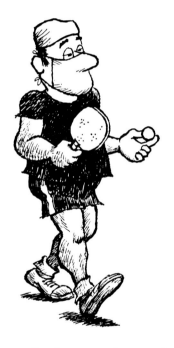

in these stores is usually far superior to the table tennis sets frequently seen in stores throughout the country. Personally I have always received very prompt and courteous help from the Martin-Kilpatrick Table Tennis Company, in Wilson, North Carolina. They will send a complete catalog upon request. This company also carries the latest books on the sport if you are unable to find them in your local book store or library. Two books in particular have been very helpful to me. They are *The Game of Table Tennis* by Dick Miles (J.B. Lippincott,

1968) and *Advanced Table Tennis* by Jack Carr (A.S. Barnes and Co., Inc., 1969).

REDECORATE

A certain degree of darkness seems to be present in this sport. For example, the dark colors of the uniform, the dark color of the table, the lack of glamour and romance, the old trade name of Ping-Pong, and the many other unexciting facets of this game. Maybe, just maybe, you are willing to go the second mile and learn to play well enough to have a great deal of fun and get a lot of exercise and feel the thrill of tournament competition, then you will help us change the image of this great game.

5

VOLLEYBALL

GEORGE E. MOORE

Volleyball was invented in 1895 by Bill Morgan at the YMCA of Holyoke, Massachusetts. Apparently his intention was to provide an interesting form of exercise for middle-aged men. The game was originally called "Mintonette," and fortunately the name was changed to "volleyball" several years later.

Volleyball can be a wonderful, exhilarating form of exercise for people of all ages—even those over 60. The game involves a moderate level of exertion with a demand for bending, flexing the torso, use of the arms, jumping, and a stimulation for enough water loss to develop the sort of after-thirst that is best satisfied while under a beach umbrella. As a matter of fact, one of the advantages of volleyball is that it can be played both outdoors and indoors. Actually that statement needs some modification since here in Buffalo there are a limited number of days during which you can play outdoor volleyball, but an excellent indoor season. The minimum requirements are a court approximately 60 feet long by 30 feet wide (Fig. 1), a net 8 feet above the floor, a ball—preferably one of the new, light, Olympic balls, and 9 to 11 friends.

There are several levels of competence required for volleyball. I prefer to divide volleyball into three levels. The first is the G level, or in other words, a game for general participants. The second level of competence might be described as the R level, or a game involving teams of a comparable athletic development. The players may be described as consenting adults. The third and highest level of competence or the X level is competitive volleyball, or as it is sometimes known, "powerball." Competitive volleyball is limited to colleges, athletic clubs,

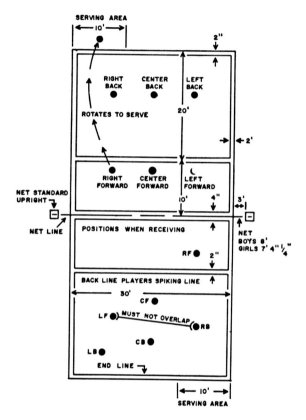

and major YMCA and YWCA teams. Competitive volleyball is an official Olympic sport (since 1964). Throughout this chapter we will refer to those rules and regulations and techniques that are applicable to these three respective levels of performance. A mixture of teams or individuals that play for the fun of it and those who play "for keeps" with strict interpretation of the rules usually ends in bloodshed.

VOLLEYBALL FOR GENERAL PARTICIPANTS

The G level of volleyball can be seen at any beach or in the backyard of any gathering of relatives or in the park where a mixture of young and old people of both sexes are engaging in a general melee, massacre, or scramble, involving a net placed at varying heights and a ball that may be an official volleyball, a rubber ball, or in fact, any kind of ball of any size; at some parties even people are used. Any number of people can play in such a game if they can stand the elbowing, the tramped feet, the dust, and the lack of rules. The only object of such a game is to deliver the ball over the net by pushing it, hitting it, or throwing it. Further, it may be passed along by one to ten people before being returned successfully to the opponent's side of the net. Since any set of rules for such a game are better left to the local mores, we will give little consideration to this sort of volleyball performance other than to suggest that it be avoided unless it is limited in scope, the contestants are friendly, someone is available to provide first aid, and one can look forward to a soothing drink afterwards. Such games, with attractive female companions, can be laughable or may be the cause for instant and permanent feuds between otherwise friendly nurses, technicians, and secretaries. There are, of course, ways of influencing the chances of winning G level games, such as choosing the side with the sun at your back, the side with an uphill rise, or even a convenient hump near the net that will add several inches to your height. Former basketball players are the best partners by reason of their height and ability to palm the ball down into the opponent's face—an illegal stroke, of course. If you must have women on your team, choose the retiring types that will be content to let you play their position as well as your own; let your opponents cope with the overaggressive types who will fight for their rights. Remember that it is always better to have fewer, better players than have to trample over excess inert bodies; be generous, let your opponents have the extra players. Do not try to re-train the players on your own side, but be free with directions to the opposing players as to how they should try to serve and return the ball in a professional style. The result is usually chaotic, because then several members must assume the role of experienced player and will infuriate the others. It is important to ensure that your own team members serve well, since in a mayhem game, serving errors will determine either the victor or the drink buyer. Only three bits of advice are necessary: (1) don't be tricky, just get the ball over the net safely; (2) serve as deep as possible; and

(3) serve a high looping ball so that there will be plenty of time for the players to fight for possession. If you have a very tall player, have him switch to the center net position from the left or right net positions after the ball is put in play. This is a legal maneuver and can be devastating if the ball can be sent to him for directed downward smashes across the net. Alternate tall and short players so that there is always one at the net. In official games only three hits are allowed before the ball must cross the net. If you have the best players, insist on this rule, but if your team is inept, plead for four hits or extra hits as a game rule.

As a responsible physician, do not let enthusiasm prolong the game over 45 minutes because most people do not use their jumping muscles every day and a serious stress of unused muscle groups will provide a painful aftermath and increase the chance of injuries.

Injuries

Serious injuries in competitive volleyball are uncommon. The most frequent and most aggravating injury is the jammed finger. Of course this may not affect the professional activities of an internist, but for anyone performing surgery, it is a one-week disaster. I suppose such an injury might also incapacitate a Freudian if it is a thumb. Like most sport injuries, jammed fingers occur when someone is just kidding around or when one is tired. I have made it a practice not to make heroic saves of the ball except with the clenched fist. Olympic rules require that the ball always be impacted sharply, thus all ten fingers must be held rigid to form a cuplike structure. The ball is hit simultaneously with the tips of the fingers. If there is any question of handling a high velocity ball, "bump it"; that is, hit it with the back of the hand or fist or with forearms held about four inches part. For a short time we treated jammed fingers with dimethylsulfoxide. The player-patients always knew that they had been treated when they started exhaling the fumes! After the government spoiled (with some justification) this exotic fling, we retreated to elevation, cooling, and analgesics—but no cortisone.

Only shatterproof eyeglasses should be allowed.

Elbows and knees get skinned infrequently in class R games, since it is usually best not to dive for most recoveries and risk giving up mobility. The dive and a position of squatting on your toes are used to "*dig*" or recover the ball before it hits the floor. These maneuvers are a necessity in competitive *power volleyball*. The Olympic champion girls team from Osaka, Japan practised for hours diving, ball retrieval, rolling and recovery, but most of us will not achieve candidacy for the Olympics.

A disabling sprained ankle injury occurs infrequently—perhaps once per three seasons. A more common problem for older players is the supraspinatus syndrome. Frankly, I do not know if careful warmup exercises and gentle initial overhand serves to prevent the onset of that awesome squeaky ache but it seems like reasonable advice. Prednisolone is the only miraculous cure for it, albeit sometimes a temporary one. Like it or not, we urge our "spikers" (strong, overhand hitters) to hit the ball gently at first and only after 10 to 15 minutes begin to hit the ball with full force.

As a physician you will be expected to provide first aid, so be sure to have enough tape and such supplies for minor emergencies, but not so much that you cannot easily ask that the player seek his own physician for further help. This ploy is particularly helpful if (1) you do not want to miss the next game; (2) you are a hematologist and vaguely remember that the ankle is a complex structure; and (3) the team has a trainer who may be very critical of your taping skills.

Provide a basketweave support and suggest elevation, an ice pack, and no more playing for at least one week. Rarely are x-rays helpful or necessary except from a medicolegal standpoint. After examining several huge, sweaty, odiferous ankles of several huge, lady volleyball players, one's appreciation of petite nonathletes increases.

Ground Rules

The volleyball court for G level games can be any size or shape, but in most other instances it is important to both practice and play on a regulation sized court. For your convenience,

a diagram of a regulation court is illustrated. Perhaps the only
unusual feature is the line dividing the playing area into a
forecourt and backcourt. Actually, it has a relatively unimpor-
tant effect on strategy even in official games, except to prevent
backline players from *spiking* in front of the line.

The most important aspects of the playing area are an adequate ceiling height, an area free of obstruction to the sides and
rear of the court, and poles and guywires to provide a very
tight net. Often the top of the net is strung on a braided wire
so that the height of the net is exactly the same across the court.
The tension on the net aids in recovery of played ball hit into
the net. Naturally those of us who are really too short for
volleyball do not mind if the net sags a little, and indeed if you
casually lean on the net a few times, you may gain a slight compensation for your natural handicap. As a matter of fact, we
little people learn to hate tall ones very early. (Some day I will
insist on adjustable floor space in the operating room. One gets
tired of climbing on rickety boxes just because the "generation
gap" is at least three to six inches.)

Serve

The serve is such a simple thing, just delivery of the ball across
the net, but many crucial games are lost by a "tricky serve."
Fashions in serving alternate between overhand spikes and a
soft delivery. The spectacular "windmill" serve is seldom used
in competitive volleyball. Each player should develop an absolutely dependable serve, and only then work on strategic ones.
A good player tries to deliver the ball into the deep corners of
the court. If possible, the ball should be hit to the corner opposite from the side of the opponent's strongest spiker. The purpose of this maneuver is to minimize the chances of the setter
delivering an accurate ball to the spiker. This ploy is advantageous because the set man must either turn so that he can
face his favorite spiker or resort to the overhead *set* which is
less accurate and more subject to *carrying*.

The experienced server holds the ball so that the stem is to one side, thus giving the ball an erratic flight; particularly it is spun by hitting the ball slightly off center. The ball must be hit while in the air rather than off the hand.

Remember, if the opposing server seems to be "hot," immediately call time-out in the hope of disrupting his timing.

Receiving

The three major actions in receiving a served ball are (1) call that you will handle the ball; (2) impact the ball sharply; and (3) hit the ball up into a high arc so that your setter has time to move under it and thus hit it accurately to the spiker.

The most frequent error in receiving is a failure to hit the ball sharply. In most instances the ball should be hit with the back of the hands, which are held together or with the fleshy part of the forearms held about four inches apart. This method is called "bumping," and it is used at least 85 percent of the time by competitive teams. I prefer to grasp the thumb of the left hand with my right hand so as to ensure that the backs of the hands will form a steady platform. The Russians and others often hit the ball with the backs of their thumbs which are kept above the clenched fists. Most beginners try to use their fingers and are immediately faulted for "carrying" or "lifting"— terms meaning that the hit was not crisp and sharp. If the set is a soft looping one, it is possible to impact the ball with the tips of the fingers but the fingers must be rigid and the fingers of both hands must hit the ball simultaneously or a "carry" may be called by the referee.

It is important to position yourself behind the flight of the served ball. The return flight of the ball cannot be "directed" or pushed to one side. The arc of the ball must leave your fingertips in a line of sight or an error will be called. Again, the ball cannot be pushed, *lifted,* or *directed,* if your are playing by official rules.

Over the years I have suggested that all players, offensive and defensive, constantly move and keep on their toes rather than have their heels on the floor. Reaction times are less if the body is not in a set position. Remember that if one intercepts a hard driven ball, the arms should not move toward it, as in tennis, or the ball may fly out of the recovery area.

Setting

The setter usually occupies the middle position along the net with a "spiker" on each side of him. He may be in the right front court so that he can deliver the ball to any one of the

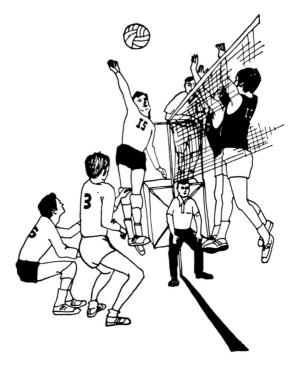

front court players. The setter is comparable to a quarterback since he determines the offensive play. He sets or hits the ball in an arc so that as it peaks just above and behind the net, the spiker can jump and forcefully hit it down over the net.

The setter must be quick enough to maneuver under the ball in such a position that he can deliver a "line-of-sight" trajectory, ending where the spiker can hit it most forcefully.

A skillful setter can deliver a reverse line-of-sight ball back over his head, but he must not either carry or direct the ball. This maneuver is useful if he sees that the opposing players are well organized to "fence" or "block" a spiked ball at the side of the court toward which he is facing.

Spiking

Spiking is the act of jumping high in the air near the net and hitting the ball with the flat surface of the rigid fingers of one hand, the clenched fist, or less commonly, the heel of the hand,

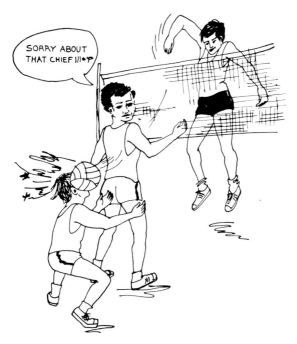

so as to drive it downward over the net into an undefended spot of the opponent's court. The hand is whipped as if it were a tennis racket with the object of delivering the ball at the greatest possible velocity. Naturally volleyball legends dictate that the speed of a spiked ball is over 120 miles per hour; I doubt it. Since the top of the net is eight feet high, men have a tremendous advantage because they do not have to make such a strenuous effort to attain the necessary height, and there-

fore usually can modify their striking positions and body directions more easily. Many spikers start their running jump from
a point six to ten feet behind the net and just outside the foul
line. Usually the ball can be hit harder from a running jump
but a whipping motion much like an overhead smash in tennis
from a standing jump is devastating. The leading spiker of the
Russian Olympic team allegedly could do a standing jump 34
inches off the floor.

The spiker may notice that his opponents have formed an
effective screen or "fence" of upthrust hands across the net from
him. In such an instance he must try to overpower them with
a hard hit ball, ricochet the ball off their hands so that it flies
out of bounds or falls close to the net, or hit a "let up" or "dink"
ball that will arc over the opponents' hands and fall behind
them.

Note: "Palming" and directing the ball are illegal. Basketball
players are frequently guilty of trying to handle the ball.

Play plans include arranging the spikers so as to take advantage of the weakness of your opponents. These are described
in the books listed in the bibliography.

The Defense

The object of the defensive team is not merely to keep the
ball in play but to handle the three successive hits in such a
way that the offensive initiative can be taken away from the
opponent. The initial receiver must try to bump the ball into
a high arc—preferably so that another player or the setter can
set it up for one of the spikers. If this is not possible, it is best
to hit the ball to one of the deep corners of the opponent's
court.

Fencing or blocking are terms used to describe the upthrust-
ing of one's hands above the net so as to deflect a spiked ball
back into the opponent's court or into a high arc so that it can
be recovered. A fence may consist of one to three players. The
fence consists of all of the front line players. A back court player
cannot join in fencing nor can he spike the ball from in front
of the *spiking line.* If one front court player is shorter than the

others, he should play in the inside position if possible and be alert for dink shots and netted balls.

The back court players on defense must not only cover any balls driven past the fence, but also be alert to receive let up shots and ricochets off the hands of the fencers. Remember that balls can be recovered from the net if done so with a clean hit. Net balls should not be hit upwards but back toward the middle of the court.

Elementary Rules and Scoring

Anyone engaging in competitive volleyball should obtain the annual rule book of the United States Volleyball Association. In brief, a successful serve must clear the net cleanly and a second serve is allowed only if the ball touches the net and falls into the opponent's court. Points are made only by the serving team. When a point is lost, the receiving players rotate one position clockwise and the new player in the right back line is the server. A game is 15 points, but if the score is tied at 14–14, two successive points must be scored in order to win. Players must be in their proper position until after the ball is put in play. The gentlemanly origins of the game are still reflected by such rules as 12.01: "When an opponent is about to play or in the act of playing the ball, players shall not stamp their feet or shout at him." Actually, whistling and waving the hands or screening the view of opposing players are also illegal.

Remember that the ball may be hit with any part of the body above the waist, but it must be hit cleanly; this is rarely possible except with the fist, arm or rigid fingers. In competitive games even the palms of the hands can rarely be used without an error being called by the referee.

Psychological Aspects

As mentioned previously, volleyball has retained the gentlemanly characteristics of its origin and continuous support by the YMCA. Thus derogatory remarks and unsportsmanlike behavior are not allowed, but shouts of encouragement are permitted.

Another source of volleyball activity is the adult physical fitness programs maintained in the evenings at the local high schools.

Less frequently, except on the West Coast, there are sport clubs who are interested in supporting a volleyball team.

In western New York we have teams from the YWCA's, sports clubs, a suburban league, and several teams developed by various ethnic or religious organizations. The teams have fanciful sponsors, for example, the "Dew Drops Sport Club," sponsored by a local tavern, the "Sterlings," representing a photography studio, and "Forbrush," sponsored by a lumberyard. Physicians should avoid sponsorship by taverns, slaughterhouses, and supermarkets.

You will encounter many "Docs," a few physicians, and a few scientists in Class A competition. Most of the "Docs" are nicknames derived from bewildering origins—first aid man during the war, "He looks like a doctor," "always wanted to be a physician," "takes care of injuries for the sports clubs," veterinarian, hairdresser, but strangely enough, no funeral directors.

A grievous error is to be anything other than a volleyball player when playing; never request or accept special favors because of your age or position.

Some of the meanest players who seemingly cannot forget their college days are ex-football players. The most aggressive player in one of our leagues—"Break their fingers"—was a high school math teacher.

The best time to establish rules and the quality of play is at the first few sessions. Do not try to enforce the rules and character of the game all at once so as to antagonize and decrease the interest of the potential players, but invite them to watch competitive teams in action and then let them play against one— and then back to the practice court.

All kinds of team play and referees are encountered.

The Roswell Park team participated in an urban league that provided referees who personally provided rules and interpretations of them according to the weather, their feelings toward the teams, and the number of accusations of foul judgment. It took us three years to develop a team that could lose gracefully in the YMCA B volleyball tournaments of New York State and another two years before we could win games from Class A teams. This kind of competition requires a minimum of practice two evenings a week plus weekly tournament play on Saturday.

We entered the annual National USVBA Tournament after holding the traditional bakery sale, or really, begging with dough. As most losers say, it was an educational experience. The shortest players on some of the California teams towered over our tallest spiker! Even the girls teams were bigger and possibly could have beat us.

Information and Teaching Aids

The sports directors at most YMCA's will usually aid in arranging for practice sessions and teaching tournaments.

Official rule books are available from the USVBA printer, Berne, Indiana, for about $1.50. The book also contains information about teams, tournment, and playing hints.

There are also films illustrating the techniques of team play as well as spiking, fencing or blocking, receiving, and serving, that can be obtained through the USVBA office, the YMCA, and private distributors.

There are many excellent inexpensive paperback books on how to play volleyball. The key reference which may not be available in a local store is: "Official Rules and Reference Guide of the United States Volleyball Association," edited by D.S. Shondell. It is obtained from USVBA Printer, P. O. Box 109, Berne, Indiana. The price for this valuable book, which is issued annually, is $1.50. It contains summaries of volleyball activities throughout the country, provides a current list of official rules and their interpretation, and lists of instructional books and movies.

I have deliberately avoided discussion of a long list of rules, since in my opinion it is better to start playing first and then gradually introduce the rules according to the level of play that is appropriate for the group. Definitions such as "A court is the playing surface divided by a net into two equal areas" are not only stultifying but usually an unattainable goal since most gyms have unequal lighting, floors, supports, ceilings, and confusing designs. Gyms that are used for many sports may provide a maze of yellow, blue, green, black, and red lines for the color-blind male.

In summary, the game provides competitive, interesting calisthenics including running, jumping, bending, and coordinated use of the arms. If one avoids playing with ex-football players, the risk of injury is slight. Volleyball can be enjoyed by men at all ages and at several levels of competence.

Volleyball can be an excellent social game for the hospital or clinic staff despite a disparity of age, and the team play minimizes the ego bruising of a neophyte or nonathlete who seeks a pleasant form of exercise.

VOCABULARY

Beach rules.
   The net is lowered to 7 feet, 10 inches if the sand is firm, and to 7 feet, 9 inches if it is loose sand.
Blocking.
   Only the front line players may block the ball by jumping close to the net and raising their hands.
Bump the ball.
   Recovery of serves or volleyed balls below the chest level by use of the forearms or backs or sides of the hands.
Carry.
   A ball that is not hit sharply or cleanly.
Coed play.
   Officially the boys and girls must have alternate positions and if the ball is hit more than once by a team, one hit must be by a girl.
Digging.
   Recovery of a ball close to the floor, often by diving or squat position.
Dink or let up.
   A spiker may elect to hit a soft shot just over the tips of the hands of the blockers across the net from him in the hope that it cannot be recovered.
Directed ball.
   A ball hit in a direction other than the line of sight of the players.

Fence.

Two or three front line players jump simultaneously and place their upraised hands close together.

Freebe.

Colloquialism meaning easy point.

Lift.

An illegal underhand handling of the ball with the palms of the hands.

Net.

The new rules permit a player's hand to cross over the net while spiking if he hit the ball while it was on his side of the net. A defending player may block over the net if he does not touch it. (These changes provide a great advantage to tall players.)

Net ball.

A served ball that touches the net and falls in opponent's court is reserved.

Power ball.

Competitive volleyball in which the hard hit or spiked ball is used. This is in contrast with "family" volleyball in which the ball is usually lobbed over the net in a low velocity arc.

Referee.

Former player.

Screening.

It is illegal for the serving team to use their bodies or arms to screen the server.

Setting.

A low velocity arching ball hit to a spiker.

Sideout. The term used when the serving team loses the ball or commits a foul and the ball is given to the opposing team. No point is scored.

Spiking line. This line divides the court into forecourt and backcourt areas. A back line player may not block the ball near the net and may spike the ball only from the backcourt.

Umpire. Old former player.

6

GOLF FOR PHYSICIANS
The Case History of a Learner Who is Still Learning

G olf has been within the physician's province since the game evolved from a pastime for bored shepherds.

It is a sport that has become a prescribed treatment. It is useful as a physician's own therapy, healing injuries of his occupational load, and it certainly has provided the physician with a fascinating study of efficient employment or misuse of mental and physical capabilities of modern man.

The physician has figured in golf from early times in the United States. Benjamin Rush, the Philadelphia physician who was a signer of the Declaration of Independence, among his extensive writings was author of *Sermons to Gentlemen Upon Temperance and Exercise.* This book, published in Philadelphia in 1772, contained the first reference to golf printed in the United States:

> Golf is an exercise which is much used by the Gentlemen of Scotland. A large common in which there are several little holes is chosen for the purpose. It is played with little leather balls stuffed with feathers, and sticks somewhat in the form of a handy wicket. He who puts a ball into a given number of holes, with the fewest strokes, gets the game. The late Dr. McKenzie, author of the essay on Health and Long Life used to say that a man would live ten years longer for this exercise once or twice a week.

There is no record that Dr. Rush played golf in the United States. He possibly did in Scotland. He went to Edinburgh after graduating from Princeton and serving six years as apprentice to a doctor in Philadelphia. After two years in Edinburgh, Dr. Rush took his M.D. there in 1768 then spent a year in hospitals of London and Paris before returning to his homeland, where at the age of 24 he began practice in Philadelphia. There in 1813, age 68, he died of typhus.

The first record in print of a golf course in the United States, serving as a golf club, was at Charleston, South Carolina, in 1786. Obviously there was delay in accepting Dr. Rush's advice about golf. The Charleston course vanished, leaving no trace on the terrain of that historic city, and not until a century later did a few courses appear in the United States.

Apparently, though, physicians in the 1890's, a budding period of American golf, recognized preventive and healing aspects of the game. The first almost explosive stage of American golf development came following the playing of our national amateur and open championships in 1895 on the nine-hole course of the Newport (R.I.) Golf Club. Newport was the summer social capital of the United States at a time when "high society" influence was spreading far and deep into the country.

Those were days and nights when many business barons both worked and played at a killing pace. Developers of our booming nation then had a regimen of Gargantuan meals, lakes of whiskey and champagne, tremendous pressures of competitive operation and growth of huge industries, no summer clothing and no air conditioning. For relaxation, the prospering capitalists indulged in romantic revels with vigorous young Broadway show girls while Mama and the daughters were at home in Newport.

Our empire builders did not have the relief of the rest and repair of the baths that high-living European royalty enjoyed intermittently at mineral water resorts, although there were several American medicinal springs, establishments at which businessmen and their families took the "cure," as it was called around the turn of the century.

The publicity given to golf at the French society resorts, Pau and Biarritz, definitely was a factor in the adoption of the game by the socially prominent of the United States in the 1890's. Physicians of the American economic royalty of that period, according to scattered references, were quick to observe that golf was the medicine for the common condition of fatigue.

It did not take long for news of the discovery of these perceptive physicians to spread. The addition of golf to the pharmacopoeia was noted by W.J. Whigham in *How to Play Golf,* one of the earliest golf treatises published in the United States. The book was published in 1897, three years after the United States Golf Association was organized. Whigham, an Oxford University graduate, won the second and third American National Amateur championships in 1896 and 1897. He was a skilled golfer, a studious observer and an able writer. He was a reporter for the Chicago *Tribune.*

In classifying golf beginners, Whigham wrote:

> The first class is composed of boys under the age of discretion, who learn games by a natural process of imitation and assimilation; in the second are found those of dyspeptic habits who have been ordered by their physicians to take a round of golf, either as a tonic or counterirritant; the third and by far the largest class includes men and women of all ages and temperaments, who by accident or intention have taken an interest in the game sufficient to inspire them with a desire for improvement.

It was not long before the golfing "men . . . with a desire for improvement" included thousands of physicians. On Wednesday afternoons in fair weather, golf courses saw medical men heeding the advice passed along by Paul, "the beloved physician" of the New Testament, "Physician, heal thyself."

To cite my own rather typical case history of a physician playing golf, I was one who eased myself of nervous and physical strain that burdens so many of our profession and may affect unhappily the physician's family and patients.

Many young physicians and surgeons of the time when I entered practice were worn by the outside work of financing themselves through medical school. I paid my way by working in a restaurant. My family was in the shipping business in Italy. As a youngster in a new country I did not know anything about American sports or about restaurant kitchens and service, but I did know very positively I wanted to be a doctor. That determination is the story of the majority of us.

When the glorious time did arrive and I was, sure enough,

an M.D., I became engaged mainly in obstetrics and gynecology in a poor and densely populated neighborhood. My colleagues who have had comparable experience know that a young doctor in such circumstances is not going to have much time or money for golf.

A druggist friend got me playing on a Chicago public course with another budding physician when the three of us sometimes were too tired to sleep, even in that exhaustion which gives youth a chance to renew itself.

From this life-saving start I came along slowly and happily as most physician golfers do. I learned a great deal of how to benefit from golf from a wonderful physician, my father-in-law, Dr. Karl A. Meyer. He for many years was the directing head and spirit of the Cook County Hospital in Chicago.

I did not realize it, but Dr. Meyer provided an ideal example of how to play golf intelligently and with consideration for your companions. Golf can be an egocentric game if you selfishly limit its enjoyment. When you consider others who are playing with you or are elsewhere on the course, you get more pleasure out of the game. That is the way Dr. Meyer has looked at golf and at life. It is a grand way to be rich in living.

Another important thing I learned about golf from Dr. Meyer was that when you are playing golf you are playing for and against yourself. If a shot is misplayed, the fault is not with the ball, the club, your professional, the grass, the wind, the soil, the sand or the water, but with you yourself. That narrows the responsibility and blasts the alibis, but it also directs you to the one and only place where your golf can be improved.

Learning the strokes and the strategy of playing courses actually is not as difficult as the high scoring average of golfers indicate. The reason so few ever play the good grade of golf of which they are capable is that it never has occurred to them they have to *learn* golf. Most players expect a satisfactory shot to result from casually taking a swipe in the general direction of the ball.

I was one of the lucky ones who discovered that effective instruction in golf is about 25 percent teaching and 75 percent learning. I started in golf without athletic aptitude or sports experience. I tried to make up for a late start by taking lessons from a number of professionals, reading golf books and articles until the literary load was something like the mountain of medical magazines the physician and surgeon tries to read and absorb.

I practiced, too—or thought I did. I stopped at driving ranges and hit hundreds of balls as a refreshing interlude between my responsibilities.

Despite that program my golf showed no improvement.

As every other aspiring golfer does, I continued to search for the "secret."

Eventually I found that the secret is found via exactly the simple policy and procedure we all must follow in medicine and surgery; we have to learn to learn. Our most valuable teachers are those who taught us to learn. Their techniques could be taught to a degree but mainly had to be learned so the pupil could adapt and apply them.

When I got my investigating organized and my experimenting intelligently employed, I began to play satisfactory golf. I will never become an expert, but I have improved enough to have won Illinois senior events, to have qualified for the United States Golf Association senior championship, and to play to my low handicap against prominent professionals and amateurs. That is about all a man whose career involves something other than golf needs to be able to do to make the most of his golf as a pleasant, relaxing pastime.

Several years ago after I had played with Tommy Armour, we were discussing the problems of acquiring a good golf game. I told Tommy that I never made any progress in golf until I had switched from hoping to be taught and began thinking about learning.

"Neither did I," Armour told me. "I took more golf lessons, in person and in print, as an amateur and professional, than anyone else I have known."

"It took me hours of intensive planning when I was in a military hospital then plenty of money playing with the greatest artists in golf before I learned that golf education was a two-way deal with the best thing a teacher could do was to get the pupil thinking clearly about what needed to be done. Then the technique for achieving the objective could be explained so it would sink in and stay."

As students, all physicians, young and old, have benefited from and passed along what we have learned from experts in doing things simply.

It takes most golfers years to learn the simple way. Most of them never do. They get so confused by "tips," that they cannot get back to the basic simplicity of the game.

My case history is typical. In two years I knew more about golf than I was able to use. Then for several years I had to try to escape the confusion of all the tips I had read about and been offered. I had to train myself to concentrate on the comparatively few essentials.

Out of hundreds of golf books and lessons, all there is to learn falls into the following categories:

1. How to hold the club.
2. How to stand in relation to the ball.
3. How to organize the swing so it will happen spontaneously without being choked or directed by tension.
4. Timing (which is mainly protection against impatience).
5. Putting, which is merely rolling the ball the correct direction and the adequate distance.
6. Course tactics in seeing the course so clearly that subconsciously your eyes direct your performance, and you "think" the stroke to a result that makes the next shot, if needed, easy.

Learn those stages and get them organized so that they are fitted into your routine of playing golf, and you will eventually discover that you are indeed a golfer. I did, and I once thought I was hopeless.

I will cite the scholarly Armour: "I've seen a lot of golfers score well with good grips and faulty swings but I've never seen a golfer who's any good with a beautiful swing but a bad grip."

The difficulty of learning a correct grip is that it feels virtually reversed for the average right-handed player. He instinctively and incorrectly holds the club strenuously with his right hand. That causes him to pick up the club with the right hand, deliver the blow prematurely from the top of the swing by a right hand flip, and never get or retain essential control of the club with his left hand.

Golf is a bilateral game, as the physician golfer eventually discovers when he learns how to play well.

The left hand, arm, and generally the entire left side, are for control. The right hand, the right forearm and the right side—conspicuously the thrust of the right knee—are for power.

That goes for the long shots. If you weaken with the left hand grip or if the left arm bends, you are ruined on any shot. The right side may get vigorously strong into the stroke as long as the left control does not weaken, as long as the left hand does not lose security of the connection and the left elbow does not bend.

Those delicate little pitches and chips around the green that the ordinary golfer often chops pathetically are misplayed because the left hand connection does not stay strong and swing through the stroke. The right hand takes command in error. The balance is lost. The sensitive touch of the right hand finger grip is missing. The right hand grip becomes stiff and numb.

There is not too much you can be taught about the grip. You can be shown, in a general way, the way the club grip should lie from your hooked left forefinger diagonally across the palm, and how it should lie at the roots of your right hand fingers. How the butt of the right thumb should be snugly over the left thumb and the V's of the thumbs and forefingers should point about to your right ear are routine doctrine which you are told by your instructor. Then you have to provide higher education for yourself by experimenting.

At that stage the competent, experienced professional becomes the partner of the pupil rather than the primary grade teacher. That is a relationship in the development of the golfer that I have never seen mentioned in any of the golf books I have read.

From what I have seen, heard and experienced about golf education, the successful instructor is not especially talkative during the lesson, but discerns significant positions and actions and then comments on them so the pupil is helped to work out his own answers. After all, the instructor is not going to be around when his pupil is playing. Then the pupil is on his own and the lesson is just as good as the pupil, not just as good as the teacher.

What did not get through to me early is that a productive golf lesson is a team performance. A bond of understanding must be established before the pupil is in condition to learn. Outstanding golf instructors are talented in establishing that rapport. So are our great teachers of medicine and surgery. It appears that professional golf needs considerable attention to this phase of its teaching pattern which has not had much change in many years, other than more use of visual education equipment.

When time permitted, the old "playing lesson" was effective. It trained the pupil to concentrate on a definite objective instead of merely hitting balls as I did when I thought I was practicing but found that I did not progress.

When I was going through the motions of what I considered practicing to attain correct muscular habits I did not know how a good shot should feel. No wonder I did not improve my game. As a matter of fact, some details of my game felt most comfortable when incorrect. That was especially the case with the grip until I learned what I should have in clubface position, secure and flexible connection, and confident control of the club at all stages of the swing. Then I learned to "feel" the clubface with my fingers.

Feel is something you must teach yourself. There is an efficient medium between the strong connection and the flabby one; you must have a grip that allows the wrists to hinge correctly and which is not so taut it restricts functioning of your muscles from your back clear down through your fingers.

It took me many, many hours of studied trial and error to learn that the easier my grip felt to me while I retained control of the clubhead, the more energy and precision I was able to exercise with the clubhead.

When I did learn the muscle tone that gave me the best results I acquired an essential of good golf that nobody possibly could teach me.

The typical golfer probably expects too much of his professional. The competent instructing professional can determine the correct positions for the individual's grip, stance and swing and to some extent the route and timing of the swing. He knows how to supervise practice and observe and direct correction of obvious errors. What may baffle him are significant details that frequently are hidden so they are difficult to locate, explain and work into the feeling of the effective stroke.

Especially is this the case in the grip; anyway it was in my experience. Diagnosing my faults of hand and finger position, points of accented pressure, feel for direction and security and coordination of my hands was an interesting but fairly long study before I reached the point where I taught my hands habits that helped to "think" the shot.

Among sources I consulted in working on my grip was industrial insurance giving high rating in payments for injuries to thumbs and forefingers. This conflicted with Ben Hogan's statement that it is ruinous to accent the thumb and forefinger in holding the club with the right hand. Others, back as far as Vardon, named the right thumb and forefinger as main elements of the grip. Armour stressed that the lower third of what he called the "trigger finger" of the right hand functioned importantly in whipping the club through the shot.

Eventually I got my confusion cleared away. The forefingers and thumbs of both hands are mainly the "feelers" in controlling the club. The middle two fingers of the right hand are the holding fingers on that hand.

There are only a few authorities who say the left hand hold concerns the forefinger and thumb. The majority recommend that the last three fingers of the left hand and the heel of that hand press together in establishing a secure and supple grip. I found that a positive hold with the three last fingers of the left hand worked for me.

Time after time while I was working toward an effective grip, I was reminded that there seldom is "too much right hand in the shot," but usually the trouble with the grip (and which by chain reaction effects much of the rest of the stroke) is a weak hold with the left hand.

You hear or read about the golfing specialists discovering a flaw in the grip. A little deviation from a correct situation in the grip creeps in and makes a big mistake in the stroke. That goes for any stroke from the power drive to the two-foot putt that is missed because of "carelessness," which generally is a sloppy grip.

My experience as a learner showed that when the right answers were learned with the grip, I acquired a pattern of study which I applied in determining and absorbing correct methods in address and swing.

In the address, for instance, position with reference to the ball and the character of the desired shot involves accurate aiming of the club, then coordinated arrangement of the feet, the body, arms and hands.

That is pretty much kindergarten stuff about which there seldom are differences of opinion in the books and articles of the experts, but it is amazing how the average golfer neglects the organized application of these fundamentals. He is like a child trying to learn the alphabet out of order, learning L-T-S-A one time, then B-R-N-Q.

The simple task of acquiring the habit of arranging myself to make a golf swing did not come easy. It never comes to those who rarely break 90. They do not seem to be able to know clearly what they are trying to do. In my case, I was slow to become aware that I was supposed to hit the ball at the bottom of the arc of the swing so the leading edge of the club got under the ball and hit it in the "sweet spot" of the clubface. The exception is the case of the teed-up drive that should be hit as the upswing begins.

After I formed a vivid mental picture of how the club should swing into and through the ball, I managed to get my feet set so I could stay down to the shot and stay in good steady balance all through the swing.

An apparently casual matter such as having the right foot at a right angle to the direction line or turned outward as the left foot is began to make sense when I discovered that on the short strokes that call for very little body turn, the right foot could be at a right angle; however, when I needed to wheel around on a stroke, the right toe turned outward gave me a lot more freedom.

Look at golfers on the tee of any private club or public course and you need not know much about golf to see that comparatively few of them look like competent golfers, even before they begin to swing. Compare them in attitude with the golf experts you watch on television. These experts stand up to the ball so they give you the definite impression of (a) having a target in mind, (b) being so well-balanced they can turn the body freely without moving the head off a vertical axis, and (c) being arranged so they can swing and whip the clubhead to its work without wasting energy. Not in one of these respects does the golfer who scores 90 or higher even vaguely look as an able performer should.

As we get older, it gets more difficult to imitate the appearance of a golfer who knows what he wants to do and how to do it. Joe Novak, for many years professional at Bel Air Country Club in Los Angeles, says that his best pupils have been Hollywood actors and actresses because they respond without reserve to direction, and when a picture gets into their minds, they replay it. They are educated to imitate. But the rest of us have not had such professional training.

Through written or oral direction, we are told a thousand things about how to execute the simple performance of a golf stroke. Golf has to be essentially simple, we as physicians know, or it would not be a game. A game, after all, is only a development of a self-preserving practice of a "dawn man."

What should be simpler than standing up to the ball with the club after we have learned how to hold the club correctly? Yet look at the variations on the first tee at your golf course. What is the best way for you? Nobody can teach you how to perform an address as well as you can teach yourself. In a minor way it is comparable with learning to operate. You can watch master surgeons operate, but you have got to work yourself up to that confident, proficient stage by yourself.

Seldom does a golfer appreciate that many requirements of a first class stroke are attained standing still. When he hears a companion say, "You looked up," he probably is not aware that he never looked carefully enough to take a "bead" on it as he addressed the ball. His left arm possibly was bent at address or the club was not soled back of the ball so that a radius of the swing was established. Or consider his other errors before he even begins to swing.

His elbows probably were spread apart instead of being held close together so his arms could work in coordination. His right elbow, instead of being close to his ribs and pointing at his right knee, already was pointing outward so it was almost impossible to get the needed turn of his shoulders.

And speaking of the shoulder turn that is required on every shot; the delicate chips and pitches often are ruined by a wristy chop instead of an easy turn of the shoulders and the arms swinging the club. Many times the ordinary golfer has his chin against his chest so he cannot turn his shoulders. He is trying to keep himself from looking up, and so he overdoes the job.

I recollect that it took me too long to learn that swinging the golf club is primarily accomplished by the left shoulder turning down and around under the chin and keeping the left arm straight.

A few years ago I read a book by Julius Boros, that admirable gentleman and expert with a classic unhurried swing. The play boiled down to turning the shoulders. He arranges himself so that it is easy, then lets nature take its course.

I began to see the light of a good smooth swing when I started to swing my straight left arm from the shoulder joint, keeping my right elbow down and close so my right forearm hinged up as my body turned around and my chin kept pointing a little bit to the right of the ball.

That is about all involved in getting the club swinging back and up to where the wrists cock spontaneously. There you can look at the ball over your left shoulder, take aim, and by setting your left heel firmly on the ground so the hips get sliding a bit to the left, you get your down swing going.

Before I acquired a decent swing, I had to learn to stand so that I could turn my body easily. That meant being unlocked at the knees and with the behind stuck out so that my first impulse was to turn the right hip around a little and get a good solid foundation on the right foot. I learned how to turn so I would establish an axis for the backswing just as one has to get set for throwing a ball.

There was no appreciable trouble or stiffness about keeping

the head still. Let it turn a little easily but not sway off center. If you swing with your left arm, then hit with your right forearm and hands, you will find it easy to turn in making a stroke instead of swaying to the right then throwing yourself to the left. I wish I could say that I learned that job of turning around on the shot as easily as I have just been trying to make it read here.

To keep from getting tight! Who can teach you that? And especially on those short shots where you read that you must keep your body out of the stroke. After some years and hundreds of misplayed shots, I learned I had better have my knees loose enough so I would not freeze on what should be a fluid action.

Another thing which I, as most other golfers, had to learn for myself, was what you can see on every fine stroke you watch on television: the right knee obviously is a significant element. When that knee thrusts into the shot the shot is good. If the right knee is frozen, the stroke is not 100 percent correct.

Who can tell you about timing except to say that you should not hit from the top? The best I was able to do for myself was to get a mental picture of having the straight left arm and the club shaft at about a right angle until the hands got somewhere down in line with the ball, then whip away. Can you imagine who could teach you that timing? You have to learn from experience.

Regarding the fine art of putting, I still think that Tommy Armour said about all that could be said in counseling to keep the head dead still and the face of the putter square to the line. That "square to the line" meant you would have to keep the putter low swinging back and low going through toward the hole, too. And it also meant a firm but delicate grip.

One time Armour and I were discussing putting and he told me about conditions of important putts he had made and some he had missed.

"The cases seem to point to critical putting being a matter of avoiding the emotions and being completely concerned with the mechanics," I ventured.

Tommy reflectively remarked: "You may have an answer I could have used more. I didn't think of anything except how to stroke the putt when I holed critical putts that won me championships. Go with the mechanics, not the emotions. You are right, Horton Smith was the best uniformly mechanical putter I ever saw. If the rest of his game had been as good he would have won many of the 'big ones.' Yet the only mechanics he ever stressed was a warning against ever allowing the left wrist to bend inward so the knuckle would get ahead of the forearm and to be sure to keep the back of the left hand moving squarely across the line of the putt."

The physician has most of the answers to the mechanics of golf. What he knows about the golfer's use of anatomy and the nervous system actually is much more than a golfer needs to know. How to employ that intelligence without interfering with the instinctive performance of hitting a ball toward a hole is a frustrating, entertaining challenge.

As a physician listening to golf professionals and expert amateurs discussing technicalities of the game, I sometimes wonder if we of the medical profession make good use of our own specialized learning in benefiting our golf.

We all know that the successful golfer must have a sound mind and body as well as a good swing. We know, too, that a well-balanced diet is a requisite to desirable condition and coordination of mind and body.

Yet, when we consider lunches we and our companions eat at our clubs before we go to the first tee, we may be inclined, on the second guess, to shudder. It would be amusingly presumptuous for a fellow who already has volunteered to give expert advice to professionals in a sport, to extend dubiously helpful service to congenial peers and superiors in his own profession. It is a risk cheerfully accepted in the brotherhood of aspiring golfers. All I dare do is suggest that three or four strokes per round could be saved at lunch.

We as physicians suspect, even admit, that improvement is possible. But as normal mortals we could not care less. Thus, again my experience may be of value only in encouraging my colleagues to remind themselves of what they already know.

I discovered that there was definite and quick value in diet supplements for golfers. The investigation would not qualify as research, but it was pleasant and seemed to improve the golf of myself and companions.

A diet supplement which I learned was useful to myself and others was alpha-tocopherol vitamin E. What had impressed me was learning that astronauts had returned from outer space with a 20 to 30 percent reduction in red blood cells because of vitamin E deficiency. When vitamin E was replaced in the diet, the red count became normal.

Something else that reminded me that adjustment of vitamin supplements might be helpful to the golfer were experiments of the athletic department of the University of Illinois. Two groups of athletes were tested. One was the control group. The other received vitamin E. The vitamin E group increased test performance 51 percent, indicating greater muscular stamina from the supplementary vitamin E. Any of us in medicine, as we look around our locker rooms, see diet correction indicated.

Golfers themselves seem to sense that need. One of my clubs has a membership exclusively of men. It is one of the most delightful clubs imaginable; I cannot imagine a gathering of a more pleasant group. Yet even here I find myself, with my practice being in obstetrics and gynecology, serving as a locker room consultant, and immensely interested in the responsibility because these are my kind of people.

So I come to my club to escape concern and discover myself worrying about my good companions. Then I wonder if one of the benefits of golf might not be that of getting every player to think about physical condition. I hope so.

My friends are a happy essential to my golf. I find myself thinking of them as a physician would consider them and not solely as golfing comrades. I hear them register their aches and pains as excuses for increasing handicap allowances or as explanations of unsatisfactory performances.

I know what they mean. I am one of them. I am one of the age group with a skeletal system losing calcium. But I am not going to volunteer a locker room office call to inform them that with loss of calcium, vertebrae and other muscular attachments become weaker and more vulnerable to the strains of a golf swing even though a golf swing is supposed to be very mild exercise.

Calcium loss accounts for the more frequent backaches of the older golfer. I suspect that if this were generally realized, the winning careers of excellent golfers might be lengthened.

I have been interested in what Hans Selye, an authority on stress, has had to say about the steroids preventing the escape of calcium to the soft tissues. Possibly it will have a bearing on a diet to have the older golfer more supple as he swings. That deserves speculation. We certainly are in a period of change.

Soil deficiency, improper food preparation, highly refined foods and the pollution we are told is killing all of us, call for applying all we can learn about diet supplements of vitamins and minerals. As physicians we probably would have to admit that we are not distinguished for taking good care of ourselves. What golf has done for our physical and mental health is considerable, though we seldom consider these benefits.

It is laughable how a golfing physician will experiment with a suggestion to improve putting but will brush aside a suggested experiment far more important to him. I had such an experience when a colleague prevailed on me to supplement my diet with vitamin E and a balanced preparation of chelated vitamins and minerals chosen for their more effective absorption and assimilation. My putting and long game improved. Of course I felt more cheerful and vigorous. The experiment was not scientific. Or perhaps it was: the results were the treatment for me.

Another phase of the physician's association with golf that I believe may be due for more attention is the field of allergies. I have been told by veteran golfers that one of the potentially great ones, Harry Cooper, had his game wrecked when goldenrod was blooming. Sports page stories about Billy Casper's allergies to Florida insecticides and to certain foods figured in having this able and admirable player nicknamed "Buffalo Bill." Possibly there are mystifying slumps many average amateur golfers might have correctly attributed to allergies.

Physicians as golfers have done the game an immense good. There comes to mind the valuable service of the men in industrial medicine who got sodium and potassium out of steel mills and other intensely hot work areas onto the golf courses for protection against too much sun.

Golf to the physician is far more important than a mere sport. His mental as well as physical exercise are involved, and golf gives him a refresher course in intellectual discipline with the concentration and coordination, the introspection and escape that he needs.

I personally know what golf can mean to a doctor. At times I have been so fatigued, concerned and perplexed that I may have been sicker than some of my patients. Then I have gone to my golf club and hit balls on the practice tee, and let solutions of problems come as naturally as I began to relax. Through dark clouds of worries came the sunshine of happy answers to things much more important than golf. I thank the good Lord for the wonderful medicinal value of the game.

The physician learns that his country club is a delightful place for his family to play, dine and relax together. There the family has the togetherness that a busy and often overworked physician needs so much for family love and mutual interest and understanding.

At his golf club the physician can "let his engine cool off" with colleagues who are talented and compatible and in mutually helpful relationships with other valuable, pleasant men and women of the community.

7

LAWN BOWLING: THE SPORT OF A LIFETIME

THOMAS N. DAVIS, III

Can a sport be fun to play day after day, year after year, decade after decade? Yes—if it's lawn bowling! But let me hasten to say that lawn bowling—also called "bowls" or "bowling on the green"—is not just an outdoor version of alley bowling. There are no pins!

No sport surpasses bowls for a lifetime of fun. I have seen, on the same green, bowlers ranging in age from the teens to the nineties. I met a Canadian who had lawn bowled 75 years, beginning at age nine. I have also seen a teenager playing in the same competition as his father and grandfather. What a happy way of closing the generation gap!

Bowls has little or no resemblance to tenpins. The winner of the 1970 Illinois State Singles Championship in tenpins, John Berry of Chicago, says enthusiastically, "There is no comparison between the two sports. Lawn bowling is much more challenging and more joy. I've had more joy from four years of lawn bowling than from 15 years of alley bowling!"

Most everybody who tries bowls for a time long enough to experience its challenge, exclaims, "How fascinating!" And when they have played it enough to encounter its many variables, they say, "I wish I had started ten years ago!" Bill Hay, of Los Angeles, gave up golf because of a spinal injury. He tried bowls and became an enthusiast. He commented, "I was only sorry that it did not happen 25 years sooner. Though I have played nearly every sport there is, the happiest days of my life have been on the bowling green!"

I was more fortunate than Bill Hay—I did not incur an injury before I discovered bowls. I became so infatuated with the game that after three seasons I sold my golf clubs.

There are about 10,000 lawn bowlers in this country, and so it is not well-known here. It has never been promoted commercially. If it were promoted as golf is, it would soon be very popular. Indeed, even without commercial promotion, it has become the most popular participant sport in England, Scotland and Australia. Glasgow, Scotland has some 200 bowling greens, as does Sydney, Australia.

There are many appealing features of the games of bowls. It is a participant sport very challenging to neuromuscular skill and a wonderful team sport (though great as singles, too). It is a game of give and take, one of strategy. It has fine traditions of sportsmanship and camaraderie. Because it is so enjoyable at most any age, I like to say that "lawn bowling is the most fun per lifetime of any sport. And because so many can play it at one time in relatively little space (up to 64 bowlers on a green 40 by 40 yards), I can also state that lawn bowling provides the most fun per square yard of any sport.

How do you play bowls? Your target is identical with a billiard ball and is called the "jack." The object is not to hit the jack but to roll your "bowls" closer to it than does your opponent. It is like horseshoes in this and in certain other respects—in the alternating of play, in the scoring, and in the fact that the distance a bowl rolls is as important as its direction.

Modern bowls are about the size of a grapefruit and made of hard plastic. They have a unique feature that is the key to the sport's fascination—they are not spherical but are slightly lopsided or "biased." This shape causes the bowl to swing laterally as it loses momentum. There is "English" built in, so to speak. If it rolls approximately 110 feet, it may "draw" or "pull" six feet or more to one side. This means that ordinarily you do not bowl directly at your objective. If you want a bowl to come to rest at the jack, aim several feet to its side.

"Bias" greatly increases the skill needed. It makes possible a great variety of shots. And it makes strategy an important part of lawn bowling. You can curve a bowl's pathway to the right or left (depending upon which way you hold the bowl). Or you can make it go straight by using enough force. If rolling a lopsided ball to the vicinity of a small object at least 75 feet away is challenging—and it is—then keeping it there against skilled opponents can be even more challenging.

The following are the more usual shots in a lawn bowler's armamentarium for outmaneuvering his opponent:

1. *Forehand draw.* Curves to the left (for a righthander).
2. *Backhand draw.* Curves to the right.
3. *Wresting-out.* Displaces a previously delivered bowl.
4. *Yard-on.* Knocks away another bowl and rolls on about one yard.
5. *Drive.* Very forcefully knocks away another bowl or the jack (if it hits it). A drive can scatter many bowls and the jack with one blow! (But woe be to the driver if it hits the wrong bowls!)
6. *Trail.* Nudges the jack to a new location. This can be a brilliant

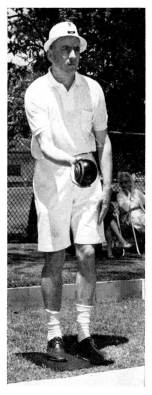

Figure 7–1. Dr. Tom Davis is taking aim to deliver his bowl. A lawn-bowler does not aim directly at his target because of the bowl's "bias."

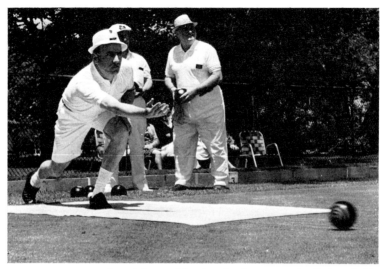

Figure 7–2. Davis has delivered his bowl, playing at the Lakeside Lawn Bowling Club in Chicago's Jackson Park. The target is not pins, but a "jack."

tactic that can change the lie completely, say, from three shots "up" for one side to 4 "down," a turnover of seven points!

7. *Block.* A front positioned bowl guarding another bowl or the jack.
8. *Back bowl.* Positioned as a potential scorer if the jack is trailed.
9. *Wick.* Caroms off another bowl.

Here is how the first "end" (inning) of a singles game might go:

You and opponent are on a green 120 feet long in a beautiful, outdoor setting. The green is like a giant billiard table. You play a game of 21 points—the first to score this total is the winner. You each have a set of four matched bowls. Let us say you win the toss of a coin and opt to play first. You stand on a mat at one end of the green and roll the jack at least 75 feet but less than 120 feet. (Make it your best length or your opponent's weakest.)

Now roll your first bowl. You want accuracy of both length and direction. Remember the bowl's bias. Do not aim at the jack, but at a point perhaps five feet to its right. Coordinating eyes, arm, torso and legs in a smooth swing, roll your bowl without throwing, bouncing, skidding or wobbling. Did you give it the right "weight"? Chances are you were too "heavy" and went past the jack. Also, you were probably "narrow" and ended up to the left of the jack. Let us say your bowl stopped six feet behind and two feet left of the jack. Now it is your opponents turn. Let us say that his bowl draws or comes to rest "jack high" but is one and one-half foot narrow.

Now it is your second shot. Try a repeat of your first, using less weight and more "grass" (the angle between the jack and point of aim). Your second shot ends up two feet short of the jack and one-half foot to the left. Your opponent now bowls a foot "wide" (to the right) and one-half foot past the jack. Your opponent now lies two shots, both of his bowls being closer to the jack than are yours.

You have two more shots this end, and so does your opponent. You have several possibilities for beating his shots. One is simply to draw closer to the jack. Or, you could diplace his bowl with a wresting-out shot. Best, if you could do it, would be to trail the jack back to your first bowl. (Remember, your first one went six feet behind the jack and two feet narrow.) If you succeed, you could not only get the jack near your first bowl to lie shot, but your trailing bowl could stay with the jack. Then you would lie two up rather than two down. Moreover, if fully successful, your trail shot could finish so as to leave your advantageous lie protected by three front bowls—two of yours and one of your opponents.

But a word of caution—your attempt to trail the jack to your bowl could backfire, i.e. the jack could go to your opponent's bowl.

These, then, are some of the many possibilities. And how really possible are they? Their success depends upon several factors, including skill and luck, and the quality of the playing surface. Drawing to within a foot of the jack occurs perhaps once in five or six attempts. Knocking a bowl away succeeds perhaps 40 percent of the time. Trailing the jack succeeds probably less than 10 percent. It is good strategy to "play the percentages."

I hope this discussion gives you an inkling of the rich variety and subtle skills in lawn bowling, including give and take and strategy; despite the fact that the sport is so simple in principle it can appear deceptively dull to a casual observer. The strategy in lawn bowling rivals chess. And the luck, uncertainty and suspense are like a card game.

As a British student of the game says, "You are not merely trying to deliver one ball to another. You're attempting to master the playing surface, the sun and wind, and above all, the play of an opponent. You're seeking to discover his strengths and weaknesses, likes and dislikes, faiths and fears, his temperament, reaction to the various techniques that have been learned over the years. It is a friendly yet complete battle of physical and mental skills. At higher levels of skill, bowls is a constant battle to produce your best shots while setting up situations, positions and pressures that hinder or prohibit your opponent from doing likewise."

But back to how the game is played. When all eight bowls in an "end" of a singles game have been played, you or your opponent—never both—score one to four points, according to

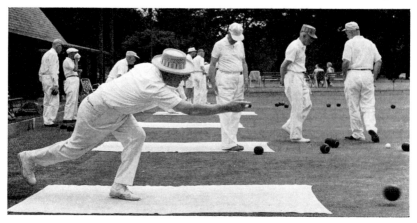

Figure 7–3. Lakeside Lawn Bowling Club, Jackson Park, Chicago, Illinois.

how many bowls one of you has closer to the jack than does the other. The winner starts the next and by rolling the jack and first bowl. The direction of play is reversed. (There is considerable walking—a minimum of 120 feet per end.)

In a well played singles game, usually only one or two points are scored per end. Scoring a three or four can have psychological impact, like boosting one player's confidence and unnerving the other. There is no sport in which there are sharper reversals of fortune. You can be behind 20 to 0, in a 21 points game, and still have a chance of winning. I saw the finals of a national doubles tournament in which one team was winning 14 to 1. They were playing "short jacks," but then they lost control of the jack's distance and they never scored again!

Bowls is wonderful as a team game—doubles, triples or fours. Each player has four bowls in doubles, three in triplets, two in fours. As strategy and team play are so important, each player is directed by his "skip" or captain, who is the last to bowl and who stands behind the jack when he is not bowling. The skips call the shots. Ideally, he is an expert shotmaker and strategist, able to "read" the green's idiosyncracies, able to evaluate the strengths and weaknesses of both teammates and opponents. Most of all, he is able to inspire his team to play

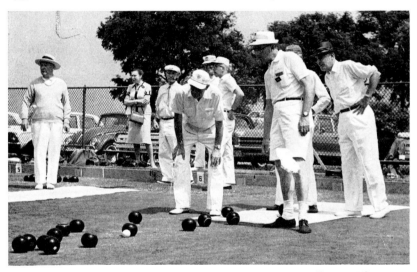

Figure 7–4. Lakeside Lawn Bowling Club, Chicago, Illinois. This competition was between South Shore Country Club and Lakeside Lawn Bowling Club. This is a well-guarded "shot" touching the jack.

its best. Good team play and a happy feeling of harmony go together.

Many enthusiasts, including myself and other doctors, believe that lawn bowling is not only a thrilling sport to play but it is beneficial to health and longevity. I have corresponded about its probable health benefits with Dr. Paul Dudley White, the eminent cardiologist. He wrote me, "I heartily agree with you concerning lawn bowls . . . I am heartily in favor of it."

Dr. Harvey Maxwell has written that it is the ideal physical exercise. He says, "Lawn bowling not only offers the finest form of moderate outdoor physical exercise of any game in present outdoor sports, but it presents it in the form of one of the most fascinating games ever devised by man."

Another doctor who writes enthusiastically about bowls as beneficial to health is Murray Blair, a Vancouver internist.

A Milwaukee internist, John Huston, estimated that in an average doubles game of 21 ends, a player gets two hours of rhythmic arm and body exercises, he walks about a mile, bends over at least 160 times, lifts some 300 pounds of bowls, and propels them nearly two miles.

After I became involved with lawn bowling, I lost 15 pounds excess weight and three inches excess waistline. Of course, the exercise in lawn bowling burns calories. And when I am not able to play frequently, I am motivated to take other exercise in order to stay in good condition for lawn bowling competitions. Furthermore, the joy of playing the sport relieves tensions which lead to my excess eating.

There are few ways of relieving tensions that are healthier and more fun than playing bowls. Certainly excesses in eating, drinking, smoking and televiewing are not the best means. I have discussed in a paper read to the Northern Indiana Psychiatric Society how bowls relieves tensions. It is an ideal outlet for excess aggressiveness and competitiveness (especially when you knock your opponent's bowls away). It enables busy professional men to forget their responsibilities. For those with more leisure, it relieves boredom. (Though you can learn the rudiments easily, it takes years to master the fine points.) Lawn bowling's strong traditions of sportsmanship, respect and camaraderie have been compared with group therapy. A saying is, "You have won the best of all victories if your opponent of today becomes your friend of tomorrow."

By the way, many of my best vacations have been lawn bowling trips—to Canada and Scotland as well as within the U.S. I have always found lawn bowlers friendly and bowls competitions challenging.

Physicians have always been among bowls enthusiasts— probably because of its health benefits, but certainly also because of the fun and joy involved. Also, they recognize its adaptability to individual needs and preferences. (You can play it as seriously as any other competitive sport—or leisurely and socially. Youth can play it at a fast tempo, older persons more slowly.) Some of England's and Australia's top competitors have been doctors. A recent president of the worldwide International Bowling Board was a physician. A British psychiatrist has written three books on bowls. Health columnist, "Doc" Brody, has frequently advocated lawn bowling.

Dr. Harvey Maxwell published a *Lawn Bowler's Guide,* full of enthusiasm and valuable information. He says:

> Lawn bowling offers more than the ideal physical exercise, it offers a better game! Come by our bowling green and you will meet a roster of members who once excelled in strenuous sports and who will now tell you, enthusiastically, 'this is the best game of them all.' No game has more sustained interest. This is a competitive man-to-man struggle . . . this is a duel, a contest where every bowl is a competitive give and take, and a perfect play can be spoiled by your opponent, even as you would do to his. The cares of the world are forgotten as the first bowl rolls down the road. It is no mystery that hundreds of thousands of lawn bowlers all over the world are lured to spend hours every day in healthy exercise out in God's fresh air and sunshine—bowling on the green is one of the finest games in all the world.

The history of bowling on the green is almost as intriguing as the sport itself. Ancient British kings banned it from the common people, whose fascination with it interferred with their practice of archery, which was the principle defense of the realm. The kings and nobility reserved this royal game for themselves, but magnanimously let their servants play it on Christmas day. The most famous bowls contest in history was played in 1588, by Sir Francis Drake and Sir John Hawkins. Drake refused to fight the Spanish Armada until he had finished his game.

Bowling on the green reportedly was introduced to America in 1607, at Jamestown, Virginia, and thus was the colonists' first competitive sports event in this country. Things had not gone too well in the colony that summer and they had a lawn bowling tournament that fall which is said to be one of the earliest recorded instances in which competitive sports were called upon to sustain public morale.

Bowls was probably the most popular sport in colonial America. A section of Manhattan Island and several towns were named Bowling Green, including ones in Indiana, Kentucky, Maryland, Missouri, Ohio and Virginia. Dr. Neil Benjamin of Australia, an international authority on the game, has written that George Washington loved to bowl on his green at Mount Vernon. But the sport suddenly died with the Revolution. "Washington patriotically, if not enthusiastically, dug up his green. A leaden statue of George III, in New York's Bowling Green, was toppled in 1776, and molded, so record has it, into exactly 42,000 bullets, to be fired at the accursed British. For amusement, the Americans turned to skittles (alley bowling)."

Was bowls banned because, as in earlier times, the fascination with the sport interfered with the defense of the land? Or perhaps it was a symbol of British rule and feudalism that needed to be destroyed. (If it was the latter, I say it is high time we forgive the British and resume bowling on the green!)

By the way, the Bowling Green Building, 11 Broadway, New York City, has a stained glass picture of lawn bowlers before the Revolution.

In the meantime, bowls almost died out in England because it had acquired a bad reputation in association with gambling and drunkenness at "pothouses." But it was saved by the Scots, who took up the game and improved it. They devised the rules that are the basis of bowls today and Scottish emigrants introduced it to other British Commonwealth countries.

An English physician and legendary cricket player, Dr. Eugene Grace, revived bowls in England around the turn of the century. He converted grass tennis courts into bowling greens.

So much for historical highlights of the "ancient and royal game of bowls." How do you get started playing it? You can try it at a resort, such as Spalding Inn, Whitefield, New Hampshire; The Inn, Buck Hill Falls, Pennsylvania; Williamsburg Inn, Virginia; Pinehurst Country Club, North Carolina; Gulf and Bay Club, Sarasota, Florida. There are a number of lawn bowling facilities in Florida and California.

If you do not know of a green near you, write to the American Lawn Bowls Association, or to *Bowls* magazine.

Do not wait for fate to get you acquainted with this wonderful participant sport. Do not miss the benefits lawn bowling offers you—new friends, fun and fitness—for a lifetime.

REFERENCES

1. Publications of the American Lawn Bowls Association, 10337 Cheryl Drive, Sun City, Arizona 85351.
2. *Bowls* magazine, 401 South Roxbury Drive, Beverly Hills, California 90212.
3. Davis, Thomas N. III: The ideal sport for emotional health: lawn bowls. *Journal of Indiana State Medical Association,* August, 1966; Lawn bowls. *Parks and Recreation,* November, 1967; Chapters in *Encyclopedia of Sports Medicine,* Larson, Leonard (Ed.): New York, MacMillan, 1971.
4. Maxwell, Harvey C.: *American Lawn Bowler's Guide,* published by the author, P. O. Box 824, Laguna Beach, California 96252.
5. Esch, Harold L.: *Lawn Bowling Handbook,* published by the author, P.O. Box 3304, Orlando, Florida 32802.

8

CURLING FOR WINTER ACTION

THOMAS N. DAVIS, III

If you are a golfer or a participant in some other summer sport, what do you do all winter? If you want to continue the joy and healthful exercise of sports participation, I enthusiastically recommend curling, the favorite sport of Canadians, who know well how to make the most of long winters. Curling is even more popular in Canada than hockey and golf. The interest in it there gets quite febrile and equals or exceeds our excitement about basketball! Although it is not considered a spectator sport, 54,000 Canadians have sat in a stadium watching the National Curling Championships! Indeed, curling is said to have united Canada in a way never possible through economics and politics.

Curling is also becoming very popular in parts of the United States. In the Chicago area, the number of curlers has increased from 40 to over 4000 in the past 30 years. Currently, there are about 25,000 curlers in 26 states. Though generally it is best known in the states bordering Canada, it has been enjoyed as far south as Florida, Texas and southern California. The fact that curling is played on ice is no deterrent in this day and time for enthusiasts in sunny climates. In Europe, it is played as far south as Italy.

There are two causes for the growing popularity of curling— which is occurring without the push of commercial promotion. First, it is a wonderful participant sport that can really get you involved. Compared to a truly avid curler, an enthusiastic golfer is practically casual in attitude. Second, bringing curling indoors, even though it is played on ice, has saved it from frustrating vagaries of weather.

Curling is a kind of shufflleboard played on ice—though curlers dislike this description because it is much more challenging than shuffleboard. No skates are used. Players wear rubber soled shoes or rubbers. Two kinds of equipment are needed: (a) standardized, highly processed, hard granite stones, shaped somewhat like a kettle, weighing 42 pounds and having a goose-neck handle; (b) brooms for vigorous sweeping of the stones' pathways on the "sheet" of ice, which is 138 feet long. Although 42 pounds are heavy, delivery of a curling stone seems effortless once a player learns a proper delivery and is accustomed to being on ice. The stone is never lifted straight up but is swung back and then forward as it is slid on the ice.

Curling is always played as a team game with four players per side, each player having two "rocks." The play alternates between the two sides, the first player of side A delivering the first stone, and the first player of side B the second stone. Then A's second stone, then B's, and so forth. And so, each "end" (inning) consists of 16 stones delivered by eight players. The direction of play alternates back and forth after each end. The winner of an end starts the next end. A game usually lasts 10 ends or about two hours.

The object of the game is to score points by delivering stones closer to the "tee" than the opponents. The tee is the center of a circle of 12 feet diameter called the "house." Only stones within or touching this circle are eligible to score. In principle, scoring is quite simple and is similar to that in horseshoes and lawn bowls. One point is scored for each rock closer to the target than the opponent's nearest one. In theory, as many as eight points can be scored in one end, but such an occurrence is rarer than a golfer's hole in one. Usually, only one or two points are scored, sometimes none at all.

A good delivery involves control of both distance and direction of the stone, and many variables can affect both of these elements. For instance, the ice can be "fast" or "slow," depending upon how frozen it is and how smooth the surface. The "speed" of the ice often changes during the course of a game.

One of the most interesting and challenging features of curling is that a stone tends to deviate to one side with a swinging

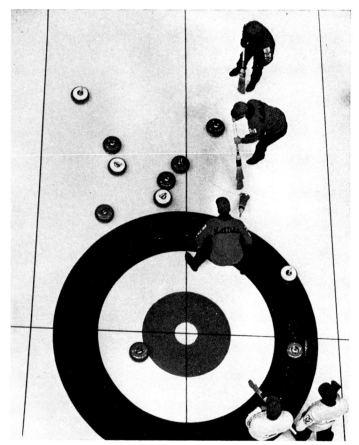

Figure 8–1. 1970 U. S. championship tournament, Utica, New York. North Dakota is playing against California.

or curving motion. This is what gives curling its name. A stone going 120 feet may deviate several feet to either side. There are different opinions as to why it curves, but the simplest explanation is that it is due to spinning by the rock. Give it a slight clockwise spin and it curls to the right—this is called an "in-turn"—for a right hander. A slight counterclockwise spin results in curling to the left and is called an "out-turn." If no spin is given to a sliding stone, most likely it will spontaneously start rotating one way or the other. If the rock is delivered with enough force, it will go straight.

As in lawn bowling, the "drawing" or curving motion of stones calls for greater skill. It makes for a variety of shots, and it makes strategy an important part of the game.

A curler's armamentarium includes "in-turns," "out-turns" and "take-outs." It is relatively easy to get a stone near the target, but keeping it there is another matter. A "guard" is a stone positioned in front of another one and protecting the other. A "raise" is the improving of a stone's position by nudging it with another one. A "wick" is the caroming of a stone off another one. A "freeze" is a stone touching another so that it cannot be knocked away if hit by a third one. There are other shots, too, such as double take-outs and even triple take-outs. Indeed there are about as many varieties of shots as in billiards and pool.

The last player on each team to deliver his stones, the "skip," is in charge of his team's strategy. In fact, the two skips are in charge of the entire match. The ideal skip is highly skilled at shotmaking and strategy and he is able to assess the peculiarities of the sheet of ice. He recognizes and takes into account the strengths and weaknesses of the players—both teammates and opponents. Most of all, he is a leader who communicates clearly and who inspires his team.

One of the most striking features of curling is that the sheet of ice is swept with brooms in front of the moving stones. This custom makes curling a truly colorful and unique sport. Why is it done? The reason is simple: to make the stone go further when it is delivered too lightly. The sweeping in curling is about as old as the sport itself—at least four and a half centuries. To ardent curlers, the sport would not be curling if there were no sweeping. Many claim that good sweeping makes a stone go as much as 15 additional feet! And machine testing has shown that it can indeed make a difference of at least five or six feet on level ice.

Why does sweeping add distance to the stone's travel? First, it cleans away any debris and frosting that would impede the rock's movement. But more than that, sweeping is supposed to melt the ice a bit and thus provide some lubrication. Of course, the sweeping has to be vigorous and forceful to make a differ-

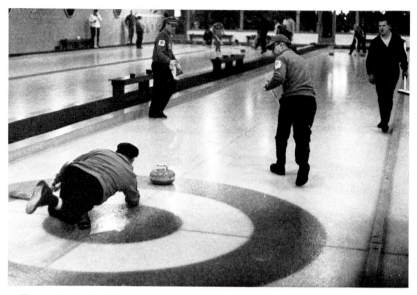

Figure 8–2. A Wisconsin team in action—ready to sweep—at a "bonspiel" at Exmoor Country Club, Highland Park, Illinois.

ence in this respect. It should also be done rhythmically and as close to the stone as possible—just in front of it but without touching it. Whether or not any melting actually does occur, a polishing effect of the ice probably does take place. Still another reason, at least in theory, is that rapid sweeping causes a partial vacuum which helps pull the stone along.

But regardless of the actual value in adding distance to the stone's journey, sweeping is an important element of curling, for it is great exercise and is emotionally satisfying. I have seen teenagers sweep in a cadence rivaling dancing for rhythm, harmony and exhilaration. And the sound that can result from sweeping the ice vigorously with a special broom can rival that emanating from a teenager's guitar!

The sweeping helps to make curling a team game par excellence. When to sweep and when not to? Split second decisions have to be made. It is up to the skip to command "Sweep" and "Brooms Up" according to his judgment. Every curler has his broom handy. The skip, when not delivering his stones, stands near the tee and holds his broom upright as an aiming sight for

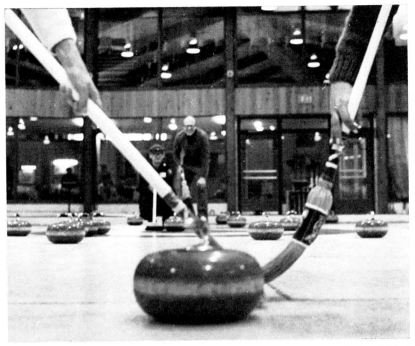

Figure 8–3. Sweeping a stone's path. It is heading toward the "skip" in the background, who directs the sweeping while the opposing "skip" looks on. This picture used with permission from *Sports and Travel*.

the player delivering the stone. And the player delivering holds his broom in his left hand to counterbalance the stone in his right hand. At the same time the other two players on the team stand poised, ready to sweep at their skip's command. It is a real pleasure to watch two skilled sweepers performing harmoniously and enthusiastically. Even though only one player delivers a stone at a time, his three teammates are occupied at the same time in team play with the skipping and the sweeping.

Another colorful feature of curling is the slide delivery. In this move, the player gets down very low and holds onto the stone during his follow-through instead of releasing it promptly. The result is that his body slides along on the ice with the stone as far as 33 feet. Indeed, the longest slide on record is the whole length of the ice sheet—126 feet to the tee! A Canadian schoolboy accomplished this feat, and as a result, a rule was made limiting the length of sliding permitted. The slide is very popular with younger players, and it is claimed to increase accuracy. Yet it is not necessary to skilled play and many players do quite well without it. And so its value to skill is controversial, but there is no doubt that it adds to the color and fun of the sport.

Curling is a splendid means of winter exercise as well as just fun. The exercise comes from the body bending in delivering the stones—with or without the slide—and from the walking back and forth after each end. And most of all, from the sweeping. The degree of exercise put into sweeping can vary considerably—from none at all to really vigorous movements of the entire body. In fact, the brooms of champion players in top competitions may last no longer than two or three games because of breaking! And at the other extreme, the broom is used for support rather than action!

This adaptability to almost any gradation of active exercise makes curling a superb participant sport. It can be played by most everybody from about 12 to 90 years. Truly a lifetime sport!

Of course, the value of any participant sport is directly related to the fun it provides, and curling is unsurpassed in this respect. Its features include the challenge of mastering the canny neuromuscular skill needed to control both the distance and direction of an object that does not move in a straight line, the competition, the give and take between the two teams, the strategy, and especially the team play. (Nothing is more important to success than team harmony.) The strong traditions of sportsmanship, camaraderie and amateurism all contribute to making curling a magnificent participant sport. (Many of these fine features are also found in lawn bowling. In fact, the two sports have a somewhat common heritage.)

Curling is such an ancient sport that its origin is obscure. There is some evidence that it may have started in Holland. But it has long been closely associated with Scotland, which has always supplied most of the world's curling stones. A curling stone was dredged from a lake bottom there bearing the date 1511. Until recently it has been almost exclusively an outdoor game there and in other European countries.

Curling has always appealed to doctors. In fact, the earliest curler of whom a genuine record exists was a Scottish physician and surgeon, George Ruthven. He and his curling stones are mentioned in a poem written in 1620, and in modern times some of Canada's and America's most enthusiastic curlers are physicians. Several have been state champions and thus contenders in the U.S. National Championships. Dr. Frank Crealock of Seattle won the Nationals in 1961, as well as the Washington State Championship. Other doctors have won the state tournaments in California, Massachusetts, Nebraska, New Hampshire, New York and Wisconsin.

An editorial in *Massachusetts Physician,* April, 1967, entitled "For Arteries and Fun," was about curling; and it recommended the sport as a good conditioning game which can be played all through the winter season, a game which can restore a satisfactory bloodflow through constricting arteries. The editorial described the rudiments of the game and then mentioned that one of the pleasant aspects of it is that the novice gets as much pleasure as the expert. It is a game whose fundamentals are easily learned, though its strategy may take years. The editorial concluded that "one of the dangers of the game is the possibility, even the probability, of becoming an addict, but the addict will be a healthy one."

A doctor is the current president of the world's largest curling organization; Dr. Maurice Campbell of Quebec heads the Canadian Curling Association, which has hundreds of thousands of members.

An enthusiastic group of American physicians organized the American Medical Curling Association and held its first annual "bonspiel" or tournament in November, 1970, at the Curtis Curling Center in Wilmette, Illinois, near Chicago. It was a mixed event, great fun, and resulted in many favorable comments. Articles about it were featured in *Medical World News* and *Rx; Sports and Travel.* Physicians wanting information about this doctor's association should write to the A.M.C.A., 200 South Main, Hillsboro, Illinois 62049.

Of medical interest are discussions about the probable health benefits and possible harm of curling. There is no doubt that curling makes a wonderful lifetime participant sport. There is almost no absolute contraindication to it except confinement to bed. People have played with such handicaps as a prosthetic leg or confinement to a wheel chair. Accidents and injuries are very rare, expecially when players receive instruction. The late Dar Curtis, of Winnetka, Illinois, taught the game to more than 2300 players and none of his pupils ever had a serious accident on the ice.

The Curler, a magazine published in Toronto, had an article discussing the effect of the sport on the curler's body. The editors corresponded with a number of curling physicians in Canada and the United States. The consensus was that the low tension and the rhythmic and continuous motion involved in delivering a stone do not strain the heart. On the other hand, the short burst of rather violent movement involved in sweeping can provoke a rather severe oxygen deficit. Some of the doctors recommend a conditioning program for curlers who are over-weight, over 40 and sedentary. This should include pre-game warm-ups, as well as pre-season conditioning.

Of particular medical interest is the Coronary Curling Club, an international organization whose membership is limited to persons who have had a coronary attack but who still enjoy curling. Dwight D. Eisenhower was an honorary life member. According to Lucius T. Hill of Boston, the founder and secretary, the majority of the members are pretty active curlers. But, he says, vigorous sweeping is out. "Most of us just massage the ice gently." I have read of Canadian coronary victims who curl with their physician's approval but who do not sweep.

By the way, country club members will be interested in what curling can do for their club's financial problems. Many golf clubs have found that curling enables them to operate 12 months a year and with startling results. As an example, the North Shore Country Club, near Chicago, found that during any given week between November 1 and March 31, they will serve more curlers than they do golfers during the busiest week of summer! Equipment used for air conditioning in the summer can be used for making curling ice in the winter.

How do you get acquainted with this fascinating winter participant sport? Until recently, I would have answered this question by referring you to Mr. Dar Curtis, who sold his business and spent the last 30 or 40 years of his life promoting curling as a full time, nonprofit hobby. He visited prospective curlers throughout the United States and Europe. He gave lectures and demonstrations, showed films, published an excellent booklet on curling, and helped to start more than 25 curling clubs. He gave $400,000 to build a model curling facility in Wilmette, Illinois.

The Curtis Curling Center is becoming a mecca for the sport, under the management of Gerry Duguid, who is from a famous Canadian curling family. Next time you are in the Chicago area, you should visit this facility. The game has no better teachers than Gerry Duguid and his wife, Betty. The center's address is 726 Ridge Road, Wilmette, Illinois 60091.

Much of the late Dar Curtis' promotion of the game is now done by the American Curling Foundation, which is "Curling's clearing house, providing stones without charge to newly organized clubs, producing and distributing motion pictures, handling other curling films and publishing books, directories and other informative materials." To learn of, or to utilize its services, write to American Curling Foundation, in care of *Curling News*, 723 Milwaukee Avenue, South Milwaukee, Wisconsin 53172.

In summary, curling is a wonderful participant winter sport. It is a lifetime sport featuring a challenge to skill, give and take, and strategy, and a team sport par excellence with strong traditions of camaraderie and sportsmanship.

REFERENCES

1. *Curling News* and Publications and Films of American Curling Foundation, 723 Milwaukee Avenue, South Milwaukee, Wisconsin 53172.
2. American Medical Curling Association, 200 South Main, Hillsboro, Illinois 62049.
3. Davis, Thomas N.: For winter fun and fitness: curling. *Journal of Indiana State Medical Association*, December, 1967.
4. Curling: hottest sport on ice. *Today's Health*, November, 1969.
5. Curling, *Rx Golf and Travel*, November-December, 1968.

6. Curling puts doctors on ice. *Medical World News,* December 11, 1970.
7. For arteries and fun, *Massachusetts Physician,* April, 1967.
8. Curtis, Dar: *Curling: Fun For Everyone.* Winnetka, Illinois.
9. Letter about Curling from Chicago District Golf Association to its Member Clubs, October 19, 1966.

9

HANDBALL

ALEXIUS RACHUN

Handball is a game played by hustlers as well as gentlemen; by city street urchins; by millionaire Hollywood celebrities; by oddballs; by perfectly sane people. Even doctors play at it—some are crackerjack performers. Like squash, it is a game in which a brisk workout can be obtained in a short period of time and it is much more fun than jogging. As it is a pastime played by men well into their 60's, it rates well as a "lifetime" sport.

There is also something nice about the game's simplicity. All you need is a small rubber ball, a pair of gloves if you are playing with the little black regulation ball, some gym attire, and a handball court. The single-wall game is usually played outdoors, mostly by the humble and downtrodden who have not the wherewithal to gain entrance to the scarce four-wall courts scattered among the various Y's, elite sports clubs and the better-financed universities.

In New York City, where I learned the game, the walls of warehouses, fire stations, and school buildings were widely used in the 1920's and 1930's for handball. Came the WPA in the 1930's and single-wall courts sprouted up like mushrooms in every neighborhood park. Up to this time, if you were interested in playing the regulation single-wall game, you jumped aboard the subway and hied yourself to Brighton or Manhattan Beaches, or perhaps to Coney Island, where the game was played from sunup to sundown by fiercely competitive, bronzed young athletes. No small wonder that so many of the national single-wall champions came from New York City. Of quaint historical interest is the handball bum of invincible playing ability, who roamed the neighborhood parks and the mountain

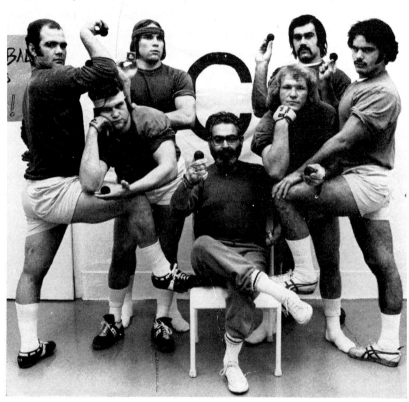

Figure 9–1. Undefeated Cornell University Handball Club and coach, 1971.

and beach resorts, taking on all comers for sizable bets—and never losing.

Handball came to our country from the British Isles where the English call it "fives." It was the Irish immigrant who, at the turn of the century, introduced the game over here. It took root in the metropolitan centers along the eastern seaboard and gradually spread westward where it gained popularity among the universities and where its value as both a recreational and conditioning sport were recognized.

As regards the game itself, which closely resembles squash, the idea is to keep a fast-bouncing ball in play by striking it with either hand against a wall and keeping it within the confines of a court as an opposing player alternately attempts to return it to the wall, under prescribed rules. The four-wall game in which caroming side-wall shots come into play is trickier and harder to master. In this game, the skilled oldtimer can often make mincemeat out of a well-conditioned, young tyro by controlling his shots in such a way as to make the youngster run all over the court barely retrieving the ball while the ancient one carefully preserves his limited stores of energy by playing "position." Doubles is played in both single and four-wall games.

Good hand–eye coordination is a distinct asset for a prospective handball player, and athletes who excel in other sports, such as baseball, usually make fine handball players. I can imagine what an ace Brooks Robinson would become were he to take up this sport seriously.

Another requirement for successful performance in handball is ambidextrousness, acquired only by long hours of practice with the weaker hand. Among top-notch players, it is difficult to distinguish the dominant from the weaker hand, the difference in their dexterity being so slight. The beginner is well advised to develop his weaker hand by using it as much as possible during a game.

If you are interested in getting into shape for whatever reason, handball is a good game to pursue. Many professional athletes and college football players keep in trim during the off-season by daily stints on the handball court. A workout of one hour is enough—this, followed by a hot shower leaves you with that good feeling of physical accomplishment.

After some experience, you will learn some of the strategy of the game, such as hitting the ball where the other guy ain't; you will learn to kill the ball by hitting it so low against the front wall that it rolls off without bouncing; and you might even learn to hook the ball on the serve so that it takes a crazy bounce to the right or left, thereby throwing your opponent off balance as he seeks to return it.

In a sport as vigorous as handball, injuries of various types occur. Obviously, you do not play hard at the game if your physical condition is not good. Just as in jogging, a rare physical fitness enthusiast has collapsed on the court. An injury unique to handball and baseball is the so-called bone bruise over the palm of the hand, which results from striking the ball repeatedly, and especially when it is cold. Over a period of time the hand toughens and the pain disappears. Severe injuries of the eye can take place, and it is absolutely imperative that you never—but never—turn your head around as your opponent behind you is hitting the ball. Among some other injuries that I have personally experienced or witnessed are acute low back strain, fracture of the carpal scaphoid, rupture of the biceps brachii, partial rupture of the gastrocnemius and an assortment of strains and sprains.

Having survived many of the above-mentioned injuries, I, at the age of 60, continue to look upon handball as the best of indoor sports.

10

AN AVOCATION IS GOOD MEDICINE: QUAIL HUNTING IS A SPORT PAR EXCELLENCE

JOHNNY A. BLUE

"All work and no play makes John a dull boy," is an old axiom proven true.

Even though one should learn to play when young, it is never too late to start some sort of diversion to rest and refresh the mind and body. Quail hunting is par excellence as such a sport, and it can be pursued in some phase in any stage of life.

Having been endowed with an appreciation for outdoor sports by a sportsman father and a nature-loving mother, and then taught to hunt by a kind brother-in-law, I was instilled with the thrills and deep satisfaction of dwelling with nature, and so naturally I was inclined to develop hobbies along these lines.

I recall as a small boy deriving much pleasure and satisfaction and feeling rather "grown-up" on being asked by one of our "country doctors" in a small town where I was raised, to accompany him on some of his calls into the country. While on these calls, we would view the countryside and look for quail. If a covey ran across the road we would stop and Dr. Findley would get out his double-barreled shot gun and unleash his faithful bird dog, Ida. I would take care of the team of horses and the rigging, and he and Ida would pursue the covey. He never paid much attention to singles, confining his time only to the covey. When he had killed enough for a "mess," he would unload his gun and put it in its case, put Ida in the

95

buggy between us, and drive home. This was very exciting and stimulating to me and taught me much. I was associating with a person of high standing in our community and I was learning the ways of nature, game conservation, and good sportsmanship.

Hunting puts one in touch with kindred spirits whose paths, in all probability, would not otherwise have crossed. Close contact with nature helps men think straight. Chaucer once said that "nature is the vicar of the Almighty."

Nature is kind and it is cruel: it is always honest.

PURSUING AND HUNTING THE ELUSIVE AND CRAFTY BOBWHITE

The aspect of quail hunting that is so thrilling is that it helps one to better communicate with nature and the outdoors. To breathe the fresh invigorating clean air, to view the autumn landscape and brilliant array of colors. There is great spiritual and moral gain to be had from an appreciation of the relation of one's self to the natural environment.

When a Bobwhite less than one year old is crafty enough to outmaneuver and outwit hunters with the best of equipment, the finest bird dogs, and 30 to 50 years of experience hunting quail, it inspires a great deal of genuine respect and admiration and shows us that we are not really supreme.

There is no better way to get away from it all than to visit and hunt with fine hunting buddies, out in the open spaces with fine bird dogs. After 60 years of bird hunting, I still get a little buck fever on a covey rise. The whirr of fast-moving wings like a thousand small airplanes excites me.

The quail is a noble, beautiful and unique bird and it seems a shame to shoot them, but when you look at the situation in a relevant way, it is not so brutal after all. Because a quail rarely lives to be much over one year old, and seldom gets any further than a half mile from where he was hatched, you can get a fair idea if he is older than this year's hatch by examining the wing feathers. If they are frizzled and worn, they are over a year old. The speed that these feathers have to endure puts a lot of wear and tear on them in a short time.

I know of only one instance where a banded quail was discovered 20 miles from where he was released, five years after his release; he just kept going upstream.

As a matter of fact, a quail covey needs to be stirred up quite a bit each hunting season because quail as a rule do not mate within the covey. By stirring them up it makes it easier for them to find a mate from another covey. This is nature's way of preserving the quality and strength of the species.

There is a stanza in the original Oklahoma State song that I learned in grade school that reads, "Oklahoma . . . where

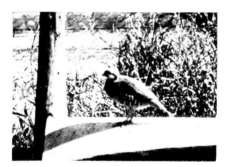

Figure 10–1. The Bobwhite quail.

the quail whistle low in the grass." There is a sort of "call of the wild" in a quail's whistling that awakens a queer sort of feeling in me—a feeling of respect, admiration, and a burning desire to get out into the field and woods and commune with nature. That whistle has a number of tones and I am sure that each tone means something to the other quail. They sound a different note when they are scared, on the move, trying to locate the covey, and even when they are saying that they are near by and need company and they want to mate. It is a great thrill to sit down or hide and whistle a quail up to you, noting his change of notes as he gets nearer. The so-called "Bobwhiittee" is the mating call and is only heard in the spring and early summer. It always represents a lonely bachelor looking for a mate. So when you go hunting in the fall, do not try calling quail by the Bobwhiittee call unless you want to scare them away or mate with one. When one hears a hunter whistling "Bobwhiittee" in the fall, you know that he is not well-versed in the characteristics of the quail and may run off more quail than he will find. He may also frustrate the dogs.

Quail do not live alone; they pair off in the spring and summer and then become "attached" to the covey and always act in unison with the covey.

Quail hunting is one of the most pleasing and gratifying outdoor sports. There are so many varied facets of pleasure and enjoyment that most anyone can derive satisfaction of some type from it, whether one is a good shot or not. In the first place, it gets you out into the fields and woods when the autumnal colors are at their richest shades. Watching the intensity the great drive and desire and actions of a fine bird dog at work is a thrill that no one can deny. The great bond between the hunter and dog is almost unbelievable. The spine-tingling, thrilling, heart-in-the-throat sensation experienced when a covey takes to wing will touch and excite the best of those who take to the field in pursuit of this greatest of game birds.

Shooting quail is an art that takes time to acquire. Like any other sport, if you want to excel in it you must spend a great deal of time at it. It takes quickness, good judgment of time, spaces and speed. You may anticipate which way a quail will fly, but do not always depend on it. He will seldom fly into a strong wind, but will go straight up and double back over your head in most instances. If there is a bush or tree nearby, you can be assured that he will get this between you in the quickest way possible.

One needs to study the quail's trails and habitats and learn where he is likely to light and hide so that you can direct your dogs into that area.

The time of day makes a difference in where you may be likely to find this crafty bird.

Having a knowledge of what a quail eats will help in locating him when he is feeding. Quail love a field-corn patch, maize

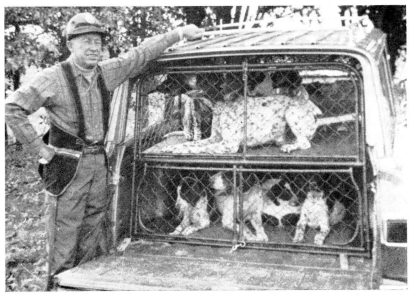

Figure 10–2. Caged and ready to roll. Note the hunting jacket.

and small grain, such as maize lespedeza, all grass seed, rag-weeds, and acorns. They love sunflower and pigweed seeds, and you will generally find them around such places in mid-morning and late afternoon. I examine what is in the craw of the quail I kill and find out what they are feeding on and then watch out for such food.

If you are having trouble finding quail, watch the migratory hawk. If you see him diving and squealing, he will have a quail shortly and fly away. The rest of the covey will stick so tight to the cover that you can hardly kick them out after the dogs point them. Instinct has taught them that if they make the slightest move, the hawk, with his telescopic eyes, will see them and will be on them in the flash of an eye. Although the quail is a fast flyer for a short sprint, he is no match for the hawk who pursues him and will seldom let him escape.

Quail are peculiar in some respects, namely they cannot survive alone and a lost chick or a bachelor will be adopted readily into another covey. That is the reason you hear hunters say they saw a "second-hatch covey." I have seen two coveys become locked in combat, a single or two or three will often be accepted in the covey.

The rooster is an honorable fellow. He chooses his mate and stays with her during the mating and egg-laying phase and helps her hatch and raise the covey while he stands guard entertaining her nearby.

When I was young, quail were plentiful and we would find a nest and take the eggs home and sit them under a fussy little bantam hen. She would hatch them out and then fuss with them while they were growing. They would become quite domesticated until they got full-grown or a little past. Then one day in early fall, despite the little bantam hen's fussing, the "call of the wild" became too strong for them and they would drift away and become wed to the covey, each devoting the rest of his short life to the welfare and protection of the covey and vice-versa.

When I was a boy, we would watch a quail light and it was a cinch that he would be there when you walked to the spot, but modern-day quail in Oklahoma have changed. After they have been toyed with a bit, as the season wears on they will light and then run for a long distance at times, especially if the cover is thin. I have watched my dogs trail them for over a half mile before they sought cover and stopped long enough that the dogs could come on a solid point.

Why have the quail changed this way? It seems logical to me that it is a survival of the fittest. The dumb or lazy ones light and stay put to be found by the dogs and killed by the hunter. The smart, wily ones run and keep moving and hide like the Mexican blue quail, and outsmart dog and man to survive and reproduce his kind. One has to admire and respect such instinctive tendencies as this.

I never use a so-called flushing whip to flush birds by beating the brush or cover to flush the quail, either while hunting or in field trials I find that this often confuses the dog, and they are afraid you are thrashing at them, so some of them will break their stance and lie down. I have seen a lot of good dogs ruined this way. When they start doing this it is hard to get them to stand up again. Picking them up and dropping them on all four feet will often get them out of lying down squatting, but you will have to be very gentle with them.

I like to use the toe or stomp the brush to flush the quail. I let the dog go with the flush so that he can see the quail down if dead or crippled.

I never come up from behind the dogs when they are on point. This causes them to look back and so distracts their attention from their object; come in facing the dog and he will remain steady and maintain an intensive point. Never run up behind a dog or hurry around too close to him when he is on point, or he may break his point and flush the birds.

You may hear hunters talk about leading the bird so far on a right or left shot or shooting him if going away and so on; I do my shooting instinctively. If I lead them, or close one eye, or keep both eyes open, I do it subconsciously. If you hunt often, it will come naturally. It is somewhat like golf, if you try to think of too many "dos" and "don'ts," you often become so confused that nothing goes well.

One of the main things I try to refrain from doing is getting mad and trying to shoot the bird after he is out of range, or shooting too quickly at close range and tearing up the bird so that he is unfit to eat. This is bad in several ways: it destroys game; it is bad on your dogs because when they retrieve a badly shot-up bird the taste of blood and raw meat makes them want to maul the bird, and if very hungry, even eat it (I always feed my dogs something at noon. I have noticed that they will be softer mouthed if they are not hungry.); you might hit him light enough to allow him to keep going and die over a hill later on, and a quail has been wasted. This last is one reason I let my dogs go with the rise and chase the birds. Many, many times my dogs will come in bringing a bird that has been crippled unknowingly and has fallen out of sight. When a dog does this, he is a really fine retriever: he not only conserves game, but reminds you to watch a bird after you have shot at him. If he starts sailing, he may be hit. If he keeps his wing beat balanced and rapid, it probably was a miss. If he goes straight up, he is shot in the head; if he wabbles, he is badly hit; if he drops both legs, he is finished after he hits the ground.

It is always well to mark a bird down by picking a bush, weed, or high grass clump, and hurry to that spot. If not your judgment of distance is sometimes inaccurate and you will miss him. If you wait too long you will give him time to recover from the initial shock and run away or dig under heavy cover and escape. There is nothing more distasteful and wasteful to me than to loose a crippled quail. One drawback to rushing to a downed bird is that it is better for your dog to pick up and retrieve all dead or crippled birds; do not compete with him in this manner.

Choosing the time of day to hunt is very important. I have had little success in hunting very early in the morning, because the quail have not started moving around yet so early. They come off of the roost shortly after daylight, according to the weather. By about 9:00 A.M., they begin to move about to feed, leaving their scent so that the dogs can smell them better. If it is wet or there is a heavy dew, it washes away the scent and makes it harder to find. When they are out of the covey to feed they are scattered out wider, and this makes them more vulnerable. After they are through feeding, around 11:00 A.M., they seek shelter according to the weather. If it is cold they will get on the leeward side of a hill, the edge of timber, a thicket or briar patch, or tall grass. If the weather is nice they will see a place to sun and wallow in the dust and a shady place when the sun becomes hot. They start feeding again about 4:00 P.M., then go to water. At about dusk they fly into a low grass spot out of the wind and get into their circle roost with tails together and all heads pointing out so that they all are on guard and their droppings are piled in one small pile. This fly-in keeps other creatures from trailing them. If not molested, they will return to this same general area several times according to the weather, but always in a different spot. Being able to judge the freshness of these droppings and the freshness of the tracks will enable you to judge whether he is close game or not.

If water is available, such as a pond or a creek, they will water about midday and late afternoon. But a quail can survive without water from the moisture he gets from the bugs, grasshoppers and worms he eats.

Bird hunters in the first half of the century had a number of unwritten codes that they followed, and these codes were adhered to very closely. For instance, one never thought of hunting on someone's property without asking for permission; when he was granted permission and the hunt was over, he generally went by the house and offered to share the game with the owner.

When you are in the field and quail would flush, if you were on the right, you shot at the quail on the right and vice-versa. You never shot at a bird which another hunter had shot or was attempting to shoot. There was very little double shooting in those days. These rules are gradually passing out of use and some hunting on public lands is not only dangerous, it is downright greedy in many instances. Getting the bag limit has almost become a status symbol, and sportsmanship and politeness have been replaced by this sort of greed and ego.

Once while hunting in the Oklahoma panhandle, I had an experience that made me have a great deal of respect for nature and wildlife.

This happened in an isolated flat river bottom. I had shot a bird while hunting without a dog, and it fell some distance away among some large cottonwood trees where the ground was covered with dead dry leaves. I marked the spot and walked to the area and began looking around for the dead bird. I was not having much luck finding the bird, when all of a sudden I heard a faint rattling sound that had a familiar ring. Now I am not the kind of person who panics when they see or hear a snake; though I am afraid of them, I do not stampede, especially if I can see them. I remained still and diligently searched the ground all around me. The sound was repeated. On looking down, almost under my feet I saw an object that somewhat resembled a cornstalk leaf lying in the leaves. Knowing that there was no field corn grown any where near, there I took a closer look. The rattling was continuing intermittently. As I looked closely, what I thought was a corn-stalk leaf began to show a resemblance to a large snake partially covered by dry, dead cottonwood leaves. He had flattened himself out on the ground which camouflaged him amongst the leaves. I immediately began to look for his head and tail, knowing that I could readily detect a rattlesnake by the blunt appearances of the rattles on the tip of his tail and the broad jaws. After what seemed to me like a long, immobile lapse of time, I saw some leaves move at one end of the object and heard the familiar rattle. Then I detected the very sharp tail end of a snake that was without rattles. With a sigh of relief, but still not moving, I stood there observing this creature mimicking one of his more deadly and feared brethren by vibrating his tail in the dry leaves, thus producing a rattle resembling that of a rattlesnake. This bluffed me and almost panicked me into hasty retreat. Of course my initial instinctive urge was to blow him to pieces with the shotgun, but I could not overlook such an ingenious, or perhaps instinctive movement of nature to protect itself. After a few moments of reverence and due respect, I took the gun barrel and lifted up the large, harmless bull snake or chicken snake and gently put him across the fence out of my way. I retrieved my dead bird and went on my way knowing that I had come out second best in another encounter with nature, but with profound respect for the craftiness, perseverance, and cunning of many of the things in this life we call creatures and varmints.

SECURITY WITH THE HERD

Once while hunting in the Oklahoma panhandle I had another very impressive experience that demonstrated how nature protects itself by the instinct of the herd.

The ranch where we were hunting was on Coldwater Creek, a hugh layout of 11,000 acres with a beautiful cold, clear stream running though the middle of it, a rare thing for this panhandle with Calichi Cliffs surrounding it. This rancher positively did not allow any hunting, but he had granted me the privilege because he was grateful to me for managing his asthma which had threatened him with the thought of having to quit ranching. This was a hunter's paradise and we were really enjoying it.

That day our host could not hunt with us, so my hunting buddy and I were hunting when I saw one of my dogs, Chiefy, come down on a classy point near a large tumbleweed. I called to my hunting partner and signaled that we had a point. The other dogs were "backing" some distance away (which is another *must* to qualify as fine bird dog. When backing, a dog stops as soon as he sees another dog on point and does not run up in front and flush out the birds. This is called "backing" or "honoring a point." We were all set for the covey rise when I kicked aside the large tumbleweed. But to our surprise there came a startling "Baaaah!" from a black object lying still on the ground. It was a prized black Angus calf whose

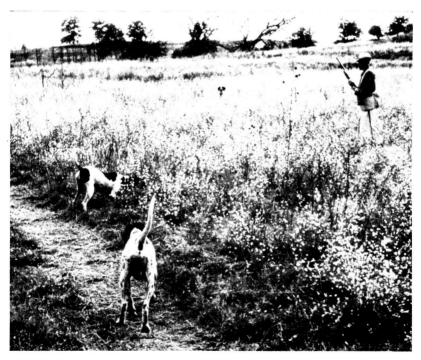

Figure 10–3. Perfect style pointing and also proper dress for the hunter. Note dog backing in background.

mother had neatly tucked him under the tumbleweed, well hidden, and had gone nearby to graze. Of course Chiefy, not knowing what this was, rose to what he thought was a challenge and "took him" right away. This elicited another distressing bawl, and the mama cow answered.

I yelled for my partner to grab the calf while I was grabbing dogs. A great fear gripped us that the prized calf would be injured and our hunting privileges lost. While this commotion was going on I looked up and saw the rancher coming

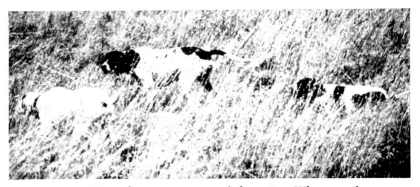

Figure 10–4. Note the intensiveness of the point. When quail are very close and dogs are afraid they might flush, the tails are not high, but they warn the hunter to be ready immediately.

in his pickup and my heart sank. I looked back behind me and there was a herd of about 50 black Angus cattle with their silver chains about their necks and the metal clip in their ears, indications of the high-bred registered stock, with their eyes shining and their nostrils open, just about ready to charge. The rancher, contrary to our fears, did not seem disturbed, and he called out to us to release the calf and dogs and quickly move away. As we did, this herd led by the mother cow let out some bellows and came charging forward. The dogs scampered past us with their tails tucked away and the little calf, walking very near the mother's legs, became engulfed by the herd.

We went our way, thankful that nature had demonstrated very beautifully how the banding together of some animals into a herd was a protective measure against the pack of wolves and other predatory animals they had had to face throughout the centuries and also that the beautiful little calf had not been hurt and the rancher was not going to run us off his place or shoot my dogs. He laughingly told us that this was a common occurrence and that it took a pretty good pack of dogs or coyotes to match a charging mama cow and the backing herd with their sharp hooves and butting heads.

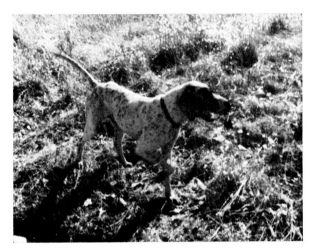

Figure 10–5. Doc on point.

CHOOSING YOUR BIRD DOG

There is nothing more pleasing or stimulating than to own, train, hunt, and work with a good dog in the field. As Huckleberry Finn says, "There ain't no harm in a hound anyway."

One should use a lot of thought and caution in choosing a hunting dog. Just because a dog has a pedigree of national reputation in field trials does not mean that he will make a good hunting dog. Bird dogs are like people: there are both exceptional and rather ordinary ones and like people, they have personalities; whether you develop or suppress these personalities depends on what kind of a dog you desire. Remember, when you choose a dog you should be with him enough so that you love and admire each other. Some dogs are lovable and others are not. When you choose one, you more than likely will be associated with him for six or seven years because one becomes so attached to his dog that it is hard to part with him no matter what his bad traits.

The more you live with your bird dog, the better your communications will be with him. There is a common practice of boarding dogs out and never visiting them until a few days before quail season opens. Under these circumstances, to expect the dog to be perfect is unreasonable. It is very depressing to go hunting and see your dog take up with another hunter and leave you flat. If you want your dog to be obedient and stay with you, you had better get acquainted with him and make him want to be with you, and not just trust his hunting instinct. When I whistle or call my dog in, he knows that I will give him a kind word or pet him for responding or that there is something exciting going on. Dogs have poor eyesight but a very keen sense of smell and hearing, so use the same whistle all the time. No two whistles have the same tone; *you* may not distinguish between them, but a dog can.

If a hunter is a slow plodder, then he needs that same sort of a dog so that he will cover less ground and stay close in. You may not get as many quail this way, but you will enjoy it more than you will if you have a big running dog that runs and leaves you for a long time. If you are a good walker, you can handle a wider range dog. It is difficult to break a big running dog to stay in close; when you do that you take something out of him and he is less efficient as a hunter. You want your dog to hunt as if he is thrilled to death to be out just for the sheer joy of hunting, finding, and handling game. A dog that tags along at a hunter's heels or stays so close to you that you are almost stepping on him will not put much game in your sack. A dog that does this has been mishandled or treated too roughly or just does not have it in him to hunt. Then, too, watching a fine, talented, bird dog work is a big part of the thrill of the sport.

Just one trial does not prove a dog. The more a dog hunts in the field with other dogs, the better, wiser and more competent he becomes. There is nothing more helpful than actual experience under proper guidance, and actually finding game is a stimulus for a dog to hunt harder. Always correct your dog when he makes a mistake, not by beating him but by letting him know he is doing wrong and that it displeases you. Some dogs can take a little rough treatment and some cannot, so try being kind but stern first—"Honey attracts more flies than vinegar." If this does not work try the old top sergeant tactics. If you punish your dog, do not remain mad at him; later on give him a good petting, because like people, a dog does not like for you to be angry at him, he loves praise. A good dog wants to please, but he has other instinctive driving forces within him that he has to overcome. I like and admire an ambitious and aggressive dog, though not a pugnacious one. It has been my experience that this sort of dog makes the best hunter and is generally more intelligent. My dogs raise a racket when man, beast or varmints approach my home or vehicle, and they generally mean business and will back it up if not restrained.

My dogs are mainly one-man dogs. I never have any trouble with them straying off or joining another hunting party. When they get separated from me they get worried and start looking for me. Most of them steer clear of strangers and will not let other hunters get close to them when out in the field. I like this because I have never lost or had a dog stolen in this way.

Dogs, like young children, do not understand words very well, what they do understand is tone of voice, harshness or gruffness, softness, pleasantness, and they respond in like manner. When you see a dog cower all the time, you can feel assured he has been mistreated.

When I start handling a new litter of pups, I have a regular grading sheet for keeping tally on them. I watch for the good and bad traits that their forebearers had. I rate them on the following points: aggressiveness, intelligence, appearance, style, hunting ability, ruggedness, retrieving, and backing. Of course, love of gun and game is always essential.

If you should be fortunate enough to have a dog that rates high in all of the above categories early, then you have literally found a "birds' nest on the ground"; this is very unlikely to happen. There are a few of the above traits that you can develop in your dog and there are some you cannot change. You can do very little about his intelligence. You can make him wiser by giving him more experience, but his native intelligence cannot be improved. His style cannot be much improved. If he has a straight tail, you will not likely change it to a high tail. If he whips or breaks his tail with a classy rhythm when he runs and hunts, that is a part of him and you will not be able to change it or teach a dog to develop it. If he stands high with head up on point do not fool with him, just admire him. Many a good dog has been ruined in this manner by too much fiddling with or talking to him until he lays down or squats down; once he starts this, it is hard to overcome.

It is upsetting to hunt with someone who is continually chatting, whistling, hollowing, and commanding my dogs; when my dogs are spoken to, it means something to them. Idle chatter worries a dog and he finally disregards everything. I do not hesitate to tell such a person to let me give the commands to my dogs, since "too many cooks spoil the broth."

You cannot make a rugged dog out of a meek one, but you can do the reverse by being too strict with such a dog.

Hunting ability and aggressiveness can be improved. I have noticed time and again that when my dogs recognize a superior dog and play second fiddle to him, they are relatively useless until you separate them and give each dog a chance to develop his own traits and stop watching the other dog. If you don't he will be backing all the time instead of finding game himself. No dog ever put much game in the sack or won any prizes by just backing along.

When you own a pup, do not pass final judgment on him too soon. He may show a lot of good qualities and bad qualities when young, and a lot of factors can suppress or bring out either trait. A bird dog never reaches his full potential before he is nearly two years old. A great deal of experience and patient handling and work will often correct a bad fault in a dog that otherwise would cause one to get rid of him.

Some hunters abhor the sight of their dogs chasing rabbits,

and do all kinds of antics to break them from it, from whipping them over the heads with the dead rabbit, to tying it around their necks. I have always contended that if you are where there is an abundance of quail you will not have to worry about your dog chasing rabbits.

I never restrain my young dogs from running anything that flies or runs, from grasshoppers and butterflies to crows and rabbits. They soon learn that a quail smells better and it is more attractive than anything that moves.

When you select a collar for your dog be cautious that you check the tightness occasionally; never have a collar that is too tight. There are several reasons for this: in the first place, if it is too snug it is uncomfortable and will choke the dog to some degree. Keep the collar loose enough that it can be slipped off with a little difficulty. This is helpful at times and may save your dog from a fatality. I have seen dogs helplessly tangled up in fences and rubbish. If they had been able to slip their collars, they could have freed themselves without much difficulty. Then, too, it enables a dog to free himself if some stranger gets a hold of him or ties him up. If a dog is unruly enough to put up much of a struggle when his master or trainer has him on a leash, then one should use a choke collar. However, never allow a dog to run loose with a choke collar on.

Puppies outgrow a collar fast, therefore the snugness should be checked frequently. If their collar is leather, then litter mates will chew it off in a short while. I therefore like a chain collar that will not rust or stain the dog's neck and is not too heavy. This can have a snap on it that can allow adjustment in size as is needed.

Some dogs are natural retrievers and soft-mouthed. These dogs are invaluable and often have other good traits. If your dog is aggressive and loves to get the dead bird and run around with it and maul it, you need to work him by himself. Work with a retriever that has tacks on it, even use a choke collar or an electric collar gently, and he will generally come around if you do not push him too much or handle him too roughly.

If you shoot a bird up quite badly, get to it quickly before the dog has time to maul it. The native instinct of a dog is carnivo-

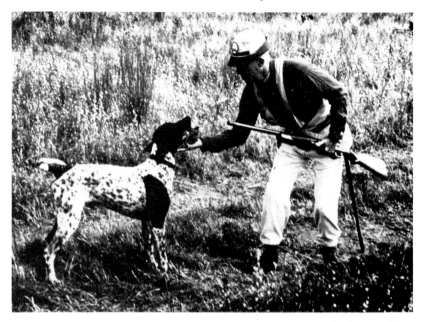

Figure 10–6. Dr. Blue displays one of his prized bird dogs, Classy Ebony, on a perfect retrieve. Note the proper quail hunting attire. Also notice the two dogs in the background, on point.

rous, and the taste of blood and raw meat plays hard on such an instinct, especially if he has gone without food for some time.

A lot of my dogs have backed instinctively; if they do not, I work with them gently. They can all be taught to back if you let them know what they are supposed to do. You may have to use a choke collar or the electric collar, but do not be too rough. This backing, though, is a must in quail hunting. There is nothing more trying to quail hunters than hunting with a friend who has a poorly trained or undisciplined dog, so that when your dogs come down on a classy point, the undisciplined dog runs up and busts out the covey before you get in gun range. You may notice your dogs making the same mistakes later and sometimes good friendships are strained in this way.

Being "steady to wing and shot" is pretty and a must in field trials—this is not the case in real quail hunting and shooting. I like my dogs to go with the covey rise, then if a bird is crippled they will have a better chance of picking him up and retrieving him. If they do not and you waste several moments reaching them and touching their collar and commanding them to go, the bird will have had time to escape, to die later and be wasted.

I have seen several potentially fine bird dogs sacrificed because they ate a quail. It is believed by some that once a dog eats a quail he can never be broken from the habit. This is not true. I have seen at least three of my dogs eat a quail but it was always my fault. He was either underfed, the quail was shot up badly, or there were other dogs trying to take the quail away from him. When these circumstances were corrected the dog did not eat the quail. This reminds me of a doctor friend of mine, Dr. Stillwell, who was an outstanding field trial man and an ardent quail hunter, one who believed in sharing the kill with his dog. One day he was hunting with a friend of ours who did not know about this. While hunting, this fellow knocked down a quail and Dr. Stillwell's dog got the bird and

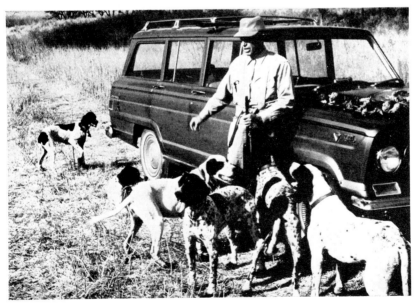

Figure 10–7. Loading up after the hunt. Note the quail (bag limit) on the car hood.

ate it. The fellow was perturbed but did not want to upset Dr.
Stillwell by compaining about his dog, so he kept quiet. After a
while the same thing happened again; this time the hunter told
Dr. Stillwell that his dog had eaten two of the hunter's quail
and the doctor responded, ". . . you should see [him] hunt after
he has eaten one or two." So if your dog eats a quail, do not
dispose of him until you have surveyed all the angles.

FEEDING AND CARE OF YOUR DOG

I think it is criminal for a hunter to keep a dog caged up all
year and then when the season opens to take him out and hunt
him all day or until the dog gives out. A dog is like an athlete,
he needs to have a scheme of exercise training that gradually
builds his muscles to where he is capable of performing all day.
I have seen dogs who were out of shape have severe cramping
of the muscles and be unable to walk and eventually die in
agonizing cramping pain, or be shot by some ignoramus who
thought the dog was having fits.

The same can be said of feeding your dog. A dog does not
sweat, and his cooling system requires frequent water both to
drink and wallow in, because he has to slobber to cool off the
heat generated by the enormous amount of energy expended
by a hard hunting dog.

A dog should not be hunted all day after an early morning
ride and a long trip home after several small findings. The old
idea that a hunting dog should not be fed prior to or during a
hunting has been thoroughly disproved by scientific investigation. If a dog is run on an empty stomach, he becomes exhausted
quicker and has to call on his liver for stored glycogen and
when this is depleted he gets hypoglycemia, weakness, and can
die from this. A hard running dog requires four times more
calories than one at rest.

I always carry water in the car and some plastic-wrapped dog
food in cake form which is a dehydrated, yet soft concentrated
protein that is light to carry and easy to feed. I give them a portion each (2 is supposed to be a meal) when I arrive at the

hunting ground, one at noon and one when we load up to go home. They line up in the cage and await their turns. This helps me remember which one has had his share and permits one from hogging it all.

Then when we get home they get a real two-course banquet which consists of a large portion of a good prepared dog food with some warm gravy made from meat scraps and suet. When it is very cold I add a little more fat of some sort. I prefer the above because it is clean, simple, easy to transport and prepare and gives the dogs a well formed stool instead of the thin, frequently messy stool.

I do not let my dogs run loose, but neither do I keep them caged up in a small enclosure. The bigger the space in which they run, exercise and play, the happier and healthier the dogs will be. I am careful to protect them from intestinal parasites, flies, fleas, and ticks. I examine them frequently and inspect their external ear canals and ears for ticks and mites, and their paws for thorns and stickers. I look at their gums to see if they are blanched—a sign of anemia. I watch them when they are (on "kennel point") urinating and having a bowel movement. I have often performed emergency surgery on my dogs, allowing them several more good years of hunting.

YOUR DOG'S BED

Even though a dog can sleep almost anywhere, his bed is very important to him and he will protect it with great fierceness.

A dog's house should have a small door that faces away from the prevailing wind, with a small porchlike shelter above the door or a cloth flap to keep out the cold and rain and to allow him to look out. If he is in a small pen, he should have a flat-top house or some object he can get up on and lie down and view his surroundings from above.

What a dog sleeps on is very important to him. If he does not like it he will scratch it out of his den. If the dog is a young pup or a bitch about to go into labor, I put an old pair of my hunting pants or some clothing that has my scent on it. This seems to settle him down somewhat.

I like wheat or oat straw with some cedar shavings for dog bedding. It cleanses their coats and keeps down fleas and ticks. But one does not want to leave it in long enough for it to become powdery or they may breath it and get pneumonia, or even contract an eye irritation from it. This bedding is fine in the winter, but they may scratch it out when the weather is hot. I often tack down a rug on the floor, but this too may prove hot and they may tear it out. As a matter of fact they sometimes tear it out no matter what it is or what the weather is.

I once noticed my dogs sleeping on the ground outside their ordinarily cozy, warm, comfortable house. On inspecting the inside thoroughly, I found that the cottonseed hulls which I had placed in there had degenerated or molded, and had become repulsive to the dogs. When this was cleaned out and fresh bedding supplied, they went back into their house. I have one dog house that has two doors and will hold eight or ten dogs. They seem to like to bed up in real cold weather, but they like to have room to stretch out and sleep in warm weather or when in a warm house.

One of the best houses I have found for dogs is a 50-gallon oil drum with a flap cut in one end; this flap is lifted up and used as a sort of porch. Bury the belly of the barrel in the ground about 6 or 8 inches and put about the same amount of dry dirt inside. Then use whatever other bedding you desire. This holds in the generated heat. It gives him good protection in a den which is very warm and dry and from which he can look out and defend himself from any intruder. They love them, especially in cold weather, and they cannot chew them up like they do wooden structures.

I always have an abundance of cool, fresh, clean water. A dog will drink anything that contains water when he is hot and thirsty, but he is a great lover of just cool, fresh water.

I housebreak all my dogs when they are puppies, so that we develop a very close relationship. By this close association they become one-man dogs and as long as this close relationship is maintained, this tie is never broken.

MAN'S BEST FRIEND

The old saying, "A dog is a man's best friend," is a true statement in every respect; the converse is also true. Numerous incidents come to mind that will express the mutual feeling between man and his dog. I recall an incident when Duchess, as a puppy was stranded on an ice flow after almost drowning in an icy, swollen river, and was snapping at everyone and everything who tried to rescue her but me. My hunting buddies and I risked our lives to rescue her by a human chain from a swift current stream full of barbed wire.

Everyone likes to boast about getting his limit of quail in the shortest period of time. This has served to overemphasize this fact to the point at which it is becoming a status symbol. There are so many more gratifying things about quail hunting than the ego satisfaction resulting from filling one's "sack."

It is a real pleasure and thrill to watch good bird dogs work together, especially if you have trained them yourself. There is a closeness and feeling between a hunter and his dogs, evidenced in the way in which the dog speaks or converses with his master through his mannerisms, actions, looks and motions.

I can never forget the look in the eyes of two of my dogs, Rip and Doc, and the distinct and impressive way they communicated with me one day while getting the car out of the deep sand where we were stuck while hunting. The dogs were out, and after the car started moving, I speeded up to get to sounder and firmer ground. The dogs thought I had forgotten them and was about to run off and leave them. They ran furiously by the side of the car and looked in the window and signaled me to let them in and not leave them. Their expressions left no doubt in my mind as to what they were trying to tell me.

A bird dog understands and has more bird savvy as he gains experience. One fall I hunted with a six-month-old puppy and some older dogs. She loved to retrieve, but was so gratified that she had found the bird and had it in her mouth that she wanted to parade around with it and would not bring it in on command. One of the other dogs, a fine retriever, looked on with much disdain and disgust and finally, calmly walked over to the pup, gently removed the quail from her mouth and leisurely returned it in a rather smug, superior manner.

I have hunted behind and owned many fine bird dogs in my 60 years of quail hunting. In that time I have formed an opinion of what I considered the ideal bird dog, known as a shooting dog. First I want him to be obedient and be looking for *me* in the field; I do not want to be looking for *him* all the time. I like a big, strong, aggressive dog with a large handsome high head; a big, short, fairly high tail; broad chest; big feet; strong forelegs and big hindquarters, with a short shin bone which gives him more power and drive. I like a square-built strong back; I am biased, preferring white and black ticked dogs. My dogs have to be fine, smart dogs and good champions, a one-man dogs so to speak, that will not hunt or retrieve with anyone but me. I like him to be evasive of strangers, so that he cannot be stolen easily. He must have a good nose and be a soft-mouthed retriever and a great bird-finder with a great desire to hunt as long as he is down. I like him to cover a lot of ground but be a medium ranger and always be in view unless on point. He should report in to me occasionally. I like him to respond readily to whistle, call, voice and hand commands.

He must cover all the objectives, that is he must instinctively know or have learned to what objects, terrain, or coverage a quail would most likely go to hide from his pursuers or to feed.

I breed and train my bird dogs and practically live with them; we are real pals. If you have never seen 12 bird dogs hunting in unison each respecting the other's ability and all on point at the same time, waiting for you to come up and kick the brush or signal them to tear up the cover to get the quail in the air (you would be disqualified if you did this in a field trial) or retrieve him if he is crippled, you have missed one of the greatest of thrills of sportsmanship.

Hunting with 6 to 12 dogs at once is frowned on by many hunters. If the dogs were strange dogs, it could be a hindrance, but these dogs have been hunting together for a long time and the older ones help train the younger ones. They respect each other's point and retrieving, and they comb the objectives pretty thoroughly and pace themselves so that they can go all day.

To see them all on point at the same time is worth the trip to the country itself. Innumerable times, by pursuing the quail, one of them brings in a bird we did not even consider we had hit. So being steady to wing and shot is another myth that is dispelled, if you want to fill your sack and conserve the bird crop. This rule is all right for field trials, but it wastes game when hunting in the field.

These dogs are not only valuable hunting dogs, their intelligence makes them useful and amusing in many other ways. Several of them will go one block away and bring me the newspaper. They inform me by the tone of a bark whether it is a varmint, animal, dog or man that approaches the place or premises. We have been burgurlarized several times in the past but never since we have been keeping some of the dogs at home. They know our cars by the sound at least two blocks away and can tell what I am going to do by the way I dress, and they react accordingly. If the paraphernalia is for play with them or hunt, they give the alarm to the others and head for the Jeep Wagoneer, bucking and jumping with glee. If it is street clothes or evening clothes, they line up in the front of the door on their haunches, assuring me that everything will be protected while we are gone.

For the past 25 years I have by selective breeding almost reached this ideal dog by mating several of the recognized world's greatest bird finders with proven great "meat dogs," to produce the first all-around quality hunting dog. Such blood lines as Luminary, Wayril Alleghany Sport and Jake, Cobb's Duchess, Texan Ranger, Paladin J. Blue's Salty, Un-Rap, Short grass Jeep Seairup, Warhoop Jake, Palamodium Parmadine, Pretty Ger Mae, Susy D. Tradition, Sports Ariel Jeep, Wanstonm, Warhoop's Belle. Such breeding has produced real meat dogs who have the heritage of Field Trial and Shoot to Kill winners. On August 29, 1970, in the *American Field,* I announced the showing of this new line of dogs, which I called the "Blue Line" of pointer shooting dogs.

The so-called modern Field Trial dogs are generally wide running, big ground coverers, and they take a man and horse to keep up with them. If they are "broke," i.e. steady to wing and shoot, and can find a bird occasionally, they have a good chance to be in the winning in a field trial. For hunting with and putting game in your sack, they may be failures. They seldom are taught to be good retrievers, and generally when they are put down, they keep running, expecting you to keep up; consequently you spend a lot of time looking for them This type of dog gets most of the publicity and recognition, but seldom makes a good hunting dog for the average hunter. This was the stimulating motive behind my effort to develop a "new type" of bird hunting dogs.

When one raises and trains his own bird dogs, he generally derives more pleasure and satisfaction from watching the dogs perform than from actually shooting the bird.

The dogs, like hunters, are subject to various accidents or hazards of the sport. Once, upon x-raying the hind leg of one of my most vigorous pointers (he had been limping for awhile), I found that five or six bird shot were lodged in the soft tissues of the leg, and some close to the bone with calcification spots.

I called a friend, an orthopedist, who agreed to look at the films and then examine the dog, Spunky. He felt that surgery was not necessary, but gave the dog an injection; the infection, which had been the result of the shot in the leg, was soon gone.

Before he left, my friend gave medical advice to my other office personnel who had questions about their animals' health; he even x-rayed a sore shoulder for me and administered an injection to alleviate the pain. He refused payment, of course, calling his assistance a matter of "professional courtesy." It was a profoundly rewarding experience for me to have had a professional colleague graciously come to my aid for this particular, somewhat unusual, circumstance.

All of these dogs have rewarded me a thousandfold for this attention—with their profound devotion, obedience and great effort to please. They tell me by their actions when the other dogs have run away, or when the puppies have found the house door open and shredded the place; they let me know when things are not going right.

When my dogs get aged I do not relegate them to a small pen for the rest of their lives. I try to pay them more attention:

treat their ailments, see that they get a few extras in their diet, taken them hunting for short spells, let them in the house to lie on the rug by my reading chair, and give them a lot of petting. I see that they are not exposed to inclement weather and severe cold and try to protect them from the other dogs and see that they do not get into a fight (their spirit is still there, but the body is weaker).

HAULING YOUR DOGS

Many of my hunting friends haul their dogs in crates in pickups, in their trunk compartments, in the back seat of the car or on the floor boards of the front or back, or in trailers attached to the car.

Many a fine bird dog has been sacrificed by being put in the trunk of the car with the lid partially opened. If the exhaust pipe is not just exactly right, the vacuum at the rear of the car will back the exhaust fumes up into the trunk and the heavy, constant accumulation of carbon monoxide gas will asphyxiate the dogs in many cases. In some cases where the dog cage is enclosed with only a small opening at the end of the truck bed, a similar thing will result.

I train my dogs to get on the floor board or lay on the seat, if I let one inside the car. I seldom let one in unless he is old or sick or crippled so that he has trouble in the cages with the other dogs.

I do not like to pull a trailer, so I devised a double-decked cage that fits into the back of the jeep against the back of the rear seat and extends to rear-end gate, allowing enough room to reach in and open the rear end. One can close it completely or ventilate it by lowering the rear or side windows as you see fit. I can haul five large dogs in each compartment without much crowding. My dogs lay all over each other anyway and are generally content to endure such closeness since they know that they are going to be well rewarded for any discomfort they encounter, by a good long gratifying and happy hunt. In the evening when returning, they are generally so tired and sometimes cold that they do not object to such coziness. By hauling them in two compartments, I can hunt them in relays of five or hunt the whole pack for a while together and later cull out the older dogs and those that are a little crippled. I let my dogs empty out and never feed them just before caging them for a trip, and they rarely have a bowel movement accident while in the cage.

SELECTING YOUR EQUIPMENT

I select my gun for shooting and not displaying. I use my gun and I do not want to be worrying or fretting because it may get a little scratch on it. I try to keep it clean and in good order and I keep it in a case when not hunting with it, even on a short trip. I do this to protect it from dust, grime and grit.

Presently my favorite gun is a 12-gauge, glass barrel, aluminum body, three-shell affair, and I use an open cylinder or a modified cylinder for quail.

I prefer #8 bird shot, rather than chilled shot. The former will splatter when it hits its mark and one shot can bring down a quail. The chilled shot do not splatter and will go through leaving a smaller hole, which may permit the quail to fly on for some distance before he dies and is lost, or it may only cripple him and he gets away. This is a waste of game.

I do not use graphite in my gun because it is very wearing on moving parts. I use a little oil or grease because if too much is used it will pick up dust and grit, and gum up the parts, thereby causing the gun to hang.

When one chooses a gun with which to hunt quail, he should take into consideration his strength, how strenuous and prolonged he intends the hunt to be and whether he is hunting for sheer sport and pleasure or for meat, so to speak. A good marksman can use anything from a 410 to a 12-gauge. One should choose a gun that feels good, is well-balanced, and that does not "kick" so that he will flinch just before he pulls the trigger.

If you are hunting in close-range territory such as brush, a light load is preferable to the heavy load, a longer range shell for the open spaces and fields. I prefer #8 or #7½ unchilled shot.

One should learn to get the gun up to the shoulder quickly, pull it tight to the shoulder, and get it on target before pulling the trigger. Be sure to instinctively watch for objects in the line of fire, because it may be the bobbing head of your hunting partner, your dog, or a horse or cow. Always wear bright clothing which reflects light. Hunting jackets, shell-holders and game bags should be selected for comfort and usefulness and lightness rather than looks.

I have the greatest respect for a shotgun because I have seen the destructive force it can have at close range. I refuse to hunt with anyone who is careless with a gun. It irks me to be walking beside a hunter who carries his gun so that you are looking down the barrel and can almost see what size shot he is using. I never walk in front of anyone who is carrying a gun. I give them plenty of swinging room to the side. When in doubt I hit the dirt. I would rather get a little dusty than beheaded.

Never lay a loaded shotgun down on the ground or lean it against a car or some flimsy object with a bunch of dogs jumping around. Those dog feet and claws can do funny tricks at times. They can knock over a gun very easily and kick off a safety and pull the trigger with ease sometimes. I have known hunters who got part of a foot shot off by such carelessness. Always unload your gun in such cases and put it up on something where it cannot be knocked over or stepped on.

Another precaution is to never remove a gun from the car or case with the barrel pointing toward you. Always point the barrel up or away from you and anyone else. These careless acts and "unloaded guns" have shot and killed many people.

When you walk all day carrying a shotgun on your shoulder with a hunting coat loaded with shells and game, the weight on your shoulder is terrific and very tiring and results in poor and careless shooting.

That is why I designed my own jacket, which consists of suspender-like straps with a waist belt to keep the weight at the waist and gives the shoulders more freedom. There is a large pocket on each hip with a zipper. Inside this pocket is a separate compartment for single shells with a zipper top. The rest of the pocket can be used for loose shells, gloves, and any other article you need handy. At the back reaching to the button is a large open sack-like game holder with a small compartment to hold a pint of water in a plastic bottle. I fill this bottle at night and freeze it in the refrigerator and put it in the holder the next morning. It will melt just enough to give you a nice refreshing ice cold drink when you become a bit tired.

CLOTHING FOR QUAIL HUNTING

When it comes to clothing I am an admirer of neatness, good grooming and style, but I prefer comfort even if I have to sacrifice sartorial perfectiveness.

The headgear should conform with the weather. You should wear a lightweight cap with a good bill to shade the eyes and of a proper size to be comfortable at all times; a tight cap or hat is a very uncomfortable thing and can produce headaches if too small. If it is too large, it is troublesome because it will repeatedly be knocked off by brush or tree limbs or be blown off by the wind; a rough material cap will do the same thing by hanging on brush.

If the weather is cold, a sort of flannel-like lined cap with ear flaps proves very comfortable. However, a quail hunter does not like to have his ears covered unless the coldness is severe, because he needs to be listening to every sound so as to hear and spot the call of the quail or other sounds such as the rattle of a rattlesnake and movements of varmints and domesticated animals.

Of all the quail hunting clothing, the headgear above all should be of bright red or yellow reflection material, so that it is visible to other hunters.

I like the clothing on my upper body to be loose and comfortable and made of material that will not pick up grass and weed and brush trash, and of a heavy enough quality that it will not snag easily in brush or barbed wire fences. The ordinary flannel-like, woven woolen shirts certainly do not meet these qualifications. I like the neckpiece to be easily opened or closed and be easy to turn up or down as the occasion demands. Windbreakers are too bulky and prevent you from getting your gun to your shoulder easily. A slick finish on the clothing allows brush and weeds to slide off easily.

I have tried all sorts of britches, trousers, pants and shapps. The heavy cotton khakis with the leather or plastic material shields on the front of the legs are very cumbersome, heavy, hot and uncomfortable and will wear one down in a full day of hunting in rough terrain. The light duck pants allow thorns, weeds, grass, and stickers to penetrate them and scratch your legs. The heavy duck pants are fairly good, but they are hot and soon wear out around the knees and lower legs and then allow thorns, weeds and stickers to penetrate them.

The best hunting pants I have ever had are made of 100% nylon facing and the body is of 100% cotton. They are manufactured by Utica Duxbak Corporation. This garment slides through brush and weeds with ease, does not snag or pick up thorns or stickers, and will wear indefinitely. They are not too heavy, they break the wind; they are comfortable and have a good appearance. I like these pants a little loose so that I can wear an angora shirt and khaki shirt if needed, and with the length long enough so that they can be tucked under at the ankles under a heavy rubber band, which prevents grass and weeds from crawling up inside your britches leg, something along the fashion of a paratrooper.

The type of underwear is very important if you want comfort. In warm weather I prefer a T-shirt and loose-fitting boxer shorts. If the weather is cool, I may wear a long-sleeve cotton jersey and balbriggan pajama bottoms or thermal two-piece underwear, large enough that they will not be binding.

During very cold bitter weather I wear Navy aviators' two-piece gloves with the long gauntlet; these have the woolen knit glove inside, with a removable outer soft leather glove that has an elastic insert at the wrists. This leather grips the gun well and is not slick and slippery as are the woolen and some heavy leather gloves.

When it comes to selecting the proper footwear, I like my boots to be light, made of durable leather that will not scuff or crack. The composition soles with the beaver tail thread will not pick up mud easily, and I like a heel. Boots should be fairly loose so that I can wear heavy socks if the weather is cold. Ordinarily I wear an athletic cotton sock with the padded woolen and cotton sole. I wear a light silk sock under these to prevent friction and the rubbing of blisters. If my boots are wet when I come in, I put the electric boot warmer and dryer in them and apply the proper dressing. In very cold, snowy, wet weather, under footing I wear a lined heavy Swedish boot, but for ordinary hunting these boots are too heavy and will tire you out.

SELECTING YOUR TRANSPORTATION

Today, in Oklahoma at least, most quail hunting is done on foot behind dogs, although there are a few hunters who drive a pickup truck, a four-wheel drive vehicle. The latter is used on rough terrain or in fields and pastures. However, most of the quail hunters who hunt for the thrill of the sport pursue the game behind their dogs, on foot.

In these days of urban America the quail have been crowded out from the periphery of the centers of population. Now one has to drive from 30 to 175 miles to reach suitable territory, where you will be permitted to hunt and where quail have suitable cover, food, water, breeding grounds and general environment—thickets, some high grass, fence rows, shelter-built trees and hiding places, briars or brush piles, and places for the quail to seek shelter from inclement weather, man, beasts, and birds of prey.

The ideal vehicle for such occasions is one which has most of the comforts of the modern day automobile, with comfortable driving ease at the established speed limit, so that one can get to the hunting grounds as fast as he can in an ordinary luxury car. Then when the destination is reached, he should be able to get off the highways onto high center roads, lands, creeks, sandhills and rough terrain in general. In order to do this, such a vehicle must have a high chassis, a rugged frame, a powerful engine, and preferably a four-wheel drive with a cable attachment so that if badly stuck you can hook the cable to a tree and pull it out that way. The tires should be rugged, heavily knobbed enough so that they will not puncture easily, but will ride smoothly on the pavement.

I am never caught out without a heavy truck jack, nor will I ever make the mistake of putting oversized tires on the rear of a four-wheel drive vehicle again. I did this once and it caused me great inconvenience and quite an expense before I learned that having the same size tires, front and back, was far more sensible.

I and several of my hunting friends have been using Jeep Wagoneers for several years with all the modern conveniences attached, we find them very satisfactory on both the highway and over rough, rugged terrain.

USEFUL GADGETS

I used to hunt with a fellow who was a perfectionist and improvisor. This game ranger really knew and enjoyed wildlife and nature, treating them with a great deal of respect. He had the greatest store of knowledge of the outdoors that I have ever seen, and always went prepared, with more little helpful gadgets in his pockets than you could imagine. He taught me a great deal about hunting, the outdoors, and wildlife.

One should carry certain pieces of equipment that might come in handy in the event of emergencies. Nylon cord and a small rope or chain often are necessary in dealing with occasional situations that the animals find themselves in. After being lost a few times, one becomes aware of the practicality of carrying a compass. An ether-aerosol can, a small container of gasoline, and a small compressed-air container can be lifesavers in dealing with car problems, as can de-icing solution and windshield scrapers. Two canteens of water and a book of safety matches are musts. Other helpful paraphernalia are flashlights, large waxed candles, pliers, screwdrivers and wrenches, and a small shovel. A large plastic sheet is helpful both in wet weather and for speading on the ground and also for use as a container for water when watering the dogs. It is wise to carry two guns, in the event that one should need repair, and a small knife and screwdriver, as perhaps the repair will be minor and could be accomplished with these two small tools. In this instance, gun oil could come in handy, too. Lastly, do carry some small change, as you may need it to use the telephone or buy a bottle of refreshing pop somewhere along the way. Firearms and alcohol can be a dangerous combination, so my companions and I avoid this potentially hazardous situation by refusing to bring alcohol on our hunting trips.

I am a true advocate and believer that a busy doctor stays a young doctor if he has the proper fun, exercise, mental happiness and peace of mind; thus an avocation is good medicine both for the patient and doctor.

11

"PULL"

ARCHIE T. COFFEE, JR.

It all started with a six-year-old, South Georgia farm boy, a double-barrelled twelve-gauge "rabbit-ear" shotgun, and a pine tree. The maker of the gun, the honorable firm of Jenssen of Belgium, no doubt never intended their fine piece to be proof-tested by such a devious method as blasting the trunk of a stationary, Southern Georgia swamp pine.

The boy, however, learned, in that split second, three indelible shooting lessons: first, the destruction was appalling at close range; secondly, one must hold tightly to his fowling-piece lest it take a running start on its way to kicking one's boney shoulder because thirdly, the stock was too long, had too much drop at the comb, and definitely was not custom-made for the shooter.

With these facts in mind and the smell of burning gunpowder for added impetus, the boy progressed to the dove fields and the Savannahs and the Tupelo bay haunts of the Bobwhite where the lessons of both lead and fast shooting were impressed upon his subconscious by informal experience. In addition, in those post-depression days, ammunition was at a premium and the need to make every shot count proved to be another important lesson. In time, the boy became a better-than-average, honest-to-goodness upland game shot.

Years away at college, medical school, the military service during World War II, followed by residency training, resulted in the finesse of that upland gunner becoming considerably tarnished. This became embarrassingly apparent one bright October day, when the boy, now a man and the author, took to the pheasant fields of a commercial game farm. The shooting was so poor that day that something drastic had to be done immediately. Acting upon the advice of a shooting friend, the local gun club was contacted. There the author was properly introduced to, and soon became addicted to, the fascinating game of clay target shooting. Many memorable hours have since been devoted in pursuit of this fine sport, both in practice and in competition.

Skeet and trap are two forms of clay target shooting popular in the United States. In trap, targets are thrown away from the shooter by a pit-mounted mechanical launching device. This device is generally electrically powered and is known as a trap. Skeet differs in that targets are thrown from two traps mounted about 40 yards apart. The targets used in each sport are identical, consisting of small saucer-shaped discs about 5 inches in diameter, formed of molded pitch, hardened by a special heat-treatment process; when centered in the effective pattern of a medium day, they scatter gun fracture into a puff of fine black dust.

Trapshooting is a much older sport than skeet, dating back possibly several centuries. Records indicating the first reference to trapshooting as a sport appear in 1793 in the old English publication *Sporting Magazine*. There the author describes use of live pigeons in competition as targets. This form of competitive shooting survives today with some modifications, as the most popular shotgun sport in Europe and Central and South America. On a somewhat limited scale, it is gaining in popularity in this country as well. Somewhere around 1831, the Sportsman's Club of Cincinnati, Ohio, used trap-released passenger pigeons as competitive targets, and hence may have represented the birthplace of trapshooting in this country. Through the late 19th century, this form of shooting was popular in the Great Lakes region in the cities of Detroit, Cleveland, Buffalo, Syracuse, Rochester and Windsor, Ontario. It was not unusual in those days for championship shooters to score 100 straight at live birds, a feat that even today with modern equipment would be exceedingly rare.

The trend to use inanimate targets rather than live birds started somewhat later and a device to throw feather-filled glass balls was developed in England and about the same time in this country. Many types of devices were developed, some of metal with wings, feathers, etc. Virtually all of these proved unsatisfactory and unpopular. Later, about 1880, a flat disc-like target composed of finely ground clay mixed with water and baked, was introduced by George Ligowsky of Cincinnati, Ohio.

These first targets were very hard and difficult to break. This idea or principle, however, seemed ideal since a target had been developed which could be uniformly produced, had little air resistance, could be thrown fast and over a long distance and visibly appeared to break when struck by shot pellets. This led to the development of mechanical devices or traps to throw this type of target, and over the years these have been improved to their present form. Most gun clubs nowadays employ automatic traps, provided with an automatic angling device to change the angle of each succeeding target thrown. As a result, a shooter is unable to predict the angle of any given target from the one thrown before. This injects an element of surprise not experienced in skeet, since in the latter the targets are thrown at a known fixed angle.

The records indicate that about the year 1915, at Glen Rock Kennels near Andover, Massachusetts, something resembling skeet was shot for the first time. The late Charles E. Davies, an excellent wing shot at the time, in an effort to further improve his prowess with a gun, began shooting practice clay targets thrown from a stump-mounted trap. By varying his position, he could vary the angle of the targets to resemble field shots. This soon led to a circle of shooting stations with the trap mounted at 12 o'clock. Later, this was modified by placement of 2 traps, one at the 12 o'clock position and another at the 6 o'clock position. In this way, a semicircle of stations produced the same shooting angles and at the same time restricted, somewhat, the shot fallout pattern.

Both skeet and trap proved excellent training for the wing shot, and subsequently gained in popularity. Skeet enjoyed its greatest impetus shortly following World War II. Military training authorities recognized this shotgun game as an excellent means of teaching aerial gunners the technique of lead or forward allowance necessary to hit moving objects. Thousands of individuals were so trained during the war years and naturally adapted to the sport when they returned to civilian life. Many became excellent instructors as well as top-notch competitors and some even continue to perform in competitive circles today. From these simple beginnings, the sport has gradually evolved to its present form. Hundreds of gun clubs and shooting facilities are in operation about this country today. Many of these hold periodic registered tournaments sanctioned by The National Skeet Shooting Association. An annual world championship tournament is held in this country each year, open to participants from all over the world. The sport has been adapted by the Olympic Games and in a slightly modified form by the International Shooting Union for world competition known as International Skeet.

Trapshooting is also enjoying continued growth and as a sport surpasses skeet in membership of registered or tournament targets shot each year. Many gun clubs have facilities for both clay target games and members which participate in either or both. An annual world championship in trap is held at the permanent home grounds of the Amateur Trapshooting Association in Vandalia, Ohio. This event lasts for a period of about seven days and 47 trap fields are utilized for the thousands of participants from the world over. International trap or international clay pigeon shooting is the Olympic variant of trap as shot in this country. This is the most challenging and to some the most fascinating of all shotgun games requiring a peak ballistic performance from the gun and the gunner as well. Targets are the same size and configuration as ordinary skeet and trap targets, but because they are thrown nearly twice the distance (80 meters as opposed to 55 yards), they must be made harder to overcome breakage from the throwing arm of the trap when released. Since the targets are harder and faster, heavier charges of shot and powder are permitted. In addition, two shots at each target are allowed, either of which may score a break. This is the most popular clay target game in Europe and South America today. One of the French team members at the recent International Shooting Union World Championships at Phoenix, Arizona, indicated there were some 5000 international trapshooters in France alone.

Skeet serves as excellent training for the aspiring wing shot, and in this regard is considered by the author as unsurpassed by any other form of competitive shooting. All competitive shooting teaches gun care, gun handling and above all, gun safety to its highest degree. It is of note that a fatal accident has never occurred on skeet or trap fields in this country despite the millions of targets shot each year in practice and competition. The skeet field, therefore, is an excellent classroom for the aspiring young shooter and either competitive or would-be hunter. The habits and safety consciousness learned there will serve him well in subsequent years of pursuing any type of shotgun sport—field shooting, skeet, trap, international skeet, international clay target or live pigeon shooting.

Figure 11–1 is a semidiagrammatic sketch of a skeet field. Traps are permanently mounted 8 feet above the ground in the high house on the left and 2 feet above the ground in the low house on the right. A squad consisting of five shooters in tournament events progresses around the semicircle of shooting stations from 1 through 8. Each member shoots two targets from each of these stations, a high house and a low house target. The squad then returns to station 1 where double targets are shot at stations 1–2 and 6–7. At that time, a target is released from each trap (the high and low house) simultaneously. The nearest or outgoing target is shot first and the incoming second. The

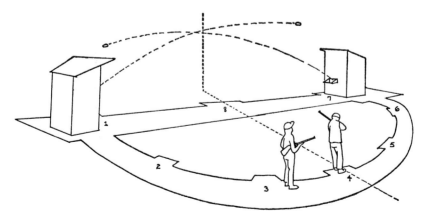

Figure 11–1. Semidiagrammatic sketch of a skeet field.

twenty-fifth target is shot as an optional one: a repeat of the first missed or lost target, or in the event the shooter has broken all 24 targets and is straight after doubles at station 7, his optional target is shot as a high or a low house target (shooter's choice) at that station.

Upon examination of the skeet field layout, it becomes immediately apparent that the various shooting stations about the semicircle provide a great variety of target angles from the straightaway or outgoing and incoming targets at 1 and 7 to the 90 degree or right angle targets at station 4. This arrangement reflects most of the angles an upland gunner or wildfowler is apt to encounter in the field with game birds. Regulation targets are thrown an airborne distance of 55 to 60 yards and are 15 feet high at the center, stake or crossing point. Their speed is about 55 to 60 miles per hour as they emerge from the trap and become airborne. Their velocity has dropped off to within 45 to 50 miles per hour at the crossing point and then diminishes quite rapidly from there onward. With the exception of station 8, the center stake is 21 yards from the center of each shooting station. Since most shooters break their targets at a distance of 21 yards or less, guns with skeet chokes or those throwing an open cylinder or improved cylinder pattern are most desirable. The full choke has no place on the skeet field except perhaps as a practice choke for the super expert. The skeet choke, incidentally, in 12- and 20-gauge guns is an excellent choice for the upland gunner, particularly for quail in the deep south. Nowadays much of the shooting has to be done in cover, and long shots at 35 to 40 yards are the exception rather than the rule.

Major skeet tournaments are usually in 400 target events with 100 targets in each of four guns. These start with a subsmall gauge or 410-gauge and progress through the small gauge or 28, the 20, and to the 12 or all-gauge. Trophies are awarded in each of these championships and to the various subclassifications in each event. The most coveted, of course, is the high overall, or the highest total score attained in all four guns. For this, scores of 395 or above are generally necessary, and this represents some rather fancy scattergun handling. Ties are

settled by means of sudden death shoot-offs. Usually there are
more 12-gauge entries in tournaments and since this is ballisti-
cally by far the most efficient gauge, there are sometimes a
considerable group with perfect scores of 100 targets broken.
Gun clubs may choose to settle such ties by shooting doubles
at all stations exclusive of station 8. This rather quickly separates
the men from the boys. Although it is a good tiebreaker, most
shooters prefer not to do it this way. Yet when several topnotch
shooters get really "hot," shoot-offs at regulation skeet may
advance far into the night before someone misses. Since a
mechanism to terminate this more quickly is needed, doubles
at all stations has been devised and despite its drawbacks and
undesirable features, solves the problem.

Figure 11–2 represents the modern trap field layout. This
consists of five shooting stations, 16 yards behind a single pit-
mounted trap. Targets are thrown away from the squad of
shooters at an unknown, unpredictable and variable angle of
45 degrees. Targets are generally broken at 28 to 40 yards distance. This requires a somewhat tighter pattern of shot, and

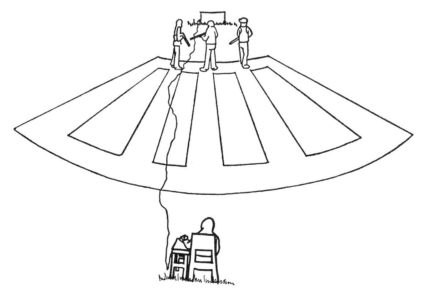

Figure 11–2. The modern trap-field layout.

hence, guns with barrels of modified-to-full choke bores are
a necessity. Singles or 16-yard tournament events are usually
shot in 100 target events, although a major tournament may
throw from 500 to 1000 singles targets over a period of several
days. All major tournaments feature doubles events where traps
are set to throw two targets simultaneously, separated by a 45
degree angle. This is a very fast-moving game requiring quick,
fast timing, and is indeed most enjoyable for those who like to
burn a great deal of powder in a short period of time.

One of the most interesting events of trapshooting is the
handicap event. Here, shooters are assigned yardages of 18 to
27 yards from the trap, determined by their known ability and
past performances. This system is a great equalizer since the
most proficient shooters are moved back closer to maximal yardage and the greater the distance, the more difficult the game
becomes. Perfect scores in this event are, as one might expect,
exceedingly rare and unusual. Most shooters, however, regardless of yardage, feel they have a fair sporting chance of taking
home the bacon regardless of who or how many notables may
be on hand. One needs only to watch this event to marvel at
the amazing degree of efficiency of modern-day shotguns and
shot shells. It is rare and unusual indeed, for maximal yardage
or 27-yard shooters to win these events, particularly when the
elements of wind, rain or prevailing light vary from ideal. These
handicap events tax the skill and ability of even the most
expert of gun handlers. Just as in skeet, the factors of concentration, quickness, smooth coordination and follow-through are
essential in putting together a winning score. The shooting
characteristics of a given gun or type of gun are much more
critical in this game than in skeet, and reach a peak in the long
yardage events. Being off the target by what appears to be 1 or
2 inches, when magnified by 40 yard distances, means the entire shot pattern may miss the target several feet. Some experts
advise use of guns which, by virtue of ventilated rib pitch and
stock comb height, throw their charges 1 to 2 feet high at 40
yards. This is ideal, however, only under certain circumstances.
Variations of target height created by wind direction and velocity become quite important. Targets thrown directly into the

wind climb sharply, whereas those with a tail wind become very flat. Crosswinds, if brisk, elevate incoming targets, depress and flatten outgoing targets. For this reason, the author feels one should become accustomed to a gun which places the shot charge where one is looking or squarely on the money when one looks flush down the rib. The advantages gained by becoming accustomed to this type of pointing or sighting are immeasurable when a shooter participates in several of the clay target games such as skeet or trap and hunting, as well.

Now let us discuss some of the basic fundamentals of gun handling and later apply these to skeet and trap. Stance and body posture are quite important in providing a stable base from which one can smoothly swing a gun. Generally, an erect posture with slight bend in the left knee and slight forward tilting of the body works best for the majority of shooters. Awkward postures, excessive bending of the knees, crouching, excessive weight on one foot, are all points which restrict and limit the range of body movement, limit the shooter's swing and follow through and add to the complexities of hitting moving objects. Some excellent shooters seem quite awkward, assuming bizarre and grotesque postures. It has always been the author's contention that these individuals would be nearly unbeatable in competition if they did not shoot under such handicaps. The author places about equal weight on each foot with a slight bend or break in both knees. Foot placement is always comfortable as though one were shooting a target over the center stake at skeet. This provides a stable, balanced base from which one may swing a gun smoothly and comfortably in either direction. It is then easy to swing back in the direction of the house from which the target will be thrown, pick it up quickly as it emerges, swing with the target and fire instantly as the sight picture appears correct and continue with a smooth, well-coordinated follow-through. This should be accomplished primarily with trunk and leg movement or by pivoting and with as little arm movement as possible. The head, neck, arms, shoulders and upper trunk should form a solid gun mount much like the turret on a battleship. The feet, legs, and hips become the pivotal base from which the smooth swing is executed.

These principles, simple as they may sound and difficult as they may seem in execution, soon become automatic and may be released from conscious thinking so one's undivided attention may then be focused on the target. These are simple preliminaries to setting up the complex reflex mechanisms of the central nervous system using auditory, visual, tactile, proprioceptive sensations as well as muscle power to place the shot charge at the correct spot in space to intercept the moving target. This latter principle is one of the most important features to get across to the student. It results in the target being broken in about the same time sequence, from the time it is picked up visually, to the arrival of the shot charge at the proper spot in space to intercept the target. This principle was well demonstrated on several occasions at the world championship tournament. Shooters having broken 250 targets straight in 12-gauge competition and participating in a sudden-death shoot-off may be seen to break targets almost precisely at the same point, indicating an almost identical system of reflexes and timing. This fact seems at variance with what one usually considers as normal individual variation in reflex time. There has to be an important message in this observation, however trivial it may seem.

Gun weight and gun balance are important considerations to be reckoned with if one is to become proficient. The human being is a remarkably adaptable individual and most of us can adapt reasonably well to the standard stock dimensions and standard weights of guns produced by the manufacturers. Some people, however, do not conform to these standards. Therefore, standard guns cannot be expected to fit satisfactorily or perfectly. This factor of correct gun fit is less critical, however, at skeet, than it is at trap. In the latter game, stock fit is most critical, particularly at handicap distances where targets are broken at 35 to 40 yards. In competitive shooting, the difference of one target means the difference between a champion and a "bridesmaid." Some guns are muzzle-heavy and some muzzle-light, while others are well balanced with an equal weight distribution in each hand. Generally, the double barreled guns fit into the latter category. These may not, however, prove to be the most popular since currently one gun, an autoloader, dominates the field and does so for a variety of other reasons. A light 160 pounder will not be able to handle a $7\frac{1}{2}$ or 8 pound gun as well as a 230 pound, muscled fullback will. However, these facts have to be taken into consideration and worked out by the individual shooter to his best advantage.

Stock fit should be such that when properly mounted and checked, one's line of sight is directly down the rib of the gun if it has one, or with the bead visible just above the top of the receiver if it does not. One crude method of checking this is to close your eyes, then raise the gun to your face and shoulder as though you were aiming it. The sight picture should then conform to the above description. Alteration in the height of the comb of the stock may be necessary to bring this about. Stock length is another important consideration to be reckoned with and may be simply altered by either adding a short section or shortening the existing stock. A coarse method of checking this is to hold the gun by pistol grip with the right hand and with finger on trigger as if to fire, and place the butt of the stock in the fold of arm at the elbow. When the length is correct, the butt of the stock should fit comfortably and snugly in the bend of arm at the elbow. If improper, this may be simply corrected by shortening or lengthening the stock as the situation would indicate, by a competent gunsmith.

Another detail of importance is trigger control. Here the ideal situation is to place the forefinger on the trigger in such a fashion that the right-hand edge of the trigger falls into the crease of the first joint. This provides positive, instant control, avoiding the soft spongy effect when the terminal part of the forefinger is placed in contact with the trigger. This is simply another small point that assists in the development of a constant and uniform time interval between the origin of the message to fire in the brain and the arrival of the shot charge at the target.

The position of the left hand on the fore-end should be comfortable and perhaps slightly to the rear of its center point, providing a bend in the left arm at the elbow. If the left arm is held too straight or extended, control of the gun is somewhat impaired. The weight and balance of the gun may dictate this to some extent, as a muzzle-heavy gun may feel more comfortable and seem to balance better with the hand a tad farther out the fore-end. Generally, a gun with excellent balance (usually commonly attained in side-by-side or over-and-under double guns) will feel best and can be controlled best when the weight is equally distributed between the hands. This feature is an inherent characteristic of a well-balanced gun.

During the past 10 years, reloading of shot shells has gained in popularity to a remarkable extent and is a story within itself. The demands of this aspect of the game have pressured ammunition manufacturers into providing shooters with shot shells formed of tough and durable plastic. With reasonable care, these will reload up to 8 or 12 times, before the shell case must be discarded. Using the specially designed tools and components available today, one may produce reloaded shells every bit as uniform in their ballistic characteristics as new commercial ammunition. Reloading presents several advantages, foremost among which is a reduction in the expense of ammunition, thereby making it possible for a far greater number of people to participate than would be the case otherwise. It has always been the author's contention that this does not measurably reduce the expense of the game, but simply makes it possible for one to participate in a great deal more shooting. Reloaded ammunition has carried many a shooter to local and regional championships. The author has been engaged in reloading for a period of about 15 years, starting with rather simple equipment in the days of the old paper shell and progressing to the rather sophisticated automatic loading equipment in use today. To many clay target shooters, this too is a most enjoyable aspect of the sport and one which can be followed when time will permit, such as in the evenings, on rainy and snowy weekends, or when a tournament is not near at hand.

This points up the fact that there are many other facets of clay target shooting which may eventually become of interest to the hobbiest. Amateur gunsmithing, stockmaking and design, gun, shell and cartridge collecting are some of the more important ones. Any one of these may absorb endless hours of spare time while providing pleasure, recreation and exercise.

Whether one approaches clay target shooting as a hunter seeking practice, a sportsman expending a few shells, a gun collector or enthusiast seeking a testing ground for his favorites, or as a serious-minded competitive clay target shooter improving his skills, there are many, many hours of pleasure, recreation and exercise for all. Since any physically capable individual may participate, clay target shooting may become a leisure-time pursuit for all family members. The female shooter is by no means excluded and may become equally or more adept than her mate. For these and many other reasons, the author does indeed recommend, even urge, that the reader visit his local gun club and become familiar with the happenings there on an average day. The odds are that you will never regret it.

12

FENCING

TIBOR NYILAS

The essence of sport activities I define as "a situation lived with great emotion." It consists of a synthesis of three elements—play, movement and above all, competition. Fencing today, as opposed to fencing in the period from the 15th to the 19th centuries is not a combat but a sport. It is a sport that ranks highest among the few so-called "ideal sports," from a medical viewpoint. It is an excellent physical exercise, it is a mode of aesthetic expression, and it has important psychological values.

Fencing permits participation of boys and girls from the age of ten to eighty, because of the rhythm of its action: short burst of activity executed with lightning speed (males from ten to thirty) or exquisite timing born of experience, intelligence, finesse (men from thirty to eighty)—a touch is scored—the action is immediately stopped by the referee or director. Now comes the physiologically important part, during the evaluation of the touch by the director and four judges. For the layman, this is "the pause that refreshes"; for the physician, the all important phase of recovery. Pulse rate and respiration return to normal, the muscle metabolism is able to prevent excessive lactic acid accumulation; and the fencers are again ready for maximum action.

A fencing bout for five touches is limited to six minutes of actual fencing time; the average is closer to three minutes. But it is followed by a rest period of anywhere between five and twenty minutes, depending on the number of contestants. The average competition will last from ten hours (local meets) to four days (Olympic games), in each of the three fencing weapons—foil, épée or dueling sword and sabre. Yet in a well-trained and conditioned Olympic athlete, the brain will tire much before the body does; and the psychological motivation, both normal and pathological, will be exhausted before the physical.

Fencing of course has the quantitative elements that appeal to the sports fan and to a certain type of sports critic interested solely in success as expressed in the score figures. But there is also a qualitative, aesthetic aspect to fencing which gives pleasure to the artistically inclined competitor or critic. Like all the arts, fencing is full of creative fantasy and reflects the psychology of the fencer as an artist and as a person in an emotional climate.

Finally, then, I come to the psychological aspects of fencing. The psychologist is not primarily concerned with what is successful or unsuccessful, with what is aesthetic or not. He is more interested in fencing as a valuable personal document which throws light on the personality of the fencer, and as a reflection of the times and an aspect of a culture.

First it must be admitted that sports have a psychologically cathartic function. Energy pent up in the course of everyday life is released and frustrations already suffered or expected are compensated. In this case, competition serves as an unavoidable defense mechanism which helps to maintain the psychophysical equilibrium. However, such a picture of competition brands it as an expression of the personality's narcissistic tendencies, an *individual-centered* function.

And yet the competitor does not always need cathartic release. Interest in sports derives also from the fact that the more well-balanced the mind, the more it is likely to welcome new experience, greater and more worthwhile self-expansion. Nothing is better than sport for achieving this. In such a case, competition is an exercise of energy within the framework of a standard of exellence and the aim is to perform as well as possible. The opponents are considered not as obstacles (as in the previous definition) but as points of reference to perfection of performance, an altruistic attitude . . . in other words . . . eminently *socially centered.*

Theoretically all competition is ideally based on the latter concept but in practice this is only seen in single historical periods or in few individuals. The explanation for these differing personal aims and their consequences is to be found in the dynamic concepts of aggression as proposed by modern psychology and in the relationship between aggression and the so-called structure of the ego, which is built up narcissistically or altruistically, depending on the individual case.

For all men for whom competition is not only a dominant personality characteristic but also an indispensable, irreplaceable defense mechanism against life's emotional frustrations, competition not only means a fight but also and above all *love of fight*. Competition as seen in sport reaches its highest value when it is a healthy catharsis of the human being's aggressive tendencies.

This does not mean that the athlete should be considered someone afflicted by painful complexes of inferiority, insecurity or dissatisfaction, nor by an aggressive need to find compensation and self-esteem. Instead it means that the athlete possesses characteristics which are typical of the personality of every human being. Thus the expression "noncompetitive sport" is meaningless. Sport *is* competitive, by definition. If competition is taken away from sport, it becomes mere movement.

The other part of the answer concerns fencing and tension. This part is easy to understand from the metabolic point of view. If fencing reduces our tensions, we have catabolism and an increase in satisfaction. If fencing generates tensions in us, we have anabolism, which is the synthetic growth process by which tissues and potential energies are not only restored, but during youth, actually increased. If anabolism in turn were not followed by catabolism (i.e. reduction of tension), brute force and pugnacity (aggression) would take over; but as we have seen, these, with the help of fencing, can be transformed or put in the service of more ideal emotional attitudes.

An ideal sport is one in which everybody should be able to participate—members of both sexes, without age limit. It should not physically harm a child or a person past middle age. It should be relatively safe from injuries. And fencing, if certain minimum safety measures are observed (good mask and jacket; well taken care of weapon), is statistically proven to be the safest exercise and competitive sport in the world. Fencing is also an all-weather sport, because it can be enjoyed indoors or outdoors, and at any season of the year. You can have one opponent or a hundred, and it is relatively inexpensive—about $20 for a complete outfit, ready to take on Zorro.

Fencing can be a most satisfying game for the natural athlete as well as the physically handicapped. One of our national champions had his right arm amputated at the shoulder. The mortality rate among fencers from natural causes is considerably below the general statistical average. One of our top-ranking fencers, who at the age of 66 competed regularly, was a recovered coronary thrombosis case. Also, fencing instruction was added to the recreational therapy of mental patients at a hospital in Kings Park, Long Island. There is a "creativeness" about fencing that fills a need in some patients. With others it develops agility, coordination and poise, and serves also as an "outlet of aggressive urgings."

Psychologically, fencing reduces tension and increases satisfaction. It is the most natural outlet for ever-present aggression. It channels the unspent part of aggression into higher emotional attitudes. A child, with the highest uncontrolled aggression ratio, will leave delinquency and other pathological manifestations of aggression in the psychiatrist's book, and express all of it in a healthy, flexible way. The mature fencer who satisfies and leaves tension and aggression in the fencing "salle" is a better family man, husband and father, or wife and mother.

Who, then, should fence? *Everybody who is able to hold a foil or a sabre!*

13

JOGGING

W.E. HARRIS

J ogging is a form of exercise that alternates walking and moderate running. It was originated by Arthur Lydiard of New Zealand, and introduced in the United States by Bill Bowerman, track coach at the University of Oregon. It has advantages in that it does not cost anything, anyone can do it, anyone can regulate the amount of exercise as he sees fit, and it does not require any special equipment or appointments.

At the University of Oregon in 1968, it began as a program to prevent and to treat heart disease patients. There is good evidence that mild to moderate exercise prevents heart disease and benefits people who have heart disease. One of the best studies (C.W. Frank *et al*) showed that people who exercise moderately have less likelihood of dying from heart disease than those who do not exercise. In our modern civilization many people do not have any more exercise than walking from the car to the office, and as a result, they are in extremely poor physical condition.

Jogging is a form of exercise that can be done any time of the day and it can be extremely mild to fairly vigorous. Many activities such as golf, bowling, fishing, hunting, handball, volleyball, tennis, and physical education classes, often have major drawbacks in respect to time involved, inconvenience, expense, reservation of facilities, possession of adequate skills, and regular participation.

Some types of physical exertion have serious disadvantages for older age groups. Competitive sports and hunting may involve short periods of intensive effort undesirable to those in poor physical condition. Other activities provide a questionable amount of actual physical exertion. Exercises that are inter-

146

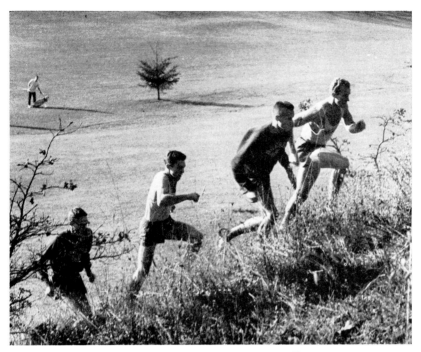

Figure 13–1. A group of joggers on a golf course.

mittent, such as golf, bowling, and fishing, may fail to provide the desirable degree of body stress found in more sustained activities, such as swimming, running, rowing, and cycling. Isometric exercise and calisthenics often are monotonous and are primarily devoted to muscle development rather than improving the function of the cardiovascular and respiratory systems.

While there is little data on the type or amount of physical activity that is optimal for the adult male, there is an apparent need for a convenient, inexpensive form of moderate regular exercise for those over 30.

Jogging is a form of exercise that consists of walking and running alternately at a slow-to-moderate pace. The degree of exertion may be varied over a wide range by regulating the distance covered, the ratio of walking to running, and the pace of the running. Alternate walking and running is of particular value in providing a graduated program of exercise that may be adapted to men of varying ages and levels of physical fitness.

Programs were held in 1965 and 1966 at the University of Oregon by Bill Bowerman, track coach and professor of physical education at the University of Oregon, and Dr. W.E. Harris. Ages of the participants ranged from 25 to 76 years.

Before starting jogging, each individual answered a medical questionnaire and received a medical examination to detect any significant disability that would contradict exercise. Separate programs were held for those who had definite heart disease and for others who had no contraindication for exercise.

For the first day the schedule was as follows:

1. Jog 55 yards and walk 55 yards four times. (These figures are subdivisions of a standard 445 yard oval track.)
2. Jog 110 yards and walk 110 yards.
3. Jog 55 yards and walk 55 yards two times.

The jogging pace was at the rate of 110 yards in about 45 seconds, and the distance was 880 yards. Of the 363 men who

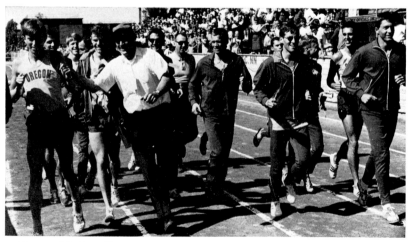

Figure 13–2. Bill Bowerman, co-author of a book on jogging, is in the center of the field in civilian clothes. He is the University of Oregon track coach and professor of physical education.

started the program, 265 completed its twelve week schedule, and 98 dropped out for various reasons.

The first day of the schedule everyone went 880 yards at varying paces, but generally at a pace that was comfortable for all. In the final week, the 36th schedule was as follows (total distance was 4 to 5 miles):

1. Jog 110 yards and walk 110 yards four times.
2. Varied pace "fartlek."
3. Jog 110 yards and walk about 110 yards.

Walk as desired between jogs (usually about 55 to 110 yards). The jogging pace was at the rate of 110 yards in about 30 to 37 seconds. "Fartlek"—slow steady running.

Flexibility of the program was obtained primarily by varying the pace of the running. A few participants in relatively poor condition were advised to progress slower by repeating schedules, and others were allowed to advance more rapidly by omitting some of the daily schedules. About 90 percent of those who completed the programs followed the schedules as outlined. During the course of the programs, seven cases of gout not previously known were discovered because of exacerbation of joint pains.

A total of 212 of the 363 participants were overweight by an average of 17.5 pounds, according to life insurance statistics. Of these overweight participants, 179 completed the programs and lost an average of 7.8 pounds without any emphasis on dieting.

Blood cholesterol readings before one program that was started showed an average of 213 mgm% out of 165 men. Blood cholesterol findings following the program were 214 mgm%. The conclusion was drawn that exercise had no effect upon the blood cholesterol.

Blood pressure readings at rest showed an average drop in systolic pressure of 11.4 mm and in diastolic pressure of 7.8 mm of mercury.

The most common reasons why people stopped jogging were soreness and aching of the ankles, legs, or back. According to track training principles used at the University of Oregon, it was considered advisable to continue light workouts in most instances. Some dropped back to less strenuous schedules, and others were placed on a reconditioning program consisting of alternately walking and slow running 55 yards on grass for a distance of one-half mile to one mile daily. These aches and pains were the most serious problems encountered in the early weeks of jogging and were a major cause of discouragement. It was necessary to encourage participants to continue despite these difficulties and to emphasize that such discomforts must be expected in those who had not been exercising for many years.

During the first program, it was found that running in groups of ten was not entirely satisfactory. Some had difficulty keeping up with the average pace, and others in better condition wished to progress faster. In the other programs, men were divided into groups of 20 and after the first two weeks were allowed to run individually or in small spontaneous groups according to their ability. This arrangement prevented excess activity on the part of those with below-average ability, but did not restrain unduly those who could proceed faster. The advantage of group participation with a leader to keep records and give advice was maintained.

Missed sessions were commonly due to travel, vacations, or acute illnesses, particularly upper-respiratory tract infections. Those who missed sessions due to travel were encouraged to follow the schedule wherever they might be. Those who were ill were advised not to jog until they had recovered, and on returning to the program, to drop back one schedule for each session missed during the illness.

Jogging has the advantage of being a sustained, pleasant, noncompetitive exercise that requires no unusual skills, since the proper running technique is relatively simple to learn. It requires no expensive equipment or special arrangements; it may be performed at convenient times such as early mornings or late afternoons; and it takes only about 30 minutes a day three or four times weekly.

Of the 365 men in the program there was no morbidity of a

serious nature. Jogging has been proven to be a safe exercise; even those with moderate heart disease may jog.

For adults in sedentary occupations, who find it difficult to engage in the usual off-job physical activites, jogging is a suitable and convenient type of exercise.

14

MOUNTAIN CLIMBING AND HIKING

TRAVIS C. GREEN

It is awesome, indeed, to view the Grand Tetons, the Colorado Rockies, or the Olympic Range in the state of Washington. The Himalayas on the northern frontiers of India and Nepal are capable of silencing the observer: the visual impact is past description. Yet as awesome and beautiful a view may be had from the *tops* of these mountains. (My "climbing" of the Himalayas was accomplished by flying over them.)

To the modern sophisticates and sedentary persons alike, climbing mountains is pure folly and a squandering of one's time. Indeed, after an exhausting climb and hike taking the better part of a day, the climber himself may have the same fleeting thoughts. But upon reaching the top at last and looking back, the sense of elation and accomplishment are quite genuine and yet at the same time intangible. Why should a person experience almost indescribable fatigue and even some degree of danger climbing and hiking through rain, snow, and ice to reach the top? It is no mystery: the answer is that it is simply fun. In my opinion, the saying "the best things in life are free" applies here fully.

Mountain climbing and long hikes demand good general health and proper immediate physical conditioning. This conditioning means tightening the muscles of the leg and lower back for lifting the weight of the body and also acclimating the lungs and heart for proper functioning at high altitudes where oxygen content of the air is sparse. (It may be recalled that at 10,000 feet altitude the atmospheric oxygen is one-half of that at sea level.) Simple arithmetic, using one's climbing weight and the vertical distance of the intended climb, will show how many foot-pounds of work the heart must do. The

demand is quite formidable; coupled with the increasing rari-
fication of air as ascent progresses, one can see that the heart
and lungs must be in top condition. Age alone is certainly not
the major factor to be considered in mountain hiking and
climbing. To be repetitious, good general condition of health,
proper acclimation, and setting one's own pace at climbing are
the major factors for safe and enjoyable climbing at high
altitude.

The equipment needed for comfortable and enjoyable
climbing and hiking are, above all, proper wearing apparel.
The boots should be of high-top variety, must fit perfectly, and
must be broken in completely before beginning the climb. The
finest and most expensive footwear is cheap at the price, for
they are worth every cent. Good boots will not cause blisters
if fitted properly and if worn with woolen socks, and they
serve as excellent protection from a sprained ankle. A head-
piece that can be made to cover the ears is necessary. In
climbing at high altitude in snowy ranges, sudden storms of
sleet or hail are common, even in the summertime. Though
these storms are shortlived (10 to 20 minutes), the ears must
be protected. Sleet and snow hitting the external ear are very
uncomfortable and even painful. A jacket should *always* be
taken on any climb. If not worn, then it should be carried in
the backpack. A zipper-fitted jacket of turtleneck design,
Dacron®-lined and weighing about 8 ounces is available. A
drawstring around the waist is very desirable. A jacket approxi-
mating the above description will keep the wearer warm at
10 degrees below zero; this is worth the investment. Even in
summer the wind factor at high altitude may cause a very
low temperature for a short period of time. Soft cloth gloves
and good sunglasses (along with a spare set) complete the
special clothing and apparel needs. Remember, do not econo-
mize on buying clothing and equipment for use in high-
altitude climbing.

When climbing by means of a trail, train yourself to take
short steps. To be specific, I mean steps that place the heel
of the leading foot no more than 2 inches ahead of the toe of
the following foot; this will permit a conditioned climber to

progress without real fatigue for as long as thirty minutes before desiring a rest period. The ideal climbing speed over a trail is about 60 steps per minute. When a halt is needed for a few minutes of rest, it is much more relaxing to the climber to remain standing than to sit. It may seem redundant to so state, but in making up a climbing or hiking party (preferably no less than three members) keep in mind that the party can progress no faster than its slowest member.

Recreational climbing and mountain hiking are thrilling adventures—what is around the next bend in the trail or beyond that big boulder up ahead? There are, however, some precautions that should be taken, for there are a few inherent dangers while in the high country. It is a matter of record that the one single cause of more mountain climbing fatalities than any other is lightning. In the high country (above treeline, which at our latitude is about 10,500 feet above sea level) of the middle Rocky Mountains almost every afternoon is heralded by a short thunderstorm between 1:00 and 3:00 P.M. If it looks like a storm is forming, the hiker should stay off ridges (not allowing himself to be the highest point); if below treeline, do not get under the largest or tallest tree. Instead, find a depression in the ground or a rock overhang. If none is available, simply sit down. A waterproof poncho should also be carried on any hike or climb into the mountains. In summertime climbing within the continental United States, dangers of frostbite or excess cold are unlikely to confront prepared climbers.

A situation which is not dangerous but *very* unpleasant is altitude sickness. This is triggered by an oxygen deficiency. The characteristic symptoms are severe headache with nausea and vomiting, and in many cases, dizziness. These symptoms will appear usually only above 13,000 feet, and frequently even a well-conditioned climber will experience altitude sickness. About the only immediate relief is to descend below the critical altitude to a point where the climber feels good again. Usually the headache will persist for several hours after the other complaints have stopped. Aspirin will relieve the headache if taken in heavy enough dosage: commonly, two aspirin tablets every two hours as needed. Abstention from smoking will go a long way toward preventing altitude sickness. If one knows by previous experience that he may have altitude sickness, he should consider taking Dramamine® or Antivert® at a dosage of three a day beginning three days prior to the planned climb.

As mentioned before, properly fitted, top-quality climbing boots are priceless on a hike or climb. You will not have blisters, and good boots help prevent sprained ankles. Another danger is of a "specialized" nature and will be pertinent to very few mountain foot trips. This is the danger of falling into a crevasse in a glacier or an ice field. A glacier is a body of ice that has a slow descending movement and has a small lake at its foot; this lake is called a tarn. A simple snow field does not migrate and usually has no tarn. Since most recreational, nontechnical mountain climbing and hiking are done in summer months, the danger of a fall into a crevasse is increased. In the northern hemisphere it is the correct procedure to descend or ascend a glacier over the right one-third. Right refers to the side of the glacier if one is at the top of the glacier and looking downward. A crevasse may be 18 inches to 3 feet wide, 30 to 50 feet deep, and covered by a thin layer of ice. This makes the danger invisible to a climber or the person sliding down the glacier. So, when traversing a glacier the hikers should be roped together with about 20 feet of rope between them. Each should carry an ice ax for belaying or breaking if a member of the party falls into a crevasse or has an uncontrolled slide. It is entirely proper and great sport (through it could result in a partial frostbite to the gluteal region) to descend a glacier by sitting and sliding downward. If each member of the hiking party is roped together, has an ice ax, and descends or ascends a glacier along the right flank, it is entirely safe.

To those inclined toward and physically capable of mountain climbing and hiking, the rewards are unforgettable, and they can be experienced as often as desired in movies or slides. The beautiful alpine flowers, mule deer, elk, and birds seen below treeline are of such variety and with such a lack of shyness that these alone make hiking in the high country rewarding. At treeline are found the beautiful columbines and the fascinating banner trees. Above treeline, one may find the ptarmigan (a chicken-sized bird) and the seemingly countless varieties of tundra flowers. The harsh climate of the above-treeline areas permits a spring (the last part of June) of about two weeks. So the lifespan of the blossoms of the tundra is very short. (Tundra is the mat of hardy plant life found in only two places within the United States: the Colorado Rockies and the plains of Alaska.) Mountains make a beautiful sight from the car on a highway, but to get to them and touch them is a thrilling adventure with nature.

The climbing of mountains by the use of pitons, crampons and the exercise with ropes called rappelling is left to the serious and not-so-numerous competent amateurs and professional technical climbers. Such climbing is an exacting science, and to accomplish this safely, one should have some knowledge of engineering and geology. It requires a long period of training and the cultivation of iron nerves. There are numerous authoritative books about the field of technical climbing; it, too, has its own built-in satisfaction for the climber. But non-technical climbing and even rock scrambling can be done by almost any interested person in good health. Some of my most valued memories, savored repeatedly and enjoyed more vividly again by viewing the movies and slides taken, have been of climbs I have made in the high country with my family. The youngest that went along was aged six years at the time of his first climb to an above-treeline summit.

If the reader has been inspired to share my enthusiasm and thrill of climbing and touching nature in her most magnificent aspect, then my aim has been accomplished. Remember, as with any recreation, safety is of the utmost importance. Memories do last forever.

15

SPRINTING

DELANO MERIWETHER

THE AMERICAN HEALTH SCENE

Back in the 1940's and early 1950's, long before I considered going into medicine, I was exposed as a child to exciting concepts of speed and fast running. In rural, semi-urban Southern surroundings, a major interest among neighborhood youths was on raw power and speed. Understandably, flamboyance and affluence (which symbolized power and achievement) held extraordinary appeal for young growing boys like me.

However, many of us could not often enjoy the pleasures of such things as specially-geared bikes, or fancy expensive speed toys, back in those days. Our families had too little money. Nevertheless, we all managed to have fun—we jumped, we tumbled, we played, and we ran. In fact, we could often be found running and racing a truck, for example; or we could be found emulating and racing the spinning wheels of a fast-moving car. So despite conditions of semi-urban America in the 1940's, fun, action and speed through running helped constitute a major, wholesome element in the lives of boys like me.

In spite of my foot races as a growing boy, I was not particularly known for my running ability during school. In fact, I ran no track in high school since there was no track team. Unfortunately, in addition, I was too skinny at 6 feet and 137 pounds to race down the gridiron. Consequently, in high school and later in college where I concentrated on preparing for medicine, I did not participate in any organized varsity sports. I had to be content with a little bicycle riding and light calisthethics. For me, my early years were to consist of

157

pleasant play and games, and of earnest pursuit of a college education and medicine.

While my years of play seem particularly memorable to me—hours of carefree play and fun—they gave way to an adult world of family, occupational, and social responsibilities. And yet, as a physician in this day and time, in this sophisticated society, I continue to concern myself with physical activity, with sports, with personally getting out there and running around a track; the reason for this, in simple terms, boils down to the following: (a) I like to run, and I recognize the fact that increased physical activity and exercise can be fun, as well as mentally refreshing and relaxing; (b) I acknowledge the physiologic health benefits of regular exercise and good physical fitness; and (c) I contend that sports offer the option of healthy physical challenge and contest in today's complex world of varied interests, various goals, and pressures.

Technological advancements in our highly industrialized society have provided unsurpassed comfort and leisure for American families. Unfortunately, however, these advancements in mechanization and automation have encouraged an inordinately sedentary way of life.

In distinct contrast to our forefathers, today's typical American man comes home from his physically undemanding, but mentally hectic job in the office, plops down in front of the television after a hardy meal, and relaxes—truly relaxes. He finds it hard, if he does not have a remote control TV, to even get up to change the television channel. Obviously, this is a sad situation for the head of the household to be in. More distressingly, this situation and this kind of behavior sets a bad example for other members of the family. Whether we like it or not, this kind of behavior can determine the present and future lifestyles of our children. Thus, when we as adults fail to set good personal examples and keep ourselves physically fit, we also fail to encourage and establish sound living practices for the rest of the family.

Abundant medical and scientific information has shown us that regular, adequate exercise promotes good health. Inadequate exercise over a period of time is associated with gradual deterioration and decrease in functional capacities of various organ systems in man. Serious reduction in physical activity along with an increase in the prevalence of obesity and habitual sedentary living among Americans has been associated with a rise in major health problems in this country—principally cardiovascular disease, arteriosclerosis, and respiratory disease. Whereas these disorders are probably multifactorial in etiology, several studies have shown that the alarming rise in the prevalence of both premature disability and death due to coronary and degenerative heart disease may be strongly correlated with inadequate physical activity.[1-6]

Epidemiologic studies such as the Framingham study have suggested that regular physical exercise (along with the maintenance of good body weight) may have favorable cardioprotective effects in man.[7] Other studies have confirmed the feasibility, efficacy, and applicability of programs of enhanced physical activity.[8,9] Consequently, there appears to be an attainable means of preventing and counteracting degenerative changes in man through regular exercise. There appears to be a realistically achievable means of preserving good health in Americans, a means through which we as Americans can fully enjoy our national dream of prosperity, high productivity, and good health.

As yet, however, little has been accomplished on a national scale to change, prevent, or correct the apathy of this country's people towards continued physical training. The President's Council on Physical Fitness, the American Medical Association and the Surgeon General of the Public Health Service have all underscored the need for health programs of exercise and diet to combat the scourge of degenerative cardiovascular and respiratory disease in this country.[10-12] The efforts of these organizations, unfortunately, have had little substantial effect on adults with regard to their participating in programs of increased physical activity.

Being a clinical and laboratory physician, I am concerned about good quality, general medical care. I am concerned about the qualitative as well as quantitative aspects of life. I am especially concerned about the preservation of health and the prevention of disease. Ostensibly, I am concerned about the health of each and every American.

Preventive aspects of health care involve efforts to discourage habits which produce ill health; they comprise efforts to promote an increase in and preservation of good health. This contrasts somewhat with the more traditional, but still all-important, therapeutic side of medicine which concentrates on treating disease once it has already occurred.

In practice, preventive aspects of medicine may be more difficult to administer since it requires effort and action from the subject at a time when he is feeling relatively well. Notwithstanding, preventive approaches in medicine are regarded not only as a challenge for the physician, but as a virtuous goal for the population at large. Preventive measures in medicine fulfill an important role in overall medical care.

Self-imposed Obstacles to Participation in Sports

Why is it that relatively few of us as adults engage in sports and regular exercise? Why is it that we feel content with our current poor physical condition and feel that exercise and recreation are the exclusive birthright of the young? The reasons are all too obvious to those over 35. These reasons appear numerous and formidable. For example, the embarrassment and self-consciousness of having to train and work out with the young folk constitutes an obstacle. Also, there are the muscle soreness and aches that inevitably accompany overzealous workouts in the early stages. In addition, we hear of cases in which there is not enough rapid progress in sports for the aggressive, successful personality such as the businessman or the leader in politics. Finally, after one or two discouraging attempts at getting back in shape, we ultimately hear too often the claim, "I'm no athlete. I give up."

Obviously, for many adults, these reasons are merely excuses, i.e. invalid rationalizations as to why they do not spend more time in physical activities. In many cases these excuses point up a lack of initiative and motivation on the part of adults with regard to increased physical activity. Furthermore, they give a false sense of security and turn out to be counter-productive to good health.

Still, these reasons successfully thwart the interests and efforts of many Americans to get out and engage in physical exercise. Unfortunately, they fall in line with the prevailing pattern of living in America which nowadays dictates that free-time be spent in luxurious drinking and eating, and in purely passive leisure. As if this situation were not discouraging enough, still other factors enter to deter increased participation in physical activity by adults. Today's labor-saving devices, today's modern means of transportation, plus that major capital offender, television, all cause man to further reduce his physical activity to a bare minimum.

With regard to television, a recent survey in Great Britain showed that TV-watching was the most time-consuming activity outside of occupational work;[13] it constituted a major pastime in Great Britain. Approximately 50 percent of the British reportedly spent up to four hours a night watching television. Britain's Central Council of Physical Recreation reported that on weekend afternoons more than 40 percent of Britishers spent significant amounts of time watching television, in contrast to 30 percent who did odd jobs, and 15 percent who went shopping.[14] Less than 2 percent of men and women participated in sports or spent their time taking walks.

Needless to say, there is little reason to suspect that Britishers differ significantly from Americans; there is little reason to suspect that they look at more television than Americans. To the contrary, there is good reason to believe that Britishers watch less television than Americans. Regardless, it is clear that television is a major force in the lives of many people. Television has significantly altered the habits and the ways of life of Western civilization and contributed towards physical inactivity.

Women in Sports

Women are often overlooked when programs of exercise and topics of sports are discussed. Whether as a result of culturally imposed restrictions, prevailing attitudes of what is fashiona-

ble, untenable physiological taboos, or disproportionate allot-
ment of time and facilities to men, women—half of our nation's total human wealth—are not receiving the benefits of
regular sports activities.

The American Medical Association's Committee on the
Medical Aspects of Sports, recently affirmed its endorsement
of several important concepts regarding women in sports. They
conceded that (a) well-substantiated health benefits of wholesome exercise are just as pertinent to women as men; (b)
women who maintain a high level of health and fitness can
better meet family and/or career responsibilities and pursue
avocational interests more enjoyably; and (c) participation in
healthful physical recreation is now rightfully accepted as contributing to the female image rather than detracting from it.[15]
In other words, participation in sound, progressive programs of
physical recreation and exercise can contribute towards increasing health consciousness in women, and effectively contribute towards developing womanhood and a more dynamic
role for women in our society.[16]

Adults Who Do Engage in Sports

At this point, one might ask exactly how many social and
political leaders acknowledge the value of exercise to the point
where they engage in sports activity themselves. How many
adults provide examples in athletics, with which others can
desirably identify? How often do men of medicine concede
the benefits of increased physical activity and put their teach-
ings into practice? Unfortunately, the answer to these questions is, "too few."

Within the discipline of medicine, there are individual ex-
ceptions—notably two physicians, in addition to myself. These
specific individuals (and to a less spectacular degree several
others) have overcome typical self-imposed obstacles and gone
on to enjoy the advantages of sports activities. They have recognized the health benefits of active physical participation and
continue to share in running and exercise as a lifelong pastime.

Dr. Roger Bannister, the world's first sub-four minute miler, is an excellent example of successful, proportionate mixture of medical and running interests. Dr. David Sime, silver medalist in the 1960 Olympics and established ophthalmologist in Miami at age 36, currently finds time from his busy medical practice to keep physically fit, to train, and to run the 100-yard dash in world-class time of 9.6 seconds. Each of these professional men help prove that enjoyable pastimes involving sports is possible. Each helps disband the false concept that professional people are too busy to engage regularly in physical activity such as running. Moreover, these examples help confirm studies[17-18] of men in various walks of life—physicians, dentists, lawyers, university professors, and nonprofessionals—that show that programs of graduated exercise are feasible for actively employed men.

Interestingly, with regard to active participation and training, medical science has shown that the trainability of middle-aged persons is considerably greater than had been suspected with regard to physical exertion and work capacity.[19] This does not necessarily depend on having trained vigorously as a youth. Like the above examples, other evidence supports the fact that adults and professionals can successfully train, develop skills, and develop motivational interests to engage in sports as adults. These examples and evidence underscore the fact that sports do serve as a potent motivational stimulus that permits healthy, efficient development of self-discipline and character.

THE CURRENT LEVEL OF PHYSICAL FITNESS IN AMERICA

In recent years, attention has been focused on the current state of relatively poor physical fitness and the need for improvement in physical fitness among adult Americans by such prominent men as Dr. Paul Dudley White, and the late President John F. Kennedy.

But what is physical fitness? Physical fitness has been variously defined. It has grown to refer to a state of good health coupled with the capacity for sustained performance of moderate to severe muscular exercise.[20] The general term implies an increased sense of well-being and reduced fatigability through an increase in one's reserve physiologic capacity. It also implies the capacity to meet unexpected emergencies safely, and to have enough energy left over from routine work and chores to enjoy leisure time.

Conditioning is a vital component of good physical fitness. Adequate conditioning not only helps improve performance, prevent injury, and insure enjoyment in sports participation, but adequate conditioning also increases the overall economy and efficiency of one's normal physiology. Voluntary muscle, cardiac, and pulmonary functions improve. Physiologic function of other body systems also improve. Rewardingly, those who condition themselves and engage in regular physical activity gradually increase their physiologic reserve and become able to carry out more vigorous activity over longer periods of time with less effort and less fatigue.

Obviously, there are varying degrees of conditioning and physical fitness. It depends partly on the initiative, interest, and motivation that one invests. Important to adults is the fact that the acquisition of a reasonable degree of physical fitness is a pleasurable experience that may require no other justification.

Having personally realized that progressive programs of regular exercise should be a part of the life of every healthy adult, I accepted my obligation in 1970, at age 27, to develop and maintain a high degree of physical fitness. I subsequently began to engage in the sport of running. It wasn't long, believe me, before I experienced and recognized the fact that my new interest added a wholesomely refreshing, new dimension to my life. Running, training, and exercising constituted a fulfilling experience in and of itself.

Nevertheless, other reasons helped influence my personal decision to devote time to running. One of these reasons relates to my being in medicine. As a physician and as a person in a position to advise patients and other people on matters of health and its preservation, I realized that perhaps I could be most effective in getting others to share in various physical activities if I personally took steps to practice what I preached.

Therefore, with this purpose in mind and my childhood love for running, I naturally selected track as the mode of exercise in which to engage.

It is not my intention to emphasize my competitive accomplishments or outline special aspects of my public success in track; these are available elsewhere.[21-31] Instead, I want to concentrate on important issues that are vital to adults who show aspirations of wanting to get back into the swing of things through sports. I wish to emphasize that through sports there is a wonderful opportunity for modern adults to engage in physical exercise and regain a respectable degree of physical fitness. I will attempt to do so with the ideal in mind that one can enjoy sports without necessarily invoking the need to excel. This attitude hopefully will help develop a lasting, mature approach to health through sports as adults.

My Current Running

Comments about my current running career as it relates to future pursuits and goals are given in the hope that they will have a favorable, and realistically sobering effect on the aspirations of adults who are thinking about getting back into sports.

First, as a pastime, I continue to sprint competitively on occasion. I do so on weekends in conjunction with my work and family responsibilities. Over the past two years, I have gained some degree of proficiency and public success at running. However, my avocational pursuit is not primarily engaged in for fame, public recognition, or reward. As we shall see, there are other more subtle, less tangible reasons why I personally devote time to exercise and running. These reasons include the simple satisfaction of being able to take time out to do some of the pleasurable things I want to do; these include the pleasure of being able to get out and run and enjoy myself.

The concept of getting out in the open air and personally enjoying myself through sports is not a totally foreign concept. We all know of, or have heard of the unusual case of the executive, the physician, the military man, or the politician—or the just plain, ordinary person like most of us—who exercises, enjoys it, and exudes the pride and satisfaction of being able to keep physically trim and fit. These individuals did not start out in sports activity for the sake of fame. They do not continue in physical recreation because of monetary or tangible reward. Neither do I.

Low Expense of Running as a Recreational Activity for Adults

As Americans and as adults, our degree of participation in sports activities is determined pretty much by such things as the convenience of facilities, the time involved, the expense, and personal skills required. They vary in time and expense, and the need for special skills. Running is a form of exercise that requires little in the way of facilities—a constructed track, an open field, or a city or country road suffices. Running requires comparatively little in the way of time—as little as one-half hour per training session is all that is needed. It requires little in the way of expense, running gear costs a few dollars and a good, comfortable pair of running shoes will do. It requires, finally, little in the way of special skills—nothing more than the fundamental ability to run.

From these standpoints, therefore, running can be an appealing sport for a significant segment of our society. But what about those who happen to have a little more time and money? Well, the sport of running permits the use of expensive facilities; it permits the investment of more hours; it permits the use of costly personal attire and equipment (for those so inclined); and finally it permits the employment of special skills such as advanced techniques in starting and distance running.

Hence, for people with the means and desire to pursue and really invest in a sport, track comfortably accommodates this segment of society as well. Of utmost importance, however, is the fact that running provides an opportunity for Americans of all walks of life to engage in physiologically and socially rewarding physical activity.

EXERCISE, FUN AND OPTIONAL COMPETITION

For the purpose of our discussion, the concept of *sports* will be distinguished from *exercise* in its strictest sense. As an example, track will be used to illustrate important distinguishing features between true sport and mere exercise. In addition, specific examples in track will show the qualities that make it a particularly rewarding and appealing pastime for mature adults.

To begin with, it is clear that track involves physical exertion. Track involves the expenditure of increased amounts of energy; actual strenuousness depends on the pace and distance, of course. But, by definition, all sports activities entail physical exertion, over and above that of sedentary living; all sports involve the expenditure of muscular energy. Yet, it is through sports like running that present day man accrues the physiologic and biologic effects of exercise that benefitted his ancestors. It is through such sports that man in today's sophisticated and highly mechanized society can still fulfill the natural biologic need for regular moderate exercise and increased physical activity.

Regarding the quality of exercise, running affords an excellent means of attaining good overall conditioning. It does so by bringing into play virtually every major muscle group in the body. Hence, running, when coupled with sensible living habits (which include sensible eating), helps maintain good muscle tone, good posture, a trimmer figure, and good blood circulation.

Still, running as a sport comprises more than mere exercise. It consists of additional elements. In keeping with the true concept of sports, running also encompasses (a) fun, enjoyment, and peace of mind, along with (b) the opportunity (optional) to engage in wholesome challenge and contest with friends. Each of these is important and has its place in sports.

The elements of fun, competition, and exercise derived from sporting activities can be seen in the following example. One of our nation's most prominent statesmen recently said, "I hate to exercise for exercise's sake."[32] Many of us share his feelings and would agree that he is right. Moreover, many of us would hasten to add that it is almost impossible to find time nowadays to engage in exercise merely for the sake of exercise. Thus, I, like several others, concede that it is going to take more than facts about the biologic benefits of exercise to get more adult Americans to participate in sports activities. It is going to take strong encouragement, and conviction in this day and time to get people to try sports.

Back to the above example, it is recognized that aspects of fun and occasional contest are features of sports that help the President keep his active interest in bowling and other sports. Fun and enjoyment also play a significant role in keeping up the interest and participation of adults in other walks of life. We all know of that occasional individual who engages in sports activities solely because he enjoys the fun and/or the opportunity for occasional contest. Perhaps some of us can personally recall these feelings from our youth. These elements constitute real phenomena. They play a powerful role in determining initial and continued participation in sports as adults.

So realistically, in spite of scientific evidence that extols the unequivocal benefits of exercise to man, despite opinions and clinical experience of modern physicians; despite the growing use by physicians of exercise in preventive and rehabilitative programs for cardiac victims and those prone to coronary artery disease, America is still a nation that responds best to incentives of fun and contest when it comes to sports.

What do we as proponents do? We acknowledge the situation, certainly. We examine adults in our society and analyze prevailing attitudes and behavior toward concepts of exercise. We face the problem; we do not give up. We, in fact, make use of concepts of fun and contest; and we persist in encouraging adults to try programs of regular sports activities.

To this end, I acknowledge unquestionably that the current interest and active participation in sports in this country is low. It is the purpose of this writing to enlighten adult Americans to a "way of life" that promotes health and good living well into advanced years. My task is to promote physical and psychological development through sports. My task is to convince adults that sports and physical exercise is rewarding and beneficial to health. My task is to stimulate adults to engage in some form of sports activity. Therefore, I will examine each of three major elements of sports—exercise, fun, and competition—and apply their virtues to helping get more adults to participate in track and other sports.

EXERCISE

An All-Important Element in Running

Running which involves increased physical activity is an ideal form of exercise for adults. It offers varying degrees of physical exertion which range from running at a pace slightly faster than walking, to running outdoors at a faster clip with friends. Ultimately, it allows the chance to race around a track in top-flight, amateur competition. But what are the advantages of regular exercise? What is the medical evidence that exercise through sports is of any benefit to the individual?

It has been shown that exercise can play an important role in the rehabilitation and preservation of good physical health. Supervised exercise has an established place in the treatment of certain diseases and in occupational as well as medical rehabilitation. Various authorities have written on the virtues of exercise. One of the foremost is Dr. Paul Dudley White, a prominent Harvard cardiologist, who has outlined six fundamental benefits of exercise to man.[33]

First, there is the establishment and maintenance of good, general muscle tone. Exercise of the leg muscles, as through running, is especially beneficial since these muscles which constitute the largest active muscle mass in the body act as natural physiologic pumps to aid the total blood circulation. Moreover, exercise is believed to increase the functional capacity of the entire cardiovascular system and make the heart a stronger functioning organ.

The second benefit, according to Dr. White, is the indirect (or secondary) effect of exercise on the psyche. This healthy relationship between physical activity and mental health should not be overlooked even in mature adults, for the ability to be engrossed in recreation is basic. In addition to relieving tension, pleasurable exercise also encourages habits of continued activity and healthy living. For many, occasional pleasant fatigue from exercise is accompanied by mental repose and peaceful sleep. Thus, in a sense there is true equanimity; there is no need for tranquilizers or sleeping pills under these natural conditions.

Another benefit of exercise, though not always appreciated, is its beneficial effect on digestion. This effect is probably mediated through the reduction of nervous tension. It can obviously be of significant benefit to Americans who spend much of their time in tense, nerve-racking work situations.

Interestingly, it has been shown that routine physical exertion does not significantly interfere with the digestive process, while strong emotion may characteristically do so. To illustrate, farmers and laborers customarily work hard immediately after meals; but it is the pressured, busy executive who classically develops the ulcers and stomach troubles. Still, with regard to athletes it is advisable in modern-day competitive sports situations (probably from the standpoint of the role of emotions) for athletes to eat pre-game meals three or four hours prior to competition. This holds true for athletes who are preparing for major competition. Otherwise, the time of day for exercise should be more in accord with one's personal inclinations, one's hours of leisure, and other determining circumstances, particularly if you are the ordinary adult who wants to merely keep fit and enjoy himself.[16]

The fourth benefit of exercise is that of helping control obesity. Overweight in our society is as much a product of sloth as gluttony. There is no longer any doubt that physical activity does play a role in weight control.[16] Maintaining a good caloric balance between dietary intake and energy output requires a sound approach to both food consumption and exercise. Still, the problem of obesity in our country is ever-increasing despite accumulating data that obesity is associated with excess mortality, morbidity, and slow degeneration in man.[7,16,34,35]

Fifth, according to Dr. White, exercise affords general benefit to the respiratory system of man. Deepening of respirations, which occurs with increased physical activity, favors optimal gaseous exchange and better lung function. Even in settings of emphysema and bronchitis which ordinarily limit amount of exercise, physical conditioning and mild rehabilitative exercises have proven to be of unequivocal benefit. In fact, nowadays many physicians agree that physical conditioning and moderate exercise is of low risk to individuals with lung disease and other forms of chronic disease. When prescribed by a physician who knows the health of the patient and is aware of potential physiologic effects of exercise, programs of supervised regular exercise have been shown to be of distinct benefit to the overall physiologic and psychologic health of the patient under question.[36]

Finally, with regard to preventive measures, Dr. White argues that the combined physiologic effects of exercise ultimately may prove important in retarding coronary and degenerative cardiovascular disease. Other physicians support this claim of cardioprotective advantages of regular, increased physical activity in man; especially since exercise has already established its rehabilitative value in such medical situations as during recovery in cardiac victims. Additionally, I personally contend that as more information becomes available, exercise will unequivocally prove in healthy persons an effective, major deterrent to coronary and degenerative heart disease and other chronic illnesses.

Exercise and Man's General Welfare

Recently, alarming emphasis was placed on possible life-threatening dangers of increased exercise. Anecdotal claims were made of mortality associated with increased, exertional exercise. While these certainly must be acknowledged, one must also realize that most of these isolated cases of mortality occurred in settings in which individuals had been exposed acutely to strenuous exercise; further, they probably occurred in settings in which individuals had not been evaluated medically beforehand.

Therefore, to help insure safe engagement in sports such as track, routine medical examination is recommended for all adults before starting a program of running. Routine medical examination is a wise precaution for all Americans. It is advised that each adult undergo a thorough medical examination to detect any disability or illness that would contraindicate exercise, or predispose to injury, or require medical management. Medical evaluation for adults ideally should include a history, a complete physical examination including weight, body measurements, and blood pressure, an evaluation of respiratory function, a standard and exercise electrocardiogram, a chest x-ray, a tuberculin skin test, and basic laboratory studies including urinalysis, blood counts, blood glucose, uric acid, and blood cholesterol and lipids. Such medical examinations, when done on a periodic basis, not only help insure safety and help detect potentially harmful conditions, but also provide assessment of the status of one's current health. Further, information obtained through periodic evaluation can be reassurring and serve to monitor physiologic changes and improvement that may result from a program of regular, sensible exercise.

Of special interest to physicians and layman is the fact that no deleterious effects have been directly attributed to regular, graded exercise in healthy middle-aged or young adults when performed under proper conditions. A joint committee of the American Medical Association and the American Association for Health, Physical Education and Recreation states that, "Precluding accidents, a healthy person of any age will do himself no permanent harm by suitable physical activity. Moreover, exercise that has been specifically selected and prescribed is needed for convalescing and disabled persons."[16] Finally, the committee states that, "Advanced age, in itself, is not a contraindication to exercise, but is actually an indication for it."

Ostensibly, the key to these significant pieces of information for adults are the concepts of graded exercise and moderation. While no deleterious effects have been attributed to sensible exercise, it is unwise to plunge a "soft," unconditioned body into vigorous exercise against someone who is substantially younger, twice as strong, or obviously more skillful than you. Let us not forget that old Indian proverb: "Running in a sense is like medicine—it is most useful when taken properly; too much or none at all may be potentially harmful."

While we do not need to baby ourselves, neither do we want to cause harm. Therefore, engage in sports activities in a judicious manner; indulge in physical activity at a level within your individual physical limitations.

The Physiologic Benefits of Regular Exercise

Proper exercise benefits the heart, lungs, and general circulation of man as well as the muscles and other organ systems[16,37] Various studies have shown that oxygen expenditure of heart muscle is reduced as a consequence of regular physical training; cardiac working capacity is improved in healthy and cardiac-diseased people.[38-47] Also, significant reductions in heart rates at rest and during exercise have been noted as the result of extended muscular exercise in man.[38,41,47-51] Mild decreases in systolic blood pressure also have been noted.[52,53] Further, investigators have observed increases in respiratory vital capacity and lung function in trained individuals.[54,55] Finally, improved peripheral collateral circulation has been seen in trained individuals as a result of extended vigorous exercise.

There is abundant scientific data in medicine and physiology that indicates that exercise through sporting activities, such as running, is an excellent means of improving and maintaining a state of good health. These data all help support the idea that regular exercise is an excellent "natural tonic" for man.

However, these physiologic benefits of increased physical activity in man, like many good things in nature, are subtle and slow to produce favorable physiologic results. In adults especially, one must only be patient, but also expend effort and energy to objectively achieve these benefits. This naturally follows, since physiologic benefits of exercise in man are actually only slow adaptive responses to increased muscular exercise. Consistent with this concept of physiology also, is the observation that the physiologic benefits of exercise are transient phenomena; under conditions of little or no exercise, they are gradually lost over a relatively short period of time. Consequently, it is important not only to participate in sports but to do so on a regular basis.

The Joint Committee of the American Medical Association and the American Association for Health, Physical Education, and Recreation recommends a program of exercise that starts at an early age and continues on a regular basis throughout life, with certain adjustments from time to time as life advances and one's needs, interests, and capabilities change.[16] The amount of increased physical activity that is desirable is largely an individual matter. Recommendations range from 30 minutes to an hour daily as a minimum. Whereas contributions of regular exercise include a sense of well-being and the ultimate development of strength, speed, agility, endurance, and skill, one should engage in hard, fast, sustained physical activity only after he has attained an appropriate level of fitness through systematic training.

To this end, my personal program of running includes a simple relaxed, but regular schedule of fast and slow sprinting. Currently, for me the following program suffices: one-half to one mile of warm-up running, plus mild calisthenics and stretching, followed by four to six short vigorous sprints and longer sprint runs of 200 to 300 yards. This is done two or three times a week during leisure. A typical session takes one to two hours.

Ostensibly, this schedule and program was devised for personal use. There is nothing magic or special about it; it is not sited as an example of an ideal running program for adults. In fact, it is not especially recommended for most adults; other schedules may be better suited.[8,9] It just so happens that my program meets my needs for exercise, fun, and occasional challenge; it happens to be the one that is flexible and convenient enough for me to fit in with my work and family responsibilities. It is the schedule that I have resorted to to help keep myself in a state of readiness and good physical fitness; it is the schedule that has helped improve my fitness and general state of well being.

The Athlete's Heart—A Myth

The notion that the athlete's heart is an abnormally and unhealthfully enlarged heart is a myth.[56] The heart of the trained athlete is now considered normal; its counterpart—the loafer's heart—is considered abnormal. According to the American Medical Association's Committee on the Medical Aspects of Sports, there is no indication that there is anything wrong with the heart of the trained athlete; there is no evidence that exercise damages a healthy heart in the properly conditioned individual.[57] To the contrary, the bulk of information supports the view that regular, increased physical activity strengthens heart musculature, and causes more efficient emptying. Increased physical activity, thereby, makes the heart a stronger and more effective organ to provide oxygen and remove metabolic wastes from body tissues.

By comparison, the loafer's heart is geared to the low demands of habitual, luxurious, sedentary living, and constitutes a potential liability to the individual. For instance, during moments of unusual stress or emergency, the capacity or level of functioning of this organ may simply not suffice. The loafer's heart, furthermore, is vulnerable to characteristic stresses of emotional pressures, as well as excessive smoking habits, and other unsound living practices which unfortunately pervade our urban way of life.

Finally, the athlete's heart, with its attendant benefits, should not be considered the exclusive property of the young varsity athlete—nor necessarily his permanent possession. Achievement of a strong, efficient heart regardless of age is to be earned through personal physical conditioning. Its attainment is possible through regular sporting activities.

Work As A Source of Increased Physical Activity in Modern-Day Society

Man during the past 100 years has made almost unbelievable advances in science and technology. This is best illustrated in our own American society—a fact of which we can be justly proud. Yet as a consequence of technological advances in mechanization and automation, our work currently is much less physically demanding than it used to be. Working conditions in our modern industrial society, generally are characterized

by a gradual elimination of physical effort along with a corresponding decline in physical fitness. Additionally, trends toward
increased leisure and decreased physical effort at work appear
certain to continue.

Because of these trends and evolving patterns of living, and
because of increasing recognition of the relationship between
health and physical activity, there is growing concern that work
in itself might no longer effectively help meet the biologic need
of man for regular exercise. Some consequently foresee the insti-
tution of special, organized programs as a remedy. Fortunately,
personal programs of regular physical training will continue to
suffice as suitable means of exercise. However, regardless of
how we get adults to engage in more exercise, the fact that some
kind of program of physical training is needed to offset declines
in increased physical activity at work is undeniable—that some
program of adequate exercise is needed (and welcomed) in
order to preserve adequate functional capacity and prolong
active, productive life as adults is undeniable.

Coronary and Degenerative Heart Disease

America is presently faced with the major problem of coronary heart disease and degenerative heart disease of almost
epidemic proportions. More than a quarter of a million people
die prematurely, i.e. before age 65, from coronary heart disease
every year.[58] Coronary and degenerative heart disease are obviously multi-causal in eiology, i.e. several factors contribute to
its cause and development. Such factors include sex, age, individual and family genetic characteristics, obesity, cigarette
smoking, hypertension, emotional stress and personality patterns, diabetes, serum lipids (and cholesterol), as well as physical inactivity.[34,35,59,60] Despite this multiplicity of factors,
physical inactivity clearly plays an important role in accounting
for the ever-increasing prevalence of cardiovascular disease in
Americans; it helps account for the current rank of this disease
as the number one health problem in this country.[16,61,65]

Are Physical Fitness Programs the Answer

In workable, everyday terms, we consider a man fit (a) if he is able to perform his chores with a reasonable degree of efficiency and meet demands of everyday living without undue fatigue; (b) if he has sufficient physical reserve to safely meet unexpected emergencies; (c) if he has the ability to recover quickly from the effects of exertion; and (d) if he has enough extra energy to enjoy his leisure time.[16] Also implicit are important factors of adequate nutrition, sufficient rest, suitable work, appropriate medical and dental care, and the practice of moderation in maintaining good physical and emotional fitness.

I think that all will agree that these are not unreasonable requisites for good overall fitness. One is really not asking too much to set out to achieve these goals of fitness and good health. One is really not asking too much to attain a basic, minimum level of conditioning that will aid in enjoying a full life.

Regarding physical fitness, there are two distinct periods in our lives when fitness and personal body image assume special importance. One is when we are vigorous and eager as kids and are expected (and encouraged) by society to actively participate in sports. The other occurs when the pressures and expectations of society are long gone; it is when, as adults, we suddenly realize that we are getting old and we had better start trying to do something about it. Sometimes it is when some physical or medical problem makes itself painfully evident. It is in this latter case that some of us find ourselves today.

We all know of physical fitness programs at YMCA's and various community centers. Some of you may have had experience with organized programs of physical fitness and exercise. Those who sought (or failed to seek) desirable levels of physical fitness through organized fitness programs did so for a variety of reasons. Some engaged in fitness programs for the exercise and its reputed physiologic benefits. In contradistinction, others failed to do so because they thought that the exercise was too strenuous and of no value. Some found fitness programs particularly enjoyable and refreshing. Still others found them boring and a waste of time. Some persisted in programs of general physical fitness because they constituted a challenge and an opportunity for comparing their own performances and body measurements. Still others abhored organized physical fitness programs because they feared that the future held little in store for them; they had already subconsciously conceded the hopelessness of the whole matter.

Regarding the above, two items deserve special comment. First, almost without exception, no one effectively engaged in sustained programs of physical fitness solely because it was fashionable or the accepted thing to do. Those who tried, did not last long. Those who had substantial reasons and lasting interests in sports, as a rule, did last.

Second, in the above example, one of the things that strikes us almost immediately is similarity between factors which determine (or failed to determine) interest in physical fitness programs and fundamental elements which effectively determine adult interest and participation in sports. Operationally, except for minor differences, these elements are the same and are effective.

FUN AND ENJOYMENT

Fun and enjoyment are a vital part of track. Without it, track and other sports would have little lasting appeal; they would become too much like work, and therefore disappear.

In my short career, I have seen sports interests among adults wax and wane, and sometimes cease altogether. In certain cases, runners trained and practiced for a short while, only to stop eventually because they lost interest and stopped having fun.

In distinct contrast, others stuck with their running programs. They clearly appreciated the fun and enjoyment and peace of mind that came with running with friends; they varied their programs so as to maintain their interest. In addition, they appreciated the sense of accomplishment that is associated with getting out and running. Enjoyment constituted the major determinant in ultimately keeping aflame their interest and participation in sports.

Distance running in the Northwest is a special example of how the pleasures of participation can sustain individual and group interest in sports activities. Running in that part of the country is a major sports pastime. Enthusiasts in the states of Oregon and Washington have shown that once you give yourself the chance to enjoy the sport of track, you really learn to like it. You learn to appreciate the psychic and physiologic benefits of getting out and running; you begin to look forward to your next running session. It is even possible that you might experience a sense of remorse whenever you have to unavoidably miss a training session or two. Regardless of other factors, running in that part of the country has proved to be a source of fun and excitement.

Antidote for Emotional Stress

Unquestionably, fun and enjoyment of sports can be effective antidotes for tension and emotional stress. Sporting activities can help reduce socioeconomic and emotional tensions. Running can help relieve pressures and anxieties of work and help take your mind off of other problems. In simple terms, running can help you learn to live better and enjoy life more fully.

Fun, as an important feature of sports, has been frequently overlooked in the past. In present-day society, however, the role of fun and enjoyment has assumed new interest, since evidence has indicated that mental and emotional stress can have significant adverse effects on normal people. Not only can mental stress evoke traditional emotional upheaval, but it can evoke physiologic changes in man as well. Adverse circulatory and cardiovascular responses to emotional stress in man are currently well recognized. Studies have emphasized that responses in man to psychic stress are characterized by "fight or flight" responses, much like those of dogs in Pavlov's historic experiments. Specifically, man's body unthinkingly reacts with a surge of neural and chemical signals to assume an immediate state of physical readiness in response to danger. These reactions to danger are deeply rooted in the prehistory of man, where they often determined survival in a hostile wilderness; in prehistoric man, the adequacy of these responses often meant the difference between life and death.

In today's environment, dangers to life are less overt. Threats of danger tend to be abstract. Threats may come in the form of unexpected bills or memos, or threats of loss of job, or in any number of other forms. Still man reacts physiologically to these threats in much the same way as did his primitive ancestors, i.e. with the same internal chemical changes and neural responses. Yet unlike our primitive ancestors, present-day man no longer dissipates these energies through fight or flight. This is unfortunate from the standpoint of physical and mental health, for man then has no releases. We are forced to stifle our rage and ineffectively repress our alarm. We do this without a specific target— except of course ourselves.

How then do we handle emotional build-up that inevitably occurs everyday? What do we do about natural physiologic consequences evoked by humoral and neural responses to danger? What are the answers? Maybe they can be found in a life of moderation and regular sports.

COMPETITION

Healthy Challenge and Competition

Good or bad, competition and challenge in today's society is a real part of everyday living. It pervades all facets of life; certainly it pervades the worlds of business and politics. It is even a part of sports, at least as portrayed on television.

Competition to some people takes on an objectionable quality. Sports in the serious context of business can take on negative, disagreeable qualities. But thankfully this situation is not true for the majority of adults who engage in sports. Fortunately for these people competitiveness, if it exists at all, takes on a totally different meaning and form.

Competition in amateur sports takes either of two forms. It may take the form of self-competition. For example, one may choose to compare his current marks and performance with those of his past or future. Obviously, he is competing with himself, no one else. No one need even know, in fact. This form of challenge is common, and in most instances is entirely accepted as healthy since it involves efforts on the part of the individual to develop and improve his skills in relation to his own desires and physical limitations.

In the second case, healthy competition may take the form of wholesome contest with others who also love the sport. Once again, challenge and contest encourage and allow one to improve skills to his own level of proficiency. Like self-competition, this form of competition provides a vital stimulus for continued participation and interest in sports.

Is Competition in Adult Sports Indispensable

What about competition in relation to the elements of exercise and fun in sports? Where does it fit in? As an element, is competition an absolute requirement in sports for adults?

It is evident from experiences of a significant number of people that the opportunity for wholesome challenge and contest adds a new, desirable dimension to the entire concept of sports. It permits development of healthy self-esteem. No doubt for many, the opportunity—self-competition or otherwise—helps increase the enjoyment and pleasure that one gets out of sports. It goes a long way towards sustaining the interest and desire in adults to engage in more physical activity.

Yet, from the workable standpoint, challenge and competition in sports is neither universally desired nor universally practiced by all adults. Notwithstanding, my personal philosophy regarding sports involves *presenting the opportunity* to engage in wholesome challenge and contest to all adults. Ostensibly, not everyone will select competitiveness as the primary element in his personal program of sports activity; but let him make the choice. In the final analysis he is the one that can best decide what makes him most happy. Let him have the option.

The key to the entire issue to competition in sports for adults lies in the concept of *option* and *opportunity*. As far as I am concerned, the option and opportunity to engage in contest and challenge make competition an indispensable element. So to settle the question regarding competition and sports, I contend, that the actual act of competing is entirely *optional*, but the *opportunity* for competition is *indispensable*.

Although my personal running efforts date back to February 1970, when I first met an accomplished 440-yard hurdler at a little local track in Baltimore, Maryland, it was not until several months later that I developed enough proficiency to engage in the thrills and excitement of competitive amateur track. Looking back, I can honestly say that I did not start running, nor do I continue to run, solely for the public thrill of running track. To me, the benefits of exercise and fun in sports are very important. The chance to engage in occasional competition is simply an added bonus. Ostensibly, most runners who truly love the activity consider all three elements important in helping get the most out of life through sports. Certainly, I do!

I have discussed several reasons why adults should participate in sports. I have given solid, rational medical reasons for engaging in increased physical activity. I have given examples of mature adults who have successfully engaged in sports and continue to benefit from all the advantages of regular sports activity. I have given insight into my personal life as a runner. All that is left now is for you to put on your sweat clothes and come on out and run!

REFERENCES

1. Yudkin, J.: The epidemiology of coronary disease. *Prog Cardiovas Dis*, *1*:116, 1958.
2. Raab, W.: Prevention of degenerative heart disease by neurovegetative reconditioning. *Pub Health Rep*, 78:317, 1963.
3. Taylor, H.L.: Coronary heart disease in physically active and sedentary populations. *J Sports Med Phys Fitness*, 2:73, 1962.
4. Morris, J.N., Heady, J.A., Raffle, P.A.B., Roberts, C.G., and Parks, J.W.: Coronary heart disease and the physical activity of work. *Lancet*, 2:1053, 1953.
5. Morris, J.N., and Crawford, M.D.: Coronary heart disease and the physical activity of work: evidence of a national necropsy survey. *Brit Med J*, 2:1485, 1958.
6. Karvonen, M.J.: Physical activity, cholesterol metabolism and atherosclerosis. *Schweiz Ztshr Sport med*, 9:90, 1961.

7. Kannel, W.B., LeBauer, J., Dawber, T.R., and McNamara, P.M.: Relation of body weight to development of coronary heart disease. The Framingham study. *Circ, 35*:734, 1967.
8. Harris, W.E., Bowerman, W., McFadden, R.B., and Kerns, T.A.B.: Jogging, an adult exercise program. *JAMA, 201*:759, 1967.
9. Hellersetin, H.K.: The effects of physical activity. *Minn Med, 52*:1135, 1969.
10. Adult Physical Fitness: A Program for Men and Women. Prepared by the President's Council on Physical Fitness. Washington, D.C., 1963, U.S. Government Printing Office.
11. American Medical Association: Dietary fat and its relation to heart attacks and strokes. *JAMA, 175*:389, 1961.
12. Advisory Committee to the Surgeon General of the Public Health Service: *Smoking and Health*, U.S. Public Health Service Publ. 1103, 1964.
13. Kiernander, B: Impact of television on medicine. *Proc Roy Soc Med, 62*:383, 1969.
14. Williams, J.G.P.: Impact of television on medicine. Direct effects. *Proc Roy Soc Med, 62*:383, 1969.
15. Committee on the Medical Aspects of Sports. American Medical Association: *Tips on Athletic Training, VIII*. Amer. Med. Assoc., Chicago, 1965.
16. Joint Committee of the American Medical Association and the American Association for Health, Physical Education, and Recreation: Physical fitness. *JAMA, 188*:433, 1964.
17. Donald, W.K.: Effect of mental and physical strain on the cardiovascular system. *Proc Roy Soc Med, 62*:1180, 1969.
18. Skinner, J.S., Holloszy, J.O., and Xureton, T.K.: Effects of a program of endurance exercises on physical work. *Amer J Cardiol, 14*:747, 1964.
19. DeVries, H.A.: Physiological effects of an exercise training regimen upon men aged 52 to 88. *J Gerontol, 25*:325, 1970.
20. Patterson, J.L., Graybiel, A., Lenhardt, H.F., and Madsen, M.J.: Evaluation and prediction of physical fitness, utilizing modified apparatus of the Harvard Step Test. *Amer J Cardiol, 14*:811, 1964.
21. World's fastest MD—just a beginner. *Medical World News, 11*:31, Sept. 25, 1970.
22. Doctor's latent track period ends. New York *Times*, Aug. 23, 1970.
23. Boyle, R.H.: Champion of the armchair athletes. *Sports Illustrated, 34*:21, Feb. 22, 1971.
24. Meet Dr. Meriwether. *Newsweek, 77*:62, Feb. 8, 1971.
25. The Dr. Meriwether saga. *Time Magazine, 98*:40, July 12, 1971.
26. Fields, S.: Doctor on the run. New York *Daily News*, Mar. 4, 1971, p. 56.

184   *Games Doctors Play*

27. Putnam, P., and Myslenski, S.: Firstest, fastest and mostest. *Sports Illustrated, 35:*18, July 5, 1971.
28. Gowdy, C.: Our Dr. Meriwether real champ. *Boston Globe Sunday Advertiser,* July 11, 1971, p. 24.
29. MD—Sprinter astonishes sports world. *American Medical News, 14:*11, Jan. 25, 1971.
30. Hersh, B.: Meteoric sprint ascent. *Track and Field News, 23:*11, Oct. 1970.
31. Reagan, F.: Physician with flying feet. *Rx Sports and Travel, 6:*16, May—June 1971.
32. Hoyt, M.F.: Washington's muscle builders. *Parade,* Boston *Globe,* Aug. 15, 1971, p. 4.
33. White, P.D.: The role of exercise in the aging. *JAMA, 165:*70, 1957.
34. Marks, H.H.: Influence of obesity on morbidity and mortality. *Bull NT Acad Med, 36:*296, 1960.
35. Shepard, W.P., and Marks, H.H.: Life insurance looks at arteriosclerosis problem. *Minn Med, 38:*736, 1955.
36. Westura, E.: Physical conditioning and the abnormal electrocardiogram. *Questions and answers. JAMA, 199:*952, 1967.
37. Hermansen, L., and Wachtlova, M.: Capillary density of skeletal muscle in well-trained and untrained men. *J Appl Physiol, 30:*860, 1971.
38. Frick, M.H., Elovainio, R.A., Somer, T.: The mechanism of bradycardia evoked by physical training. *Cardiologia, 51:*46, 1967.
39. Frick, M.H.: Coronary implications of hemodynamic changes caused by physiological training. *Amer J Cardiol, 22:*417, 1968.
40. Frick, M.H., Konttinen, A., and Sarajas, H.: Effects of physical training on circulation at rest and during exercise. *Amer J. Cardiol, 12:*142, 1963.
41. Hanson, J.S., Tavakin, B.S., Levy, A.M., and Nedde, W.: Long-term physical training and cardiovascular dynamics in middle-aged men. *Circulation, 38:*783, 1968.
42. Karvonen, M.J.: Effects of vigorous exercise on the heart. In Rosenbaum and Belknap: *Work on the Heart.* New York, Parker, 1959, p. 199.
43. Letunov, S.P., and Motylyanskaya, R.E.: Preventive significance of exercise training in elderly adults. In Raab, W. (Ed.): *Prevention of Ischemic Heart Disease.* Springfield, Thomas, 1966, p. 316.
44. Barry, A.J., Daly, J.W., Pruett, E.D.R., Steinmetz, J.R., Birkhead, N.C., and Rodahl, K.: Effects of physical training in patients who have had myocardial infarction. *Amer J Cardiol, 17:*1, 1966.
45. Clausen, J.P., Larsen, O.E., and Trap-Jensen, J.: Physical training in the management of coronary artery disease. *Circulation, 40:*143, 1969.
46. Hellerstein, H.K., Hornsten, T.R., Goldberg, A., Burlando, A.G., Fried-

man, E.H., Hirsch, E.Z. and Marik, S.: The influence of active conditioning upon subjects with coronary artery disease. *Canad Med Assoc J, 96:*758/901, 1967.

47. Jokl, E.: Cardiovascular responses to exercise concerned in rehabilitation of cardiac patients. Physiologic considerations. *Amer J Cardiol, 7:*320, 1961.

48. Holmgren, A., Mossfeldt, F., Sjostrand, T., and Strom, G.: Effect of training on work capacity, total hemoglobin, blood volume, heart volume and pulse rate in recumbent and upright positions. *Acta Physiol Scand, 50:*72, 1960.

49. Jokl, E., and Wells, J.B.: Exercise training and cardiac stroke force. In Raab, W. (Ed.): *Prevention of Ischemic Heart Disease.* Springfield, Thomas, 1966, p. 135.

50. Raab, W., de Paula E Silva, P., and Starcheska, Y.: Adrenergic and cholinergic influences on the dynamic cycle of the normal human heart. *Cardiologia, 33:*350, 1958.

51. Tabakin, B.S., Hanson, J.S., and Levy, A.M.: Effects of physical training on the cardiovascular and respiratory response to graded upright exercise in distance runners. *Brit Heart J, 27:*205, 1965.

52. Kral, J.A., Chrastek, J., and Adamirova, J.: The hypotensive effect of physical activity in hypertensive subjects. In Raab, W. (Ed.): *Prevention of Ischemic Heart Disease.* Springfield, Thomas, 1966, p. 359.

53. Mellerowica, H.: The effect of training on heart and circulation and its importance in preventive cardiology. In Raab, W. (Ed.): *Prevention of Ischemic Heart Disease.* Springfield, Thomas, 1966, p. 309.

54. Dawber, T.R., Kannel, W.B., and Friedman, G.D.: Vital capacity, physical activity and coronary heart disease. In Raab, W. (Ed.): *Prevention of Ischemic Heart Disease.* Springfield, Thomas, 1966, p. 254.

55. Balke, B., and Clark, R.T.: Cardiopulmonary and metabolic effects of physical training. *Proc. Conf. on Health and Fitness in the Modern World,* Rome, Ang. 1960.

56. Committee on the Medical Aspects of Sports, American Medical Association: *Tips on Athletic Training, VII.* Amer. Med. Assoc., Chicago, 1965.

57. Committee on the Medical Aspects of Sports, American Medical Association: *Tips on Athletic Training, II.* Amer. Med. Assoc., Chicago, 1960.

58. Fox, S.M.: Incidence, prevalence, and death rates of cardiovascular disease: some practical implications. In Hurst, J.W., and Logue, R.B. (Eds.): *The Heart.* 2nd ed., McGraw-Hill, New York, 1970, p. 567.

59. Stammler, J., Berkson, D.M. Lindberg, H.A., Hall, Y., Miller, W., Mojonnier, L., Levinson, M., Cohen, D.B., and Young, Q.D.: Coronary risk factors. *Med Clin North Amer,* 50:229, 1966.
60. Friedberg, C.K.: *Diseases of the Heart.* 3rd ed., W.B. Saunders Co., Philadelphia, 1966, p. 644.
61. Holloszy, J.O.: The epidemiology of coronary heart disease: National differences and the role of physical activity. *J Amer Geriatr Soc,* 11:718, 1963.
62. Cureton, T.K.: Physical fitness works with normal aging adults. *JA Phys Mental Rehab,* 11:145, 1957.
63. Frank, C.W., Weinblatt, E., Shapiro, S., and Sager, R.V.: Physical inactivity as a lethal factor in myocardial infarction among men. *Circulation,* 34:1022, 1966.
64. Kannel, W.B.: Habitual level of physical activity and risk of coronary heart disease. The Framingham study. *Canad Med Ass J,* 96:811, 1967.
65. Rose, G.: Physical activity and coronary heart disease. *Proc Roy Soc Med,* 62:1183, 1969.

16

MOUNTAINEERING

JOHN B. GRAMLICH

WHY MEN CLIMB MOUNTAINS

Man does not climb a mountain "because it is there." He climbs because he wants to climb. The urge to move onward and upward is an immutable instinct.

On the sharp edge of the world of man, standing on the summit which has been the vague focus of his dreams, the mountaineer feels the uplifting of his soul, his heart, his body and all his secret longings.

As far as the eye can see, a realm of forests and rocks stretches out before him wrapped in the challenge, the silence and mystery of the infinite. It is like being in a new world; the mountains seem less a part of this earth than an entirely separate kingdom, unique and mysterious, where to venture forth, all that is needed is the will and the love.

Rocks, slabs, chimneys, chockstones . . . the mountaineer has given his best to climb them. Tired, yes, but also content and exhilarated. And then he gives himself up to his thoughts, while there mounts within him a happiness such as he has not known before, but for which he has felt a strange, undefined need. His head pulses, his heart beats with emotion. The air has a sharp tang, the sun pours out its benediction, and at the end of a rope he has found a fine, deep comradeship with climbing companions.

And if mist and clouds have obscured the minds and worlds of other men, then this kingdom is his own for a brief snatch of time. He has triumphed over the ground, he has conquered himself, and here is heaven's reward for his effort.

Climbing is an instinctive thing. Children spontaneously

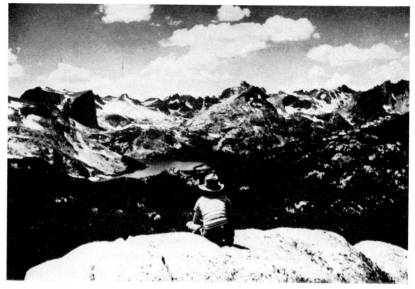

Figure 16–1. A youthful mountaineer savors his view of the magnificent Cirque of the Towers, in Wyoming's Bridger Wilderness. Credit for this picture to Wyoming Travel Commission.

climb trees, windows, walls—anything that is in their paths. The joy of climbing is the pleasure of discovery, of being able to see farther and from a greater height. This is the fundament of mountaineering.

HOW MEN CLIMB

Mountaineering as a sport is a little over one hundred years old. It was in 1852 that a clerk in the office of the Survey of India looked up from a maze of figures and announced to his superior: "Sir, I have discovered the highest mountain in the world!" The summit of that mountain (Everest, elevation 29,028 feet above sea level) was first achieved in 1953 by a British expedition which placed Sir Edmund Hilary and his Sherpa companion, Tenzing, on the top. The techniques of enjoying mountain climbing and the pleasures derived from technical proficiency have evolved and become quite refined. Mountaineering no longer need be deemed an heroic sport. Vastly improved equipment and modern materials have served to make

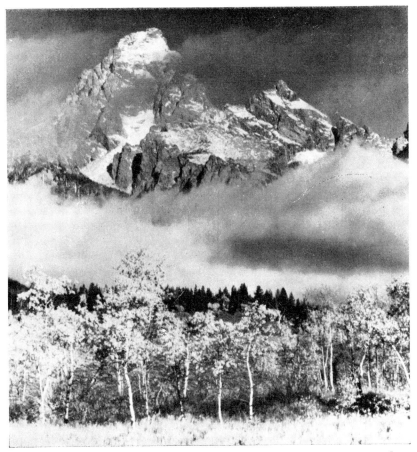

Figure 16–2. The Grand Teton in Western Wyoming. Unsurpassed in grandeur to climbers and viewers alike. Credit for this picture to Wyoming Travel Commission.

a two-day trek up the Grand Teton or a month-long expedition in the Himalayas equally enjoyable.

Good equipment is an absolute necessity. Lightness of weight and high quality of material are the fundamental requisites of satisfactory mountain gear. To simplify advice-giving to the beginning climber, three general categories provide needed information. These are: clothing (what you wear), housing (food and shelter), and hardware (technical climbing supplies). Trail hiking or back packing require only the first two. High-angle rock climbing demands an adequate supply of technical climbing equipment.

Clothing

Mountain weather is fickle. Those properly outfitted consider this part of the charm of mountaineering; the weather always changes! Mountain rainshowers are common and they are almost always cold. So the basic philosophy of clothing involves keeping the climber warm and dry.

A wool cap keeps one's head warm. The knit ski cap is eminently practical in terms of efficacy and convenience. Heavy wool mountaineer's caps are more bulky and take up more space, but are favored by some for their "climber's mystique." High-angle rock climbing requires the wearing of a hard hat.

Parkas have been vastly improved during the past decade. High-quality goosedown jackets are still necessary for severe cold weather as might be encountered on glacier climbs. But for all-around usefulness, unlined rubberized cloth parkas that breathe have been made available. These are windproof and waterproof—not just "water-repellent," which in a heavy rain shower is a soaking euphemism—and they have the added virtue of versatility. With a wool sweater and wool shirt underneath they can be as warm as down. Then when the sun comes out, the layers of clothing can be reduced to appropriate levels of comfort. This layering technique is becoming increasingly popular in average climates because warmth equal to that of down can be achieved with greater variety and less bulk.

A word about wool: no fabric, cotton and all synthetics included, is as warm as wool when wet. Probably because it is an animal fiber, wool can be soaked from rain, perspiration, or snow and still provide a degree of warmth. Even down garments, superbly warm when dry, are cold when they are wet, largely because the down becomes packed and loses the air insulation effect.

Wool is also the ideal material for pants. It is warm when the weather is cold and cool when the sun shines. Pants should be loose enough to allow easy mobility, as on a long leg-stretch. Mountains are no place for tight blue jeans. They are worthless in all respects, except possibly for a half-day trail hike in good weather. Far wiser is the common practice of throwing a pair of cut-offs or shorts into one's pack for a quick change when the going gets hot. Leather knickers are more glamorous than baggy wool pants. Disadvantageously, they are heavy and hot and they are very cold when wet. They are good for roadside rock climbing, however, since they are scuff-resistant and wear well.

Double layer cotton long underwear of the type used by skiers and hunters is currently standard. It suffers the disadvantage of getting wet from perspiration and then cold because it does not transpire and dry easily. But until something better is developed, and something surely will, it remains a necessity. Norwegian fish-net underwear, a cotton knit with wide interstices, has achieved considerable popularity because it is warm under cold conditions and cool when the weather is hot. Something relatively impermeable must always be worn outside since it functions on the principle of entrapped air insulation. Many climbers have noted, however, that when the fish-net underwear is removed, the wearer is left with a sensation of coldness of variable duration. Whether this effect is psychological or physiological has not been determined. As of now, the ideal underwear is probably cashmere, but the initial high cost and difficulty of maintenance have kept it from becoming universally used. The widely advertised double-layered nylon with dacron fill is valueless since it is bulky and constrictive.

Heavy wool socks are essential. Many climbers like to add an under-layer cotton or nylon sock for added protection and comfort. An extra pair of wool socks must always be carried in one's pack. This is so wet socks can be changed to dry at day's end and also to simplify sock-washing chores on a long trip.

Boots are probably the most important single item in the climber's armamentarium. They must be strong, waterproof, and most important, equipped with a Vibram or tough rubber-lug sole. The properly fit boot is not loose. Too much foot room can produce blisters on the approach hike and when one is climbing, he will have little rock-staying power. Boots should only be large enough to accommodate a thin sock plus a wool sock and still be comfortable. An adequate break-in period is essential and sometimes arduous. Never start out on an expedition of more than one day wearing new boots. And *never* use sneakers for anything but a short hike on a clean path. They are not stiff enough to hold on a narrow rock ledge and they allow an ankle to turn and skin and bones to bruise. The well-fit leather climbing boot is also best for a long hike.

A specialized climbing boot is useful for more complex technical rock climbs. This is a lighter, lower boot with a thin Vibram sole and is usually made of suede. It is called a Kletter Schuhe and is very popular with non-climbing college students who have anglicized the name and spelling to Klettershoe.

A *cagoule* or poncho should be carried in areas where mountain showers are especially frequent. *Cagoule* is a French word for "monk's hood" or "penitent's cowl." It is designed as a waterproof over-parka and is about knee length. A poncho is larger and is useful to cover the hiker and his pack since it is longer in the back than the front. Ponchos are available in light inexpensive plastic materials that occupy very little space. Although many foreign-made models are flimsy and not very durable, getting them torn on tree branches or rocks or underbrush does not represent a significant financial loss. A refinement in raingear, which has not achieved the popularity it probably deserves, is the rain suit. This is an over-parka and a separate over-pants set that is usually made of plastic. The pants cover the boot tops and keep water from running down into otherwise waterproof boots; they keep the legs dry from knee down, something no *cagoule* or poncho accomplishes.

Gaiters or anklets are zippered nylon tubes that bridge the gap between the bottom of the pants leg and the top of the boot. They are easy to take on and off and keep small rocks and scree, as well as snow and rain out of boot tops. Moreover, they make the wearer look like a real mountaineer.

Housing

Housing includes shelter and maintenance supplies. All items are designed to be readily transported on a climber's back.

Ingenious material and sensible design combine to make the climber's life more comfortable and even luxurious at times.

Many types of tents are available and are specially constructed for the climber. Three design principles are characteristic of the best tents: minimum weight, maximum interior space, and durability. The variables are size and special adaptation requirements. Size varies from one- to four-man types. Except for major expeditions, tents larger than a four-man are impractical. A four-man tent, complete with poles, stakes, rain fly and stuff sack should not weigh more than ten pounds. Smaller tents should be proportionately lighter. Special situation tents for use on winter expeditions or in high-wind areas and on narrow rock ledges, for example, usually require individual design and manufacture.

Since all good tents are semipermeable so they can breathe away normal human humidity, they are accordingly not waterproof and must be supplemented with a rain fly which is mounted over the tent and few inches above. Durable waterproof floors are standard in good tents. Essential also are provisions for good ventilation and for the covering of doors and windows with mosquito netting.

The little plastic-tube tent which can be strung over a suspended cord seems an attractive idea since it is light, small and inexpensive. However, it is also impervious to the occupants' expired moisture which will condense on the top inside the tube. On a cool night so much condensation will drip onto the climber's sleeping bag that it will soak through the bag and he will awaken wet and cold.

Choice of a sleeping bag is a personal matter. Although many filler materials are used in the construction of a sleeping bag, good quality goose down is certainly the best. A down bag is lighter, warmer and more compressible than one filled with any other material. The amount of down in the bag and therefore the degree of warmth provided is measured in pounds. A two-pound bag is suitable for above-freezing temperatures. Up to five pounds of down may be used in a bag designed for very cold situations. A three-pound bag is probably best for multipurpose requirements. It is warm enough for summer use in most areas in the United States and on a very warm summer night it can be unzipped when it is too hot. Every good sleeping bag manufacturer provides information concerning the care and maintenance of the bag. This advice should be followed meticulously. All good manufacturers also produce matching bags with full-length zippers which can be joined together to simulate the old-fashioned double bed. The advantages of this arrangement are immediately apparent.

The luxury of a good night's sleep is further enhanced by a comfortable mattress. A bed of boughs, dry leaves or dead grass may sound romantic but is in fact lumpy. The sensible climber carries a foam pad or an air mattress.

The foam pad should measure between one and two inches thick, twenty to twenty-four inches wide, and forty-eight to fifty-two inches long. Although both foam pads and air mattresses can be obtained in seventy-two inch lengths, the fifty percent additional length adds extra weight and bulk without corresponding benefits. Only the hips and shoulders need the mattress. Sweaters, parkas and other clothing serve nicely for padding under the head and feet. Air mattresses are traditional and comfortable. But they are a nuisance to inflate and deflate and they are prone to air leaks. On the other hand, foam pads take up more space. They are currently considered more desirable than air mattresses though, because they are warmer and less expensive. And finally, the experienced climber has long ago learned the very comfortable trick of digging shallow identations in the ground beneath his air mattress where his hips and shoulders will be lying.

Food and cooking gear have been revolutionized in the last several decades to the point where today's climber may be a neogourmet. The small liquid fuel stove of the Primus or Optimus design is light, compact, and reliable. The French have produced a butane cartridge stove (the "Bluet") which is very popular because it is efficient and clean. Both types of stove work well in wind and rain, times when a camp fire may not be so desirable.

Cooking gear has been nicely refined and follows fairly definite style patterns. Nesting aluminum pots, teflon fry pans, and provisioning tins are available at mountaineering shops. These items are relatively inexpensive and even though used only for trail cooking, they are light, compact and long lasting.

Modern mountain foods represent the greatest recent advance in trail technology. Freeze-dried and dehydrated foods are now available in an amazing array of superb quality. Meats, vegetables, fruits, salads, puddings, even cakes and pies can be purchased in taste-tantalizing quantity. Many are packaged for the appropriate number of people so that extra carrying and wastage are practically eliminated. Moreover, many items useful to the backpacker can be found on grocery store shelves. The uniform characteristic of all is that they need only addition of water to reconstitute them to a flavorful original state prior to cooking. Even though everything probably tastes a little better in the mountains, a sea level sampling will convince even the most arrant skeptic that mountain provisioning can be light to carry, easy to use, and a delight to devour.

All this equipment must be carried to the mountain on the back of man. A few years ago Kelty designed a pack frame made of aircraft aluminum tubing and so constructed that much of the pack weight could be supported on a sacral pad or alternately on a pelvic girdle strap. Shoulder straps take up part of the load and proper weight distribution then allows the backpacker to walk comfortably upright instead of bent forward as he would be required to do if all the weight were suspended from his shoulders. To this frame is added the pack bag made of high quality, heavy, tight-weave nylon. Most bags are compartmented for easy access and the frame is so organized that tie-on space is available for sleeping bag, foam pad, tent and climbing ropes. The Kelty bag is the prototype for similar backpacks of good quality, produced by many manufacturers.

With such a backpack, an adult male can carry a thirty to fifty pound load all day with a minimum of discomfort and fatigue. But the Kelty-type pack cannot be used for serious rock climbing; it is too large, high and heavy and tends to throw the climber off balance. Therefore, a smaller, lighter contour pack must be used for technical climbs. A pack of this type, usually called a summit pack, is without a frame and is slung from the shoulders. A light leather waist strap is some-times used to hold the pack from swinging. The problem of carrying two packs to the mountain is easily solved by placing something in the empty summit pack—for example, a sleeping bag—then strapping both of them into the position on the pack frame usually occupied by the sleeping bag alone. After camp has been made, the frame pack is left behind and the climb accomplished with the light day pack.

Hardware

Technical climbing equipment begins with the rope. Modern climbing ropes are seven-sixteenths of an inch thick and from one hundred twenty to one hundred fifty feet in length. They are made of nylon or perlon, and when properly cared for they are indefinitely durable. The prime purpose of the rope is for the climber's protection. Secondarily, ropes are necessary for rapid descent, or rappelling. Climbing rope should be pur-chased from a special mountaineering shop or firm.

Other technical equipment, loosely called hardware, includes carabiners, pitons and a hammer, and slings. More complex climbing requires stirrups, or light aluminum and rope ladders, and occasionally star drills and rock bolts. This latter equip-ment is used for "direct-aid" climbing and is only for the most devoted and experienced mountaineer. Special situations such as ice and snow climbing obligate the climber to be equipped with crampons, an ice-axe, and special ice screws, ice pitons and snow anchors.

Hardware and its proper use varies with the abilities of the climber and the particular terrain being enjoyed. The beginning climber must determine first what he wants to do and where. Then he must learn to do it. Fortunately, there are excellent climbing schools available (see Appendix I). The proper place to learn what one likes and wants to do is under the capable and safe tutelage of a mountaineering instructor in a good school. No amount of textbook reading can teach the beginner as rapidly as supervised field study in a rock-bound laboratory. Supplemental reading (see Climbing Schools and Services) is useful and great fun between climbs. Moreover, the mountain-

eering handbooks contain invaluable information about leader-
ship, weather, route-finding, use of the compass, and technical
tips. But one learns to climb by climbing. That this must be
done under skilled guidance cannot be overemphasized.

WHERE MEN CLIMB

The mountaineering fraternity is worldwide. There is superb
climbing in the European Alps, South America, the British Isles,
Africa and, of course, the Himalayas and the Karakorams.
Wherever there are mountains there is climbing. However, there
is enough good climbing in the continental United States so
that no climber could accomplish it all in a lifetime of ten-hour
days and seven-day weeks.

Curtis W. Casewit and Richard Pownall° observe that listing
ten of the most interesting climbs in North America would be
a subject for endless debate. Boldly, they suggest:

1. The Grand Teton, Wyoming; 13,770 feet
2. Long's Peak, Colorado; 14,256 feet
3. Mount of the Holy Cross, Colorado; 14,005 feet
4. Devil's Tower, Wyoming; 5,117 feet
5. Mount Shasta, California; 14,161 feet
6. Mount Hood, Oregon; 11,245 feet
7. Mount Rainier, Washington; 14,410 feet
8. Mount McKinley, Alaska; 20,320 feet
9. Mount Waddington, British Columbia; 13,177 feet
10. The Bugaboos, Snowpatch Spire, British Columbia; 9,600
    feet

For a beginning climber, none of these would be desirable.
He should investigate a lot, dream a little, read some; then get
outfitted, find himself a climbing school, and begin one of the
most exciting, rewarding recreations known to man.

> Nature is man's teacher. She unfolds her treasures to his search,
> unseals his eye, illumes his mind, and purifies his heart; an influ-
> ence breathes from all the sights and sounds of her existence.
>
> (*Alfred Billings Street*)

° Casewit, Curtis W. and Pownall, Dick: The Mountaineer's Handbook, An
Invitation to Climbing. New York, J.B. Lippincott, 1968.

CLIMBING SCHOOLS AND SERVICES

Here are listed some of the well-known schools and climbing services of national repute. This does not imply there are not others of equal or superior quality.

Exum Mountain Guide Service and School of American Mountaineering
Moose P.O., Wyoming 83025

Mount Rainier Guiding Service
Paradise Inn P.O.
Mount Rainier National Park, or 1525 11th Ave., Seattle, Wash. 98122

Sierra Club
220 Bush St., San Francisco, California 94104

Hans Gmoser - Canadian Mountain Holidays
Box 1660, Banff, Alberta, Canada

The New England Trail Conference
Secretary: Miss Edith N. Libby
26 Bedford Terrace, Northampton, Massachusetts

The Federation of Western Outdoor Clubs
Secretary: Mrs. Betty Hughes, Rt. 3, P.O. Box 172
Carmel, California 93921

Colorado Mountain Club
1400 Josephine St., Denver, Colorado 80206

Appalachian Mountain Club (Connecticut Chapter)
Secretary: Mrs. Charles H. Alexander
Bethmour Road, Bethany, New Haven, Conn. 06525

Sierra Club, Washington Office
235 Massachusetts Ave., N.E.
Washington, D.C. 20002

Sierra Club, Great Lakes Chapter
Chairman: Mrs. Jean Leever, 10240 Huntington Court
Orlando Park, Illinois 60462

Philadelphia Trail Club
Secretary: Mrs. Alberta M. Sargent
204 S. Marion Ave., Wenonah, New Jersey 08090

Sierra Club, Lone Star Chapter
Chairman: Orrin Bonney
1204 Sterling Bldg., Houston, Texas 77002

EQUIPMENT SUPPLY

This abbreviated list is not intended to be a measure of endorsement. Nor is it in any sense complete. It is offered merely as a starting point for a beginning mountaineer.

The Ski Hut
1615 University Avenue
Berkeley, California 94703

Colorado Outdoor Sports Corporation (Gerry Division)
P.O. Box 5544
Denver, Colorado 80217

Holubar Mountaineering
P.O. Box 7, Boulder, Colorado 80302

Eastern Mountain Sports, Inc. (formerly Mountaineering Supply)
1041 Commonwealth Ave., Boston, Mass. 02215

Abercrombie & Fitch
Madison Avenue & 45th, New York, N.Y. 10017

Eddie Bauer
417 East Pine, Seattle, Washington 98122

Recreational Equipment, Inc.
1525 11th Avenue, Seattle, Washington 98122

Scott Surgical (Climbing boots for handicapped people only)
724 E. 17th Avenue, Denver, Colorado 80203

SUGGESTED READING LIST

These are only some of many mountaineering books that are recognized classics. But reading even one of them quickly leads, through the principle of serendipity, to an appetite for others. The interested mountaineer can quickly accumulate a library of any size suitable to his tastes.

Backache, Stress and Tension, Dr. Hans Kraus. New York, Simon and Schuster, 1965. $4.50

Mountaineering: The Freedom of the Hills. Seattle, Washington, The Mountaineers. $7.50

The Mountaineering Handbook, Curtis W. Casewit and Dick Pownall, New York, J.B. Lippincott Co., 1968. $5.95

The Complete Walker, Colin Fletcher, New York, Alfred A. Knopf, 1970. $7.50

Basic Mountaineering, edited by Henry I. Mandolf. San Diego Chapter of the Sierra Club. $2.50

Be Expert with Map and Compass, Bjorn Kjellstrom, LaPorte, Indiana, American Orienteering Service, 1967. $2.95

Medicine for Mountaineering, James A. Wilkerson, M.D. (Ed.), Seattle, Washington, The Mountaineers, 1967. $7.50

Backpacking, Minneapolis, Minnesota, Burgess Publishing Co., 1967. $3.95

Mountaineering from Hill Walking to Alpine Climbing, Alan Blackshaw, Penguin Books, 1970. $4.95

Basic Rockcraft, Royal Dobbins, LaSiesta Press, Box 406, Glendale, California, 1971. $1.95

17

ALPINE SKIING

RUSSELL M. LANE

Back in the mid-1930's in Rhode Island, skiing for a young lad consisted of crude hickory instruments with single leather straps across the toes of four-buckle canvas overshoes. Ski poles were virtually unheard of and the slopes were somebody's unlevel backyard or perhaps risking apprehension on the local golf course. Snow itself was an inconsistent finding; but despite all these factors, I would have to assert, as a true New Englander, that I started skiing before my tenth birthday. Yet I probably skied no more than a half dozen times in this era of my life.

So in 1965, at the age of 37, I responded to my wife's statement that if we were going to live in Maine we should take advantage of the State's winter sports facilities as well as its summer activities. Poker clubs were abandoned, bridge partners were given over to others, and arrangements were made for our first ski holiday. From the outset it was a family affair, and has remained so for the Lanes ever since. During that initial trip we were five, but my wife obligingly conceived a sixth thereon, to add substance to some of the legends you will have heard already about fertility, the cold New England winter nights, and skiing. From that maiden ski holiday in 1965, then, our family has been on the slopes every weekend and every holiday of every winter since. And there have been a few "hookey" mid-week skiing days sprinkled in now and again when possible, and even a summer excursion this year of which I will say more later. The unmistakable point then, is that for our family, if there is skiable snow available, then we will be there using it to the exclusion of all other activities. This is the mark of a committed skiing family: some folks invariably refer to us as "ski nuts," or as "ski bums," but we feel the correct term is "ski enthusiasts." After all, skiing is basically a very healthy sport, it is one that families can participate in as a unit, it is one of excitement, fun and thrills, and since the equipment is moderately expensive to acquire, we feel that its full use is our way to justify our involvement (this logic is referred to by certain students of regional philosophy as New England or Yankee frugality).

From the outset of our family's entry into the sport to Alpine skiing, we made three basic decisions which I think are worthy of passing along to readers who may be considering taking up the sport in their family. These were our personal decisions, but we had some excellent counsel from friends with thorough background and experiences in skiing. Our three decisions were:

1. We would provide ourselves with complete and proper equipment, from skis to underwear, and it would be properly fitted and/or adjusted to its individual user.
2. We all would avail ourselves of proper and qualified instruction on a regular and continuing basis.
3. We would approach skiing as a skill to be mastered and as a sport to be enjoyed, realizing that both required dedication of effort for fulfillment.

The equipment problem never ends for the Lane Family; and we are now six on skis, as the 1965 addition has grown into full participation. It is an interesting sidelight on children and the sport of skiing that whereas "hand-me-down" clothing in the school and party categories are avoided, resisted, and sneered at, when it comes to ski clothing and equipment, these same children will argue and even battle to get only marginally serviceable "hand-me-downs." From skin to snow, the varieties are staggering and the "expert" does not exist who can provide you with all the answers. There are wooden, metal, and fiber glass skis; leather and plastic, buckle and tie boots; step-in and cable bindings galore; parkas, sweaters, warm-up pants, race pants, wind shirts, mitts, gloves, face masks, helmets, ear bands, hats, turtlenecks, insulated socks and underwear, plus the other thousand or more minor items which often seem to be most important to the children. And then you must consider that I have made no attempt to mention the transporting gear needed for your car, the storage gear needed for your attic (clothing) and your cellar (skis, poles, boots), and the waxing and sharpening gear called a "ski-preparation" kit, which is traditionally the property of everybody in the family, but singularly "Dad's job." Needless to say, my feeling is that knowledge of clothing and equipment is a very essential element to a person's or a family's involvement in Alpine skiing, and that skiers need to be as knowledgeable as humanly possible in these matters. Said knowledge is primarily a matter of experience, and of interest in learning. Borrowing and renting of clothing and equipment in Alpine skiing have never received my endorsements; I have seen too many tragedies, from injury and from improper protection from the elements of nature, resulting directly from rental or borrowed gear.

So now you have your clothing and equipment; but just as the full safety and enjoyment of your first automobile required some instruction before you drove it 50 miles an hour so likewise you will want to have some "qualified" instruction in how to handle those "boards and poles" before you point them down the hill, where they too are capable of going 50 mph. And just think how much better than your car those skis will make you feel: no registration sticker, no excise taxes, no gas tank to fill, no antifreeze to check, no exhaust fumes and oil drippings to pollute the environment, and no "jump cables" on the battery to make the car go on cold winter mornings. But your "driver's license" for those skis had better include said "qualified" instruction, since head-on collisions with frozen maple trees or granite boulders (when skiing out of control through lack of prior instruction) can be just as destructive of life and limb as any collision on our American highways. And instruction is usually available at most ski areas, even the smallest community slope. Remember you do not have to have the top racer or the top form-skier in the world as your instructor; you do have to have a qualified (or certified) individual who desires to help you, and most important of all, your instructor has to have in you a pupil who desires to learn and work towards improvement. It has been the policy of our family, since ski equipment is undergoing certain changes each year, since techniques of proper skiing are being similarly modified, and since skiing is essentially a "one-season-out-of-four" sport with a long summer layoff, that all will avail themselves of some instruction at the beginning of *each* winter ski season. I sincerely believe this is a good piece of advice to pass on to all readers of this essay; despite the fact that characteristically, "old Dad" is the hardest to get to sign up for lessons each December, is the worst pupil during the classes, and is the least accomplished skier come midwinter. But I do believe in the principle as expressed, and do hope my readers will follow my children's footsteps more closely than mine.

And now with clothing and equipment, and with some lessons in how to use them properly to your enjoyment and with reasonable safety, what do you intend to do with skiing? There are organized ski clubs in Florida and Hawaii (and they are *snow*-ski oriented, not water-ski), and I have a good friend in Daytona Beach who takes his Maine-born wife for a one-week ski vacation each year and remains an ardent winter-sports enthusiast. But I cannot quite agree with that approach and have managed to thoroughly sell my family on the exact opposite. As mentioned, we are on the snow in the fall as soon as it is skiable (sometimes this is prior to the official opening of the areas, and before the lifts start their operations), and we ski long and hard every available day until the snow becomes unskiable in the spring. We have found, however, that area managers usually keep their lifts operating for the "slush skiing nuts" about one week longer than our family can endure that mayhem. Late springtime "slush skiing," in my book is more treacherous than stalking grizzly bears with a peashooter. Nevertheless, my point is, once again, that the full enjoyment of skiing as a sport and as a skill, especially when it can be and is a family affair, requires and commands time on the slopes, dedication of effort to its mastery, and an understanding of the mechanics and physiology of the sport. Believe me when I say that the rewards (personal and collective) coming to the real ski participants are great: health fitness, relaxing diversion from life's chores and pressures, and just plain exhilarating fun.

Expressed thus far you have the Lane family's introduction to skiing and something of our philosophical approach to involvement in the sport. Perhaps now it is only fitting that I identify us and our location, since skiing is a sport that definitely does have certain regional characteristics. We are Mom and Dad, both in our early 40's; Patty and Kathy, 13-year-old twins; Michael, 10; and Nancy, 6. Orono, Maine, is our home, where I am a full-time student health physician and team physician to the intercollegiate athletic program at the University of Maine. In response to locating that "perfect" piece of land for a camp in the woods, which I am convinced is an incurable disease (note, if you will, the medical approach taken here) of the great majority of adult males in New England, last summer (1970) we had a family project of building our camp about one mile from the base lodge at "Sugarloaf U.S.A." Most of the work we have done as a family, coinciding with our approach to skiing and most of the construction errors have been "Dad's" (just as in ski technique, the rest of the family will hasten to add). Everybody outside the family on hearing of the camp wants to know whether it is a chalet or an A-frame: the truth of the matter is that it is neither; but rather a plain shack with four walls and a roof which leaks when the ice builds up more than two and one half feet at the eaves in the winter. I feel sure that the children will never declare our camp construction job to be "completed"; that just is not in their nature, nor do I really want it to be. There is always something to be adjusted or something more to be added, and we have surprising fun at these tasks; but in the way of advice to those of you considering adding a New England ski camp to your real estate holdings, let me strongly urge a few points. Do not get tied up in a high-priced camp unless you are a millionaire to start with; $15 to $20,000 will still give you a fine camp, even with today's constructions costs rising so rapidly, and a more reasonable camp attracts fewer taxmen (state and federal), fewer vandals intent on pilferage, and more potential buyers when you wish to sell in the future. Nevertheless, your camp *must* have an adequately pitched $(\frac{10' \text{ to } 12'}{12'})$ and eave-flashed roof, a piped-in water supply, a central furnace and radiators, a fully-plumbed bathroom, and a complete kitchen. Otherwise, you might just as well save a lot of money and cut your family an igloo out of blocks of snow; they are just as serviceable as a ski camp without the above. For those who may doubt my word, I invite you to consult your wives and teenage daughters; they will set you straight on these matters. Go economy on the furnishings, lumber, paint, etc.; but do not omit or skimp on the heat, bath, or kitchen. Currently, I myself have yielded to the extent of a washing machine and clothes dryer, a shower added to the bathtub, a disposal in the kitchen sink, an automatic dish-washer (with four children of our own and all of their house-guests available for the same job, no less), and a Franklin fireplace. Yet still I cannot get anyone excited about a snow-blower for my chores in the driveway. However, do not be misled by my complaints my wife will hasten to tell you that my comments are most obtuse concerning the things I enjoy most, and this is certainly true of our camp. Once again, to me, skiing is a full-time winter avocation: it is at the same time both skill and fun, it is a family-oriented sport, and the *ski camp* is very much an integral feature of this subculture of New England life.

Perhaps now a brief chronology of the Lane family's skiing history will be of specific interest to those of you who are familiar with Maine ski areas, and of general interest to others of you who are reading about how skiing develops into an all-family activity. February 1965 witnessed us traveling (as a family of five) to Vermont for our initial skiing, four days of introductory lessons for all at Madonna Mountain. This trip, stimulated in part and encouraged in full by an intern col-league of mine and his family of six skiers. We were their house guests and briefly used some of their gear in getting started. The following winter (1965–66), we commuted 45 miles from our home and medical practice in Blue Hill, Maine, to a small club area (Ski Horse Mountain) near Bangor. The new baby stayed home with her grandparents, and we skiers worked on basics at this four-trail, 300 foot-vertical area, serviced by a 300 foot rope and a 1200 foot T-bar. Winter 1965–1966 included a nine-day trip to visit encouraging skier friends in New Hampshire and a series of lessons for all there at King Ridge. By Winter of 1966–1967, I had discontinued general practice in Blue Hill and we had moved here to Orono for my university position thereby placing us about 50 miles closer to the major ski areas of Maine. Our lessons of the two previous winters had readied us for these longer and steeper slopes; so in winter of 1966–1967, we moved our skiing to Squaw Mountain in the Greenville-Moosehead Lake area, but were still daily commuters, and the youngest still stayed home with a "sitter." The ensuing three winters (1967–1968, 1968–1969, and 1969–1970) found us skiing regularly at Squaw, although we had ceased to commute, having found a cabin for season rental at Wilson's on the shore of Moosehead Lake.

An aside to our chronology is pertinent at just this point, as I relate to you our switch from "commuting" skiers to "cabin-based" skiers. Namely, that one of the facts of life, which must be accepted by any skiing family before they ever take up the sport, pertains to your automobile. It must be a large and heavy station wagon-type vehicle; you must be prepared to put about 10,000 miles of driving into it during a full, family ski season; and you must be prepared for the fact that it will be a worn-out vehicle after two, or at most three winters of skiing in northern New England. We have found our station wagons are less durable as a result of our skiing activities, than are the skiers and their ski equipment. Automobiles do not come with any hand-me-down feature as does ski equipment and clothing; and they do not similarly heal their wounds by the application of a bit of plaster, or by a summer of rest and rehabilitation, the way skiers can and do.

Our three years as renters at Wilson's and skiers at Squaw were marked by a number of features worthy of mention. We all continued with our lessons and became more proficient in our abilities. Nancy, the youngest, joined us on the slopes when she was three years old, spending mornings on skis and afternoons napping soundly in the base lodge nursery. The three older children involved themselves in a program called "Junior Masters," a superb way of presenting ski lessons in basic forms (nonracing) to the younger skiers. Junior Masters has many advantages for children over regular lessons in the ski school. In it the children work as a group, there is season-long continuity to their program, there is place for the competition so natural to all children's programs, and the program can be more economically offered than individual lessons. By winter 1969–1970, Nancy was skiing full days with the rest of us most of the time, and had joined the Junior Masters program with great pride. That season also saw the three older children request to enter some of the "sanctioned" U.S. Eastern Alpine Ski Association races for their age groups in Maine. Mom and Dad granted their wishes. Going to races can be great fun for everyone; only the car complains about the increased mileage and deterioration. The children get to visit and ski new areas, they get to be friends with children from different sections of the state and region; also, of course, being able occasionally to bring home a trophy or a ribbon adds enthusiasm to these programs that both children and parents cannot fail to understand and cherish. The Lane children proved to be no different than any other family contingent; we had some tears of joy, and some tears of disappointment, from each one of them at times. But my real disappointment of this three year period at Squaw came on December 29th, 1968, when I sailed into a bank of soft, heavy snow 15 minutes before closing time on my new Christmas skis. It was, naturally, my "last run for the day." The result was a fracture-dislocation of my right ankle, and later in the evening, an open-reduction with deltoid ligament repair. The orthopaedic surgeon's comment pre-op was, "Russ, let's just say you've destroyed your ankle joint!" I have been determined to prove him wrong ever since. That year was pretty much a loss for my skiing, but I have averaged about 45 skiing days a season in the two winters since, and even my most severe critics agree that I ski better now than before my injury.

Then we came to the winter of 1970–1971, with our new ski camp and the move to Sugarloaf, with its increases in "vertical," lifts, trails, and skiers. The three older children made their decisions to concentrate singly on racing, and worked regularly in the Sugarloaf junior racing program. Nancy, still only five years old and still a preschooler, was with the area's Junior Masters group. Patty had a tough winter injury-wise, with a medial collateral ligament sprain of the right knee in December and a "boot-top" fracture of the right tibia in February. And Mike had an acute hematogenous osteomyelitis of the upper right humerus in April, although we cannot directly relate this to a skiing injury. But the winter was a full one for the family: skiing, training, traveling, racing, and patching up "hurting" bodies and equipment. For us, it is "fun-work," and my point is to tell you that it can be equally so for your family if you so desire. There were some really exciting moments, also: (a) the Sugarloaf World Cup Races in February at which I served as a course physician: (b) Kathy's selection as 1st alternate on the state team in her age group (Eastern Class III-G), and (c) "Mommy's" *entry* into a NASTAR race in March (alas, her Cubco binding fell completely apart in midcourse, and you can imagine what mayhem then followed from all others, directed at Dad, the family equipment manager).

In the summer of 1971, we tackled skiing from a new angle, but still as a *family* venture. Traveling 2750 miles each way by auto from Orono to Cooke City, Montana, we spent three weeks skiing at the Spalding All-American Summer Ski Camp. The older children were full participants in two nine-day sessions of intensive race training and I served as camp and course medical officer. For those who are considering anything more than a strictly casual approach to racing for your children, these summer programs are essential. They are hard work for staff and racers, the clothing and equipment needs vary considerably from winter skiing, and the sun, heat, and altitude introduce new factors requiring special preparations. "Getting the poop" from an old hand at summer race training camps before going yourself or sending your children is strongly urged.

That about brings me up to the present in my chronology of skiing for our family. Currently we are spending our weekends making minor repairs and adjustments to our camp to make it ready for next winter, and we are constantly discussing next year's equipment and clothing plans. Although skiing must be limited to that part of the year when the areas are open and the tows are running, maintenance of camp, equipment, and clothing is a year-round part of the sport. And there is another form of maintenance which is year-round and which is an integral and essential link in the sport of skiing in our family's program. That is the item of physical fitness and off-season conditioning. For the children, we have chosen ballet, and they have an average of two or three classes per week. Ballet, with its emphasis on agility, balance, and quickness, seems an ideal complimentary sport to skiing, and personally we have been guided thus in our decision by having an excellent ballet school for children near at hand. In addition to ballet, we all have cross-country skis and accessory "X-C" gear, and try to get in a mile or two of "running" in the hayfield behind our house each weekday evening during the winter. Cross-country skiing is considered by many authorities in the field of exercise physiology and rehabilitative medicine to be the best single conditioning exercise that there is. Therefore, the fitness level of the Lane family is kept very good, and readers would be well advised not to slight this aspect of the total picture of the sport of skiing for yourselves or your families. However, despite recognizing the importance of fitness, and despite recognizing its year-round need, and then putting these recognitions into actual practice, there are going to be injuries from time to time. We have had our share, as mentioned already, and some of you will experience yours, also. Regarding injuries, then, my best advice would be to stay fit, choose your equipment properly and keep it operating correctly, maintain your ski techniques through periodic "qualified" lessons, ski regularly (at least two days each week during the season), and do not ski with fear (of injury)!

In conclusion then: from a Rhode Island lad on hickory staves one or two afternoons a winter in the mid-1930's, to a 43-year-old Maine physician and father, skiing about 45 days each winter and driving 2750 miles to Montana to ski in the summer also, is my story of the "game" this doctor "plays." The "game" is Alpine skiing; and it is not my game, it is that of my entire family. I enthusiastically urge it for those of you and your families, who are fortunate enough, as we are, to be in an area of the country where you can make it a seasonal sport and focal point for year-round health and fitness. At age 43, my weight is 150 lbs. (the same as it was at age 18), my resting pulse is 40, blood pressure ranges about 125–75, no glasses, no medications, and no cigarettes, and I run three to five miles daily at a pace of about 6:30 per mile. Of course, skiing is not the only answer, but I am convinced it helps to keep me "where I'm at," and it sure is one hell of a lot of fun and excitement!

18

WATER SKIING

TRAVIS C. GREEN

The "inventor" of water skiing certainly has earned a special place in the long history of recreation. The followers of this sport can be divided into the *tournament class*, good skiers who go about it in a semiscientific manner; and the *Sunday afternoon variety*, those who ski on the water for pure pleasure. The vast majority of us are in this latter classification.

It is a truism that doctors, as an occupational group, have inadequate physical exercise, yet we admonish our patients not to lead sedentary lives, to put a few demands on the "ticker" to keep it healthy, and to get away from it all for a time of mental and physical recreation.

Learning to water ski is the easiest part: any friend of yours who can ski would likely be flattered and have his ego boosted by being asked for some free instruction. A person of sound body and with a real desire to learn will be skiing within twenty minutes of the start of serious instruction. (My two teenage sons and I rarely go to the lake for a session of skiing without taking along at least one friend who likes the sport, too. We have initiated dozens of youngsters into the activity.)

I have as much fun and real satisfaction in driving the boat as I do on the ski; pulling a skier is real pleasure. Our own equipment consists of a 16-foot Evinrude fiber glass hull with inboard-outboard 100 horsepower engine. This will pull an average-weight skier with the driver and an observer in the boat at 40 miles per hour. This is at least 10 miles per hour faster than most skiers like to ride. Maneuvering on skis becomes increasingly difficult and tricky as the speed advances.

The basics of skiing equipment come in a vast variety: boat size; make and size of power source; inboard, outboard or inboard-outboard arrangements; ski design and price ranges; different types of life vests; towrope colors and materials; and other accessories of almost countless varieties. But it is fact: the better your equipment the more enjoyable the sport of skiing. Like a hunter who takes pride in his beautiful guns, attractive and high-quality equipment for skiing is a constant source of personal pride and pleasure for the owner.

Let us get into the water. With the 75-foot polyethylene towrope tied securely to the boat (with a minimum of 40 horsepower) the skier is in water at least four feet deep with a pair of skis securely on his feet. He is holding the single handle of the towrope in both hands. The boat operator carefully takes up the slack in the towrope; with both water skis partially out of the water and parallel to each other about six inches apart, the skier settles into a slight crouch. When he is ready he yells "Ho!" and the boat operator gives it full throttle. The skier of average weight (150–190 pounds) will be planing within three seconds and within a distance of twelve feet. As soon as the skier is on the water planing he may straighten his legs if the water is fairly smooth. If the water is rough from wind or from wakes of other boats he will have to maintain a position of the knees being slightly bent to give his legs a little spring for cushioning effect, the original "knee action."

After planing the skier, the boat operator throttles back to the prearranged speed or to about 28 miles per hour. The smoothest area for the skier is *directly* behind the boat where the towboat wake goes to each side of him. A skier leans in the direction he wishes to go— left or right. He can take a turn easily or he can swing out in a pop-the-whip fashion if he wishes. A slalom ski (single ski) with a concave under surface will allow the skier to corner much sharper than a flat-bottomed ski will permit.

Smooth, slick water is much less fatiguing to the skier than rough water. After about ten minutes, the skier is ready to come in for a "landing." At skiing speed the boat passes about fifty feet from the point where the skier wants to stop. He lets go of the towrope handle, coasts some forty feet before naturally coming to a stop, and slowly sinks into the water. The most spectacular and individualized spills are made during skier landings.

Figure 18–1 shows a saucer, one of the fun devices for water sports. This is a simple, polished and painted disk of three-fourth inch marine plywood 3 feet in diameter. About the maximum speed to ride is fifteen miles per hour. To launch on the saucer the rider kneels on it holding the towrope handle with both hands against the leading edge. A very slow forward motion will plane the saucer at once. After planing, the rider

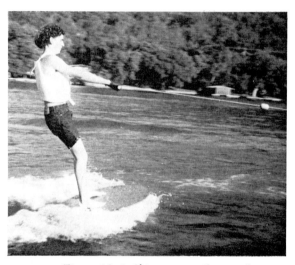

Figure 18–1. Skier using a "saucer."

simply stands up. With a little practice he can learn to rotate (saucer and all) passing the towrope handle behind his back as he rotates. Riding the saucer is an apt way for the rider to show off to the folks on shore.

In Figure 18–2 a "Butski" is shown. This is a pair of skis attached to a rigid seat. The rider sits on this seat, holds the towrope handle and, on signal to the towboat operator, planes very quickly. Riding the "Butski" on slick water is a real thrill and is completely safe. There is no critical speed limit, and it can be suited to the skier. The rider can easily swing the "Butski" far to the outside of the wake of the boat by leaning in the direction he wishes to go—left or right.

Next, of course, is the conventional pair of matched water skis. In reasonably calm water and at moderate speeds (20 to 30 miles per hour) a skier can ride these for ten miles or more without tiring. If the water is smooth, the skier can keep his knees stiff, and it is hardly more fatiguing than simply standing. But with any waves the skier has to have his knees slightly bent for a cushioning effect, and this is quickly tiring. Two skis are not quite as maneuverable as a single slalom.

An average-size man (180 pounds), when launching from deep water, will have to exert about 700 pounds pull against

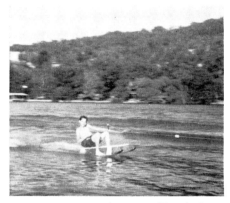

Figure 18–2. Skier on a "Butski."

the towrope for three to five seconds until he begins to plane. This is why the more powerful the boat, the quicker he planes on his skis, and it is therefore less exerting to the skier.

A shallow-water launch is really the easiest way to begin planing. The skier has on a slalom ski and is standing in water about a foot deep, his free foot on the bottom and his ski held on the surface of the water. (Be sure that the leading point of the ski remains out of the water.) There is a lot of slack in the towrope and the towboat proceeds at approximately 5 miles per hour in the intended direction of the launch. The skier himself "calls the shot" on this maneuver, and when he sees that about ten feet of slack remain in the towrope he yells "Ho!" The towboat operator firewalls the throttle. This is a rather spectacular takeoff by the skier and is also the way to launch if the water is uncomfortably cold. While wearing a matched pair of skis, a dock takeoff can be done. The skier sits on the edge of the dock and lets his skis touch the surface of the water or near the surface. The towboat operator's maneuvers are similar to those made during a shallow-water launch.

Because of the intense pull on the arms of the skier, the possibly cold water, and the general excitement of skiing, it is evident to the reader why a skier should be in good physical condition. A person with known or suspected heart disease (residual failure of rheumatic heart disease, angina pectoris, cardiac hypertrophy from whatever cause, and post coronary occlusion with infarction) should not get on water skis or on any device pulled by a boat for recreational purposes. The risk is too high for the skier with such a medical history. Safety, as previously stated, is the *first* and uppermost consideration in water skiing. This should be the guide in any recreational activity.

Injuries to a skier while in the water are uncommon but do occur and can be laid to carelessness on someone's part. An alert, competent towboat operator, an alert observer in the boat, and a healthy and watchful skier is a combination virtually assuring an unmarred skiing session. The skier should wear a vest-type flotation device rather than a ski belt. The flotation device made from rubber with a good fit is the best one. This helps protect the skier from a blow in the pit of the stomach (solar plexus) in a hard fall; and if for any reason the skier should be in the water unconscious, this type of vest will keep his face out of the water. With the exception of a skier being hit by a boat or contacting some other obstruction or object, it is *very* unlikely that he will be hurt, no matter how hard he may fall on the water.

Two or more skiers being pulled by the same boat should travel at least ten feet apart laterally so that if one falls he will not hit his partner. The other skier (or skiers) should release their towropes at once when any one of them falls. Another point of safety to observe carefully is not to get a loop or half-hitch of the towrope around an arm or finger. On one occasion, a 13-year-old boy lost his left thumb by having it pulled completely off by a small loop of towrope around it.

A word to the towboat operator: a boat always has seats. *Sit in them.* The gunwale of a boat was designed to keep out water and not as a seat. A boat operator or passenger sitting on a gunwale throws a boat out of balance and makes the person vulnerable to serious injury by falling overboard and being hit by another boat or even by his own. Another point of safety to consider is that a device such as a surfboard which is tied to the boat by a long towrope is potentially dangerous. If the rider should fall forward while riding this, broken bones, deep lacerations, or concussion could result if he is hit by the device.

Near the beginning of this chapter it was mentioned that the presentation was aimed at family fun, recreation, and good exercise by introducing the reader to water skiing. If the reader desires more information and wishes to work toward becoming a tournament-quality skier he can pursue this through several good books and, even better, through individual instruction by a competent teacher. Ski-kiting, official slalom course skiing, trick skiing, and ski-jumping are great fun and rewarding to the eager water-athlete. An excellent reference is *Let's Go Water Skiing* by T.C. Hardman and W.D. Clifford, Hawthorn Books, Inc., New York.

To equip the family or even oneself for water skiing is rather expensive. I urge the interested reader to buy the best equipment which he can afford, from boat to flotation vests. Good, prideful equipment is a genuine pleasure. The best is not necessarily the largest or most expensive. In the years ahead some of your fondest memories will be of water skiing with the family.

19

LONG DISTANCE SWIMMING: THE ENGLISH CHANNEL

ADRIAN C. KANAAR

G oing to war in civilian clothes was not what I had expected! Yet here I was, in September 1939, being rushed across the English Channel as a medical officer in charge of troops in the British Expeditionary Force before I had even been outfitted with a uniform. The crossing was undisturbed by enemy action, so I leaned over the rail for a while, thinking of happier times in the Channel. "Sea slight to moderate, I should guess," I said to myself, remembering earlier days when some such estimate was given to me daily over the telephone by a kindly official at the Air Ministry. I had waited and waited at my home in London for three and a half weeks until finally I got the message "sea slight." Then I took the first train to Dover, and at 2 A.M. I was crossing the Channel with six friends and three boatmen in a trawler with a rowing boat in tow. As soon as we made Cap Gris Nez, I stripped rapidly and covered myself with ten pounds of thick grease. Wearing only swimming trunks, at 5:17 A.M. I jumped down on to the beach and at once waded into the water. I looked out over the vast expanse of sea before me, and then struck out vigorously. It was August 30, 1933, and I was making my second attempt to swim the English Channel.

The previous year the boat had been one and a half hours late in arriving at Cap Gris Nez for the start. On that occasion Burgess, who had swum the Channel on his twentieth attempt, was there to see me off. "You'll never make it today," he said. "Do you think it's too late?" I enquired. "Yes," he continued, "you'll miss the tide when you reach the other side." "Anyway I

Most of the first section of this chapter was written in 1943 but never previously published.

218

am going to try because if I don't go today I shan't have another
chance until next year. In two days time I am to be adjutant at
a boys' camp, and when the camp is over, it will be too late in
the season for Channel swimming. I have trained for over three
months working up to a seventeen-mile swim in the Serpentine
in London's Hyde Park, and finishing my training by doing
fifty-four miles in four swims in ten days. I don't intend to
waste all this effort even if I do fail."

Burgess was right. One and one half miles from Dover, the
tides slowed me down. Another quarter of a mile and I ceased
to make any headway during a whole hour. I was thoroughly
fit, but it was impossible to beat the tide. "It will be five hours
before the tide turns," I was told by the boatman who was rowing ahead of me. I remembered Helmy, the hugh Egyptian who
was only one mile off Dover eleven hours after leaving France,
but had to swim another twelve hours before he finally set foot
on shore, at Folkestone, seven miles from Dover! Reluctantly
I decided to conserve my strength, and try to arrange for
another attempt after the camp had ended. I swam-out for
another twenty minutes from sheer bravado because I felt so fit,
then I climbed back into the boat. We had been twenty and
three quarter miles as the crow flies, but actually further on account of the tide which makes the course a zigzag one. I had
taken twelve and three quarter hours, but the last one and one
half hours had been wasted on account of the tide. So we had
been twenty and three-quarter miles in eleven and a quarter
hours.

After it was all over, I pondered those statistics. The official
record, held by Temme, was fourteen hours, twenty-nine minutes, for the swim from France to England. One swimmer had
claimed to do it in eleven hours, but his and other quick times
had been supported by too little evidence for acceptance by the
Channel Swimming Association, which was formed to see fair
play after a disgraceful episode had brought the sport into dis-
repute. Before my Channel attempt, I had told scarcely anyone
of my plans, lest I should make a fool of myself by an ignomin-
ious failure. Now, I secretly determined to go all-out for the
record next time.

I could get very little guidance about diet and exercise in training. I cycled eight miles to and from home and Hyde Park at top speed, or cycled to my medical school for classes, and experienced none of the supposed antagonism between the training of the cyclist and that of the swimmer. During each swim I kept off the meat meals which had made many Channel swimmers vomit in the water. My chief error was to overtrain for my first Channel swim. It happened because things went wrong on what was to have been my last training session. Accompanied by a rowing boat, I was swimming three times around the five-mile circumference of Dover Harbor on a cold day (water temperature 56-59°F) with morning fog. At the end of the first three hours and then every two hours I had arranged for a thermos of hot coffee to be ready at a given point, along with my other food. At seven hours there was no coffee. At eight hours I began to flop around in the water, swallowing a good deal. The boatman tried in vain to pull me out. I fought free. Fortunately we were passing along the shore and I was spotted by Temme the famous swimmer who in 1934 became the first to swim the Channel both ways (long before anyone tried to do it both ways nonstop). Temme rowed out and to my protestations affirmed, "You've done 12 hours—now come on out." His white lie and two men's strong arms got me into the boat. He rowed to land, threw my 180 pounds across his shoulders, walked across the seafront to my hotel and up the stairs, where he put me into a hot bath. There was a one and a half-hour gap in my memory when I came to in the lounge, somewhat woozy with the brandy I had been given. Uncertainty as to why I had collapsed, combined with the nearing end of the season led me to prove myself by putting in two more long training swims at only two or three day intervals—too little time for muscle recovery. The resultant strain of my groin muscles and right shoulder plagued me increasingly from then on.

Although I had been on my school swimming team, I never really learned the smooth timing of arms and legs with breathing which makes the crawl stroke ideal for long distance. Taught these refinements in 1930, within two years I had increased my crawl distance from about one-quarter mile to 17 miles at a stretch. During the winter of 1931–32 and on through the summer, I swam about two miles a week in a pool. Then from early June when the Serpentine opened to the public I did most of my training there, except for an eleven and fifteen mile swim in Dover Harbor to get used to the waves and the colder water.

My second attempt, as I feared, had to be postponed until 1933, and this was doomed to failure, too. The boatmen claimed that spring tides are essential for a successful south to north Channel swim, but the season was wearing on, and I had waited for smooth water for nearly a month, so I decided to take my chance with a neap tide. As far as was known no one had even tried to swim the Channel on a neap tide in this direction, but there was some reason to hope that it might not be so difficult as had been imagined.

Long before we reached mid-Channel we could see both coasts clearly. It was a glorious sunny day, and the sunburn on my back lasted for a year! The water was as calm as a millpond. I swam hard all day, trying to make every stroke a strong pull. At last we came in sight of the beach and breakwaters of St.

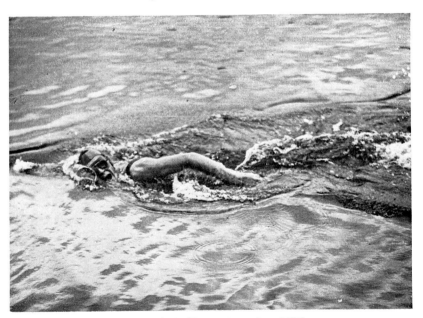

Figure 19–1. Kanaar in action, 1932.

Margaret's Bay near Dover. Through my watertight goggles I could just discern people on the shore. "How far now?" I asked. "About two and one half miles," the boatman replied. It had been slow going because of the neap tides. I had had twelve hours in the water but still felt fit. I had arranged to stop and tread water for ten minutes in every two to two and a half hours, while I had a meal consisting of hot, sweet coffee, honey sandwiches, sweet biscuits, cake and sugar lumps—all readily digestible foods providing heat and energy. Because of the apparent risk of low blood sugar, I warned my six friends that under no circumstances must I be allowed to miss a meal even if I strongly requested it. Now the beach looked so near, the tide was on the turn, and I feared that delay might lose me the record, so I announced that I would press on, and eat when I arrived. After twelve hours' effort a swimmer lacks the clarity of thought required for such a decision, and that was why I had put the responsibility on my friends. Unfortunately they were not firm with me, and I missed the meal. I began to tire, making barely one mile in the next two hours. As I flopped about in the water near Dover, a pleasure steamer brought holiday makers out to watch. As it passed by, sounding its hooter to cheer me up, its wash gave me the *coup de grace,* and I was picked out of the water in a semiconscious condition, violently expostulating against this insulting vote of no-confidence! I was one and a half miles off Dover after fourteen hours in the water. I intended to try a third time, and in 1934 I began to do long swims again, but I had only trained up to seven hours swimming when I was obliged to give it up. To avoid muscle pains I had to keep changing strokes during each swim. Eventually, the pain became intolerable, in spite of the untiring efforts of the St. Bartholomew's Hospital Masseurs, who with my colleagues and teachers, gave me their wholehearted support.

What fun those long swims were! On my second attempt, I had six friends to swim with me in turn during the last ten hours, and my brother, who was only thirteen, swam five miles. At the end I had the humiliation of being unable to keep up with him—and he nine years my junior! The only drudgery was the relentlessness of the training. I drew up a program which I attempted to carry out whatever the weather might be. An eight-hour swim on a misty, cold day in Hyde Park with little or no company was not very pleasant. In order to get used to the cold I used no grease during training, and I slept without any blankets on my bed at night. But it was all worthwhile.

Why did I do it? I have often been asked that question and felt too embarrassed to give a direct reply, but now, at this distant date, I will divulge my secret. I was a worker for Christ amongst boys, and wanted to show that a Christian can be a good sport, too. I remembered how much I had been impressed by the Christian witness of some rugby and hockey international players, and a Cambridge Rowing Blue. Boys are like that. I believe that every Christian should give his best in everything he does, not to boost his own vanity, but to win credit for the cause of the Master who is his inspiration, and thus the source of his success. Here is an aim which gives scope for lawful ambition, resource and grit, and can be applied in every sphere of life. What is more, it is inexhaustible. Distance swimming was my favorite sport, so I made every effort to achieve that record which has been the ambition of long distance swimmers from all over the world. Although I did not gain my objective, I had done my best and I gained a great deal from the discipline required in training—and from the discipline of failure too. Besides all this, I enjoyed feeling really fit and having energy to burn, as I put all I had into every stroke and every mile.

FOR THE MATURE ADULT

When training for a hoped-for third attempt on the Channel in 1934, I had a visit from Haydn Taylor, a dentist, who was considering attempting the Channel himself. I had met him earlier when we competed in 1932 at the British Long Distance Championship (5 miles) in the Thames. Now he was 45 and I 23. I told him all I knew, and outlined my "ideal" training, based on study and two years experience. He followed it closely and in 1935 he succeeded, being at that time the oldest to have done it, and only one-half hour short of the official record. Long distance swimming, like marathon running and even

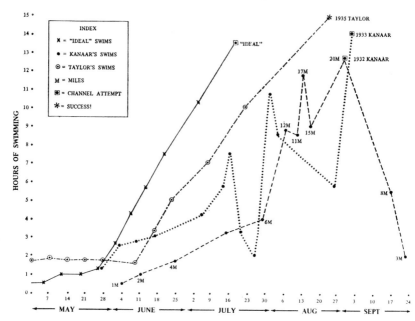

Figure 19–2. "Ideal" training chart.

mountain climbing, are activities in which stamina based on lifelong fitness[1] counts more than the spurts of speed for which youth is better suited. I have proved this myself, and at 60 still swim up to six miles against the tide in the Hudson River. I love skiing (water and snow), sailing, cycling and running, but for sheer *joie de vivre* it is long distance swimming for me. For vigor in advanced years the undisputed champion must be the 106-year-old man who was interviewed on television not long ago while working at his job as a waiter. He was still running six miles a day!

Most of those who have left fitness behind them long ago (or never experienced it) can still find the way. Barring severe physical disability, even the elderly person can start at the bottom of the scale in a carefully graduated program.[2] In sixteen weeks he may be fitter than he has been for fifty years.

A patient of mine, aged 44, has gladly allowed me to refer to his remarkable achievement. At six feet tall, his ideal weight would be about 150 pounds. However, on June 10, 1971, it was

302 pounds. Inspired by a lecture by Thomas Cureton, instructed by reading Cooper's *Aerobics*, encouraged by his physically fit wife and son, and finally challenged by a bet with a fellow fatling, he reduced his weight to 199 pounds by October 22, 1971. During the same four months he became an athlete. Swimming one to two miles a day he has covered 425 miles in the past 10 months, and now covers a mile in less than forty minutes. The cost? Only the fee for YMCA membership. The savings? A vast drop in the family food bill. His betting friend also took off about as much but had to take leave without pay for five months, and spent a fortune dieting at a sanitarium,

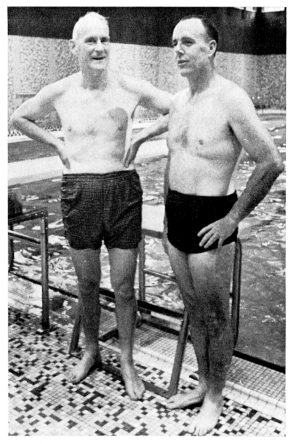

Figure 19–3. Kanaar and new, slim Prosser at YMCA, Oct. 27, 1971.

where there was scarcely any emphasis on vigorous cardiovascular-developing type of exercise. Both are lighter but only my patient has gained a plus in pleasure, adding *life* to his years, as well as removing a dangerous handicap. He intends to continue swimming at least a mile a day in the pool. He devised his own diet: a breakfast of orange juice and vitaminized cereal; a thermos flask of black tea taken at intervals at work served also as lunch; a supper (on alternate evenings only) of meat and vegetables; and *no* snacks! This keeps him in fine fettle. He puts in a full day's work as a computer programmer and has no problem with hunger.

Not only the overweight, potential "cardiac," but the postinfarction case can often regain fitness—and long distance swimming is as good a way as running, cycling or anything else. Cardiologists are increasingly recognizing that advice given to patients is often far too conservative. In fact we may reasonably say that your best—probably your *only*—hope of improving your heart and having a longer and happier life is through a progressively vigorous physical training program. Along with this, you will of course have to stop smoking completely and permanently, and keep your weight at an ideal level for your height. Too often we prescribe medication for mild (obesity type) diabetes, hypertension, high uric acid, high cholesterol and pedal edema but soft-pedal the prescription of exercise, forgetting that all of these abnormalities may revert to normal in the physically fit person, even without *any* medication. With this in mind, today's physician could parody that famous political aphorism:

> For forms of government let fools contest,
> Whate'er is best administered is best.

substituting:

> Let E.K.G.'s and other tests depress,
> *By training only*, fitness we assess.

In other words, you never know till you try.

Almost every physical fitness program requires self-discipline, but the pleasure must outweigh the boredom if it is to become a lifelong activity. This accounts for my personal preference to swimming in the sea or a lake or river, whenever possible. I can take only so much of going up and down a pool. True, one can make it competitive by watching the clock or having a well-matched pacer (if you can find one) but a distant goal and changes in scenery are more appealing. One has, of course, to face the question of danger. In my busy life, often with an 80-hour working week, I can rarely arrange for company on a swim—either in the water or in a boat. In fifty years of swimming I have only once had to get out of the water because of cramp. Twice I became unconscious, but only after eight to fourteen hours swimming. I would not go for such a long swim, especially in cold water, unaccompanied, but I do not find it feasible to keep constantly within my depth. Nor would I suggest this as a really reliable precaution. If one becomes unconscious one can drown in two feet of water. I keep reasonably near in shore, whenever convenient, but I swim around islands or across rivers or bays whenever I get the chance. Rough seas and contrary currents add to the fun. Others may take their risks in private airplanes, driving home after imbibing at a cocktail party, or jaywalking. I take mine in the water—and with sensible precautions regarding food, sleep, training, water temperature, lightning, currents, fog, sharks and speed boats. Like the 74-year-old who was leading a group of climbers in the mid-Hudson Valley in October 1971, and had a fatal stroke in the very midst of his chosen sport, I would be as content to die swimming as to do so on land.

In my work as a specialist in rehabilitation medicine I frequently recommend swimming. It is great for people with arthritis, neurological disorders, amputations and other conditions in which it is easier to exercise with gravity diminished. I recall meeting "Zimmy, the legless swimmer" in 1932. His thigh stumps were only a few inches long and he traveled everywhere on skates, propelling himself with heavy gloves. Several times he swam about halfway across the Channel!

A few personal experiences and tips may be in order for the would-be distance swimmer. At the peak of my training (at age 21, in 1932), my pulse was down to 44 in bed at night—and beat with such vigor that it shook the bed! I also had well

marked capillary pulsation in my finger nails. Both items are
quite physiological, and merely indicate the tremendous output
of the heart per beat, and the diminished peripheral resistance.
I once had my body temperature down to 84 F! This was *not*
so physiological. I had swum around Inchkieth, an island in
the Firth of Forth in Scotland, in October, 1941. It took me
over an hour. I took my rectal temperature about five minutes
after finishing. I did not really *feel* cold, but it took three refills
of a hot bath to bring my rectal temperature back to normal! I
later learned that at 80 F one is likely to become unconscious.
I have borne this in mind since then. Normally the body temperature seems to be well maintained in long swims with a
water temperature of approximately 63 F, but there are doubt-
less individual variations. Unfortunately my rectal temperature
was not tested on the two occasions in which I became unconscious in the water. I now suspect that low body temperature
may have been a factor.

Eyes and sinuses require some special care. My eyes became
so sensitive to water that even a few minutes in a pool would
make them red for two days. I therefore routinely used goggles.
The modern type of goggles which also cover the nose may help
to decrease the risk of filling the sinuses with water, especially
if one dives or does somersaults. When I was 18, I did a 20-foot-
deep dive in the clear waters of Brittany and filled my sinuses
with water, which poured out as from a faucet when I dried
my hair. Having not yet studied anatomy, I had no idea as to
where it had come from. It may have been the start of chronic
sinusitis, a problem which necessitated four major operations
and was a factor in my giving up my specialty of surgery fifteen
years later. In 1968 I uncovered another advantage of goggles,
when snorkling off St. John in the Virgin Islands. They enable
you to keep a wary eye on a barracuda. Without goggles one is
a much easier prey for a shark or other predator. One is less
likely to suspect his presence until he strikes. Jacques Costeau
and other undersea explorers have shown us in color photography
that one may brush shoulders so to speak with most of the predatory fish (the killer shark excluded) if one can see what is
going on and keeps calm. In my own case, I backed away slowly

to the shore, keeping the fish under constant surveillance, with my flippers extended toward him, for a tasteless mouthful if he wished. Curious, he swam around me and followed me right into shore, but made no threatening gestures. Now, I recommend the wearing of a knife on the leg where such creatures may be expected. At least one then feels confident.

I have limited experience of surf riding or scuba diving, but would certainly do more if I had the opportunity. The wetsuit is a great invention, largely eliminating the danger of a fall in body temperature, and making year-round outdoor swimming a practical possibility. Nevertheless, there is much vigor—mental and physical—to be gained from a brief unprotected exposure to really cold water. Members of Polar Bear clubs, and sauna club members who lie nude in the snow can bear witness to this. Probably there is a hormonal explanation—pituitary-adrenal cortical stimulation is a likely one—but there is no denying the fact. A cold shower or bath is a less exciting substitute. I recall swimming in a partly frozen mountain lake in Switzerland, swimming in the sea in Northern Scotland on New Years Day, swimming one-quarter mile in the partly frozen Ness River in Scotland, and breaking light ice in an inland lake in England. Crazy? Perhaps so, but I know of no statistics which would show the danger as being comparable to that of smoking as little as five cigarettes a day! And it provides an incomparable eye opener for a vigorous day. I would not recommend it to an untrained cardiac case, but the "shock" danger is probably an old wives' tale.

REFERENCES

1. Kanaar, Adrian C.: Life long fitness: a positive approach *J Assoc Phys Ment Rehab*, vol. 16, Nov.-Dec., 1962.
2. Cooper, Kenneth H.: *The New Aerobics*. New York, Bantam, May, 1970.

20

BLACK BASS FISHING IN THE SOUTH

W. W. WALKER

Where in the world would I begin to write an article on bass fishing? And especially about a plastic worm I created. I guess the best place to begin would be to discuss the best type of lures to use if a man wanted to catch bass.

Basically there are five better types of lures for catching bass: my plastic worms, spoons and spinners, deep and shallow running plugs, and top water plugs. These lure vary from one season to another. We shall begin with the worm season which begins when the water starts to turn warm. Some fishermen prefer to use live bait, but this method has not proved very satisfactory for me. If I had my pick for an all-around lure, I would choose the two-hook, four-inch worm. The green sparkle two-hook four-inch plastic worm has accounted for more black bass in the boat than all the other lures combined for the past five years. It simply catches bass in bunches. Bass seem to be like chickens. When you throw some bread into the chicken coop, one chicken grabs the bread and runs with it and the others follow. For some reason, and I do not know why, if one anchors his boat properly, he can completely clean out a school of bass with the green worm. Now, how could anyone make a statement like this? I have had personal letters sent to me from all over the South telling me about catching as many as thirty black bass on two of my green worms— not just one letter but hundreds—and also personal contacts and telephone calls from fishermen up and down the Catawba River. The worm seems to work just about anywhere and anytime of day you use it. I personally have not used it in a still pond, but I have had testimony that it works there, too.

I guess the reason the two-hook worm catches so many fish is because of the small size of the worm and the arrow-like shape of the hook which rests close to the worm; and the fish swallows it in one gulp.

We are attacking the fish at the throat with needle-sharp hooks, rather than using a large hook to penetrate the hard rind of the mouth of the fish. In the process of swallowing the one-gulp lure, the back hook of the worm catches the fish

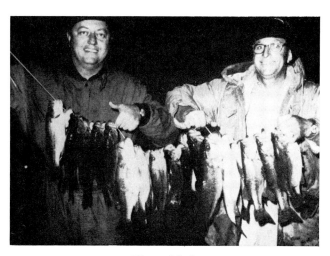

Figure 20–1.

under the lower part of his front lip. In the event the bass throws the front hook, he can still be boated with ease by the second hook, hung under the soft portion of the lower lip. One of the most important things that I have found is that your worm must be soft. We have tried hard plastic worms and find that the bass will spit them out before the needle sharp arrow-like hook can grab him in the throat. Some fishermen use this worm from the bank; some use it off piers and around boat houses, while others take it along in their boat. I have found that it works anywhere, anytime and in just about any manner you want to use it just as long as you move the worm very slowly, like a caterpillar crawling along your arm.

The worms are also available with weedless hooks.

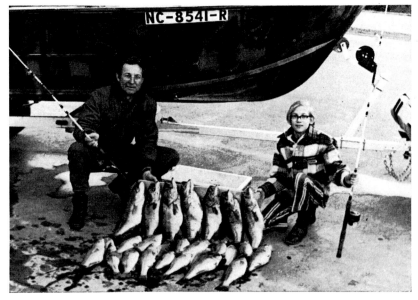

Figure 20–2.

I am illustrating a photograph of the coloring of worms that I have created, and each color seems to work at different times of the day, in different temperatures of the water, and during different months of the year. However, I have found that one particular color that I liked for spring fishing may turn out to be the hottest bait in your box in the middle of November. The bass just seem to want this worm best when the color of it is green.

I have added a sparkling substance with a secret suspension which holds the sparkle up in the material of the worm. This seems to be the most successful green worm that I have created. The sparkle substance has been added to the head and the tail of the worm and seems to give a crunch to the bite of the worm, and this crunch sets off an irresistible reaction which makes the bass inhale the worm down in the goozle. The needle-sharp hook will penetrate the fleshy portion of the throat, and it is almost impossible for the bass to throw this worm. The fisherman must carry along needle-nosed pliers when he uses this small worm. The black bass simply will not inhale a large worm with a large hook. The fisherman must set the hook as soon as he feels the strike of the bass when using a four-inch two-hook worm.

The bass seem to be close to shore in the early morning and night while moving to the deeper water when the sun comes out. I have gone along the shore at night with a gas lantern in front of a large mirror to reflect the light down during part of the year when the water had become clear. I saw many large bass in water one-foot deep almost up on the bank. I have dangled many lures in front of the mouths of these bass without success, but the moment he sees this green worm, he attacks it violently. I have not been able to find fish with a light in the winter time because of the wind and consistent rainfall which keeps the water murky, and my wintertime fishing will be described later—but back to the little green worm.

Every fishermen has his own way of fishing, and as long as the method works for him, that is fine. I will describe my way and will agree with anyone that there is no one way to do anything. The method I will describe has been used since I made the four-inch two-hook sparkle green worm some two years ago and which seems to work best in this area. The rod of my choice is the seven and a half-foot Old Pal spinning rod and an Old Pal Cougar 600 open-face reel. The reel carries twelve-pound test line and can be cast with the same ease as a smaller reel with lighter pound test. The reason I use twelve-pound test line is because I fish for large fish. When a lure is tied to six-pound test monofilament line, the line becomes almost three-pound test in the area the lure is tied to the line. In other words, a large bass can snap a six-pound test line at the point of contact with the lure as a knot tied in a line weakens the line. Try taking a three-foot strand of six-pound test line and tie a single knot in the middle of the line and then snap on both ends of the line and the line will pop with ease at the point where the knot is tied. Twelve-pound test line does not cast well on a cheaper reel, and I do not enjoy hearing the clinking of a cheap bail nor the grinding of the brakes as I retrieve my lure. If a less expensive reel works best for you, then I suggest you use it. However, when I go fishing, I buy the very best equipment available so that I do not lose my creel from using inexpensive gear.

I do my serious fishing out of a 14-foot homemade boat that sets deep in the water and does not rock (back and forth) as you move about in the boat. I have a larger boat for rough water such as the ocean and the Santee Cooper fishing area where one encounters very rough water at times. I have to do my weekend fishing with this large boat as I find I must jump from hole to hole due to the heavily crowded conditions on Saturday and Sunday. On both my boats, I have two anchors for the front of the boat and two anchors for the back of the boat. Each anchor rope is fifty feet long with a light anchor on one end and a heavy anchor tied on the other end of the rope. We use the light anchor when it is not windy and the heavier anchors when it is windy. I use fifty feet of anchor rope as we fish anchored in deep water and throw our worms onto a sunken island that is fifteen to twenty feet deep. My anchor rope is nylon winch rope that is 3/8 inch thick. It is made from soft nylon and will not rot. Each rope alone costs about $10. A small ski rope is cheaper but it cuts your hands and fingers. When my boat is anchored, the rope is tied tightly so that the anchor is straight down from the boat. The light anchor weighs about fifteen pounds and the heavy anchor about twenty-five pounds; therefore, I am carrying about 80 pounds of anchor each time I go fishing. The motor of my choice is a Mercury motor with a slip clutch on the propeller. With my green worm, all the tackle that is needed consists of barrel swivels and lead sinkers. In other words, in the season from the time the water starts getting warm until the end of November, the only thing that a fisherman needs to keep in his tackle box is a sack full of green worms (which come in five different shades), some brass swivels and slip sinkers. I bury my brass swivels so they will corrode and carry my lead slip sinkers around in an aluminum box so that they will become dull. The bass will strike your green worms better if the barrel swivels and the lead have been allowed to corrode. I have just learned this from experience, I do not know why it works.

With all the above-listed equipment, we are now ready to fish. The plastic worm is tied onto a three-foot leader with a five-turn, monofilament knot and to a #3 barrel swivel at the other end. I have found that the longer leader you use, the better the fish strike the green worm. A small slip sinker is placed on the main line, and this line is attached to the other end of the barrel swivel. Sometimes I place a middle-sized slip sinker and a small slip sinker ahead of this for added weight for strong wind. This is just one of the many trials of fate that have made my green worm so deadly. In other words, there will be times when it is better to put two small slip sinkers on your line rather than one even though it is not windy.

When a bass strikes the worm, the main line will slip through the lead slip sinker undetected by the bass. Had the lead been attached to the main line, i.e. a rabbit-ear type of sinker, the bass would have to drag along the lead as he is swimming away with the worm. If he feels the lead as the lead strikes an object such as a rock or a tree branch, the bass will spit the worm out before it has gone down into his throat enough to get hung up by itself.

This one simple correction will add many bass to your creel, that is, a #R 276 Old Pal rod which has a flexible tip so you can "feel" what is going on at the other end of the line and a stiff "butt" so you can really "sock it to him" when you set the hook, without snapping your line or cracking your rod. Sometimes it is a good idea to set your hook two or three times to make sure your hook is set, as it is possible the bass had started to spit the worm out and with this good hard set you will penetrate the fleshy portion of the rind that surrounds his mouth.

When your boat is properly anchored with no slack in the line, that is, with the anchor straight down, the boat will face the same direction all the time, and each time you cast, it will still be in the same area you just pulled your fish from. In other words, after you anchor your boat, pick out a tree or a house or a telephone pole on the shore and throw toward it. If you did not get a strike, make your next cast to the right or left of the first cast. If your boat has been anchored from both ends with a heavy anchor that will resist wind movement, you will stay anchored in the same direction and you will be casting in an accurate direction each cast. If you do not anchor your boat in this way, your boat will turn one or two feet and you will no longer be casting in the same area in which you caught your fish. As I said before, bass are usually in schools and stay in an area about one-half the width of a highway and in an area that is covered with stumps and rocks.

You may take needle-nosed pliers and turn the hooks of the two-hook worm down until you get a strike and then open the hooks on your next throw in the event you had the hooks closed too much. This is one way that I explore rough underwater obstacles. For some reason, I have found that if you tie one worm in front of another you set off a trigger mechanism which stimulates the strike mechanism of a bass and makes him want to eat even though his stomach is full of shad. I have noticed when I bring in my catch, that the bass spit out large quantities of a certain size shad. And this is what gave me my idea for my two-hook spoons which I will describe in my wintertime fishing.

If you are to be a successful fisherman, you must believe that you are going to catch bass and not be discouraged after a few minutes of fishing.

If your sinker is getting tangled up too much, you simply take it off and put on one that is lighter in weight. You may also stand up on the seat of your boat to help keep the worm coming over the snags rather than through the middle of them. Sometimes I stand up on my seat and retrieve my worm with my rod tip almost straight up. This increases the angle vector and will prevent your staying hung up all the time. One of the most important things I have learned in fishing is to be able to put my boat back exactly where I fished the day before on any given point in the middle of a river, and this is very easy to do.

If one looks down the barrel of a gun, he lines up the "V" on the stock of the gun with a point on the end of the gun. This means that when you line these two points up on a third object, you will be shooting in a straight line, so my method is simply to pretend that the boat is the target of two rifles that are about to fire at you from two directions—say north to south and east to west. You simply look on shore and try to find a telephone pole *close* to the shore and something that is in the shape of a "V" or a cross, or a power pole that is off in the distance. The further these two points are apart, the more accurate will be your relocation on the river. You simply do this procedure from two directions, and this will put you back exactly in the middle of the river where you were the day before; and if you cast your lure exactly toward the object on the shore that you did the day before, usually at the same time of day that you fished the day before, there is a ninety percent chance that you are going to catch more fish in the same area.

It is better to fish with three in the boat than by yourself, as the area can be fished out three times as fast, that is, all four sides of your boat must be fished as the bass wander around on the bottom like those chickens in the chicken coop running back and forth when they see another chicken running after a beetle or a butterfly.

From May to November, as the season progresses, the water gets colder and I find that the bass start "blipping" my plastic worm. This tells me that the bass are still in the same places, but they are no longer hungry for the soft green plastic worm, and this is when I try to outwit them. It is at this different time of the year that the bass seem to want a small dull type of spinner or spoon and here again I find the one-gulp type of lure the most effective. The best combination that I have ever found, and with which I have caught innumerable large bass, is a double crystal spoon, that is, a small two-hook spoon with a crystal finish to give a fish-scale effect. This seems to be the size that resembles the shad the bass were spitting out as I described earlier in this article. I do not find the bright shiny spoons with mirror finishes that the lure companies have worked so hard to get, as effective as a crystal spoon. The silvery crystal effect seems to be the most deadly of any of the many types of spoon or spinner ever designed.

I illustrate my one-gulp spoons. Here again I am using needle-sharp hooks—small hooks—in addition to small lure bodies, but these lure bodies are too small and light to be cast by themselves. You must, therefore, tie on a larger spoon either in front or behind these one-gulp killers to act as the vehicle to get the lure away from your boat and into the place where you think the fish are. You start off fishing the same places that you caught the fish with the plastic worm and in the same manner. This is, throw the double spoon combination into the bass areas, put your reel back in gear and watch your line as the heavier spoon makes the lighter spoon sink. If your line so much as flinches, jerk back on your rod as the bass are hitting in a manner which I call "falling back." If a lot of slack comes in your line as your lure sinks, jerk back on your rod tip as hard as you can as the bass has struck your plugs and is running toward your boat in a manner which I call "throwing slack." If you have not had a strike from the original cast, let the double spoon sink to the bottom and just sit there and play like you are fishing, that is, do not even move the rod or the line. The bass out in the hole have all gathered around this mysterious combination and are mesmerized by this thing lying on the bottom. You may slowly lift your rod tip, but be ready for a violent strike! And he may strike it in one of the two manners I just described, that is he may run toward the boat, which will throw a lot of slack into your line or he may run away from your boat which will almost jerk the rod tip from your hand. You must remember that you have *two* lures on the end of your line and that the other bass follow this bass like the chickens previously described and will hit the other spoon that was the weight cast vehicle to begin with, which means, "Get ready for another violent strike as you are retrieving the original strike." This is why I use twelve-pound test line.

I have boated forty-two bass, the least of which weighed two pounds and ten of them weighed close to six pounds, caught in this described manner. I have fished in this same manner with shiny spoons, that is spoons polished to a brilliant luster, and could only catch small bass. I have duplicated this method over and over and have found no other method that will compare to it. If the bass does not strike when you lift the line up, and you must remember they are all out there just looking at this object, slowly retrieve your double spoon combination like you did the plastic worm, and they will strike the smaller one-gulp spoon ferociously. This double combination must set off some type of trigger mechanism that makes the big bass rush in and grab the goodie before the little ones have a chance. After two or three casts, it will be plain to see how the bass want you to work the spoon combination, that is, if he hit it while it was sinking and does not hit it in the slow retrieve method just described, then it is best to simply cast and let him attack the lure as the lure sinks. If he does not strike the lure in either of these two manners, then simply throw it out again, let it sink and quickly wind the lures with your reel and at the same time, lift up the tip of your rod until it goes up to eleven o'clock and hold on tightly, he will strike at the top of your retrieve. I do not mean to confuse you with so many methods of using one lure. I simply know that these three methods will work.

Another method of using the spoon is simply to use one of the original crystal spoons by itself—slowly retrieve and let it pulse and flutter along the bottom. This is why I like to fish with two other people in the boat besides myself, so we can find out in a few casts what the bass will hit and in what manner of retrieve he is going to strike.

There are times when the bass seem to like a spinner-type of lure better, and this can be fished in the same manner as the spoons. However, I do not tie on a one-gulp spoon ahead of a spinner. Some day I may. Up until this point I have not had to.

As the water progressively gets cooler, the bass leave these deep holes and go to the bank, and this is when we take on an entirely new type of fishing. A lot of our fish are caught with a joint fina, type of Old Pal shallow running lure which will not run very deep and which can be twitched so that the head will make a U-turn and pop back up. We do this type of fishing around piers, stumps and tree tops. Here again someone else in the boat will have a deeper running lure of this type. Throw toward the shore and retrieve with the lure so the lower lip will bump against the bottom. Then let back off the rod tip to let the lure start rising, and this again is when you will experience two types of strikes. He may strike your lure and run toward your boat, and you must watch for this slack to suddenly appear in your line and jerk back on your rod; here again is where you need a rod with a stiff butt so that as you set your hook you do not get a lot of bend in your rod, and the force that is exerted will be in the penetration of the hook into the fish's mouth rather than expelled as a limber bend in your rod, while your fish is spitting your lure out of his mouth after a strike. If you have a rod with a stiff butt, simply hold your rod erect or at eleven o'clock and keep your line tight. As a big fish makes a run, simply lower your rod a little bit. Let him run and play him down. This is why you came to fish in the first place. Do not horse him in—simply let him tire himself out.

I do not recommend a net for the following reason. When I reach over to pick up my net and the bass sees this thing coming over him, his survival instinct mechanism will give him one last lunge in a desperate effort to save his own life and this has caused the loss of some of my largest fish. If you are a true sportsman, you will give him a fighting chance, as all the odds are on your side to begin with if you are properly equipped.

The shallow running type of lure is simply cast up around brush and stump areas and allowed to rest a few seconds, then twitch it, dance it, jiggle it, etc., until you find out the strike mechanism for the bass. There seems to be a given time at which they stop eating and then do not hit any more, but if a two-hook spoon is placed ahead or behind a super, blooker, type of lure, here again the bass will strike at the two-hook spoon. This type of fishing lasts on into early April when the best type of fishing of all begins, and that is top water.

This is where the two-hook spoon accounts for an incredible number of large bass, crappies, white bass, and just about everything else in the river, except carp and gar. The top water lure of my choice is a super blooker, preferably clear with a green back.

The second type is a cigar-shaped lure with a propeller at the back hook, a green back and hooks painted green. I find that sometimes the bass want to hear a blooker go, "blook, blook, blook" and at other times they like to strike a lure that goes "zit, zit, zit," the sound you get from a propeller. The darker green colors seem to work best when there is fog on the water. Here again, one must feel out the action that the bass want for that particular day and fish at a time of day during which the bass are striking. I find this to be early in the morning just after daybreak up to about six thirty or seven o'clock, and late in the evening just for a short while after sundown until a few minutes before dark.

The "blook, blook, blook" type of plug has been found to be effective in all seasons of the year and sometimes works best with the two-hook spoon tied behind it, and you must carefully check your *blooker* after you have *blooked* it to see if it twitches, which means that the bass has struck the two-hook spoon. The two-hook spoon is made with white, yellow or green maribu feathers.

In the swampy areas of the South, especially where there are miles and miles of water about waist-deep, there abound dead shrubbery and stumps for undercover. This is usually where bass are caught during the hottest part of the day—in the middle of the undercover. This requires a change in your whole fishing armamentarium.

I have caught so many fish in the Catawba River compound that I have not found it necessary to resort to this wading in waist-deep water with alligators and snakes, although this is practiced by many professional men from the Charlotte area. The Santee Cooper River compound extends for hundreds of miles of shore line of submerged stumps, logs, etc., and is subject to extremely rough water such as no fishermen has ever experienced until he has been in it. Some of them have never returned. Some have frozen in their boats or have become lost. Their method of fishing consists of using a large worm of the same soft consistency as its shorter cousin, the two-hook four-inch worm, and fished in about the same manner except the sinker is wedge-shaped and rests against the worm which contains a number 6.0 hook with the point of the hook stuck back into the worm to make it weedless. When you feel a small blip, you simply open your bail and let the bass run with this huge worm, chew it up, and then run as he swallows it. This is when you close your bail and set your hook with all your might. The guide that first showed me this method uses forty-pound test line so that he can horse these lurkers from the underbrush, and I have seen them personally get out of the boat and wade into these bushes and swim under them to stick a hand into their mouths to pull them out of the underbrush. This type of fishing simply does not appeal to me. However, these guides are the finest bass fishermen in the world, in my opinion, and catch fish consistently, every day of the year.

The next type of fishing will be that described as "weedless spoon fishing." One of the best spoons I have found is the one-half ounce crystal spoon that has been made weedless and that has green spots on its back. This spoon is used around lily pads, grass beds, stumps, and partially submerged bushes. It is most effective when a pork rind or a six-inch green plastic worm is put on the hook. The fisherman simply casts the weedless spoon over and toward the middle of a pile of bushes or the grass becs or the lily pads and starts retrieving the spoon before it has hit the water. This, in effect, keeps the spoon from sinking, and the fisherman merely skims the spoon over the surface of the grass bed with its tail dangling behind, which makes the spoon ride on its back with the hook up. One would think that this method would hang the spoon up, but you will find the spoon will dance right over the bushes and hangers. If you throw the spoon into the same area two or three times, you have the bass in that area so confused that you will usually get a ferocious strike. The same method is used when one treetop fishes. Both methods can be used at just about any time of the year as the bass seem to work in and around these areas summer and winter.

In treetop twitching, you simply throw your jointed plug

into an open area between limbs of a submerged tree that has fallen into the river and twitch the joint fina with short jerks. The joint fina does a beautiful job of doubling back on itself and diving; and if one repeats this process two or three times in the same area, he will usually get a strike.

There is a type of fishing down South called "jigger fishing"; I do not recommend this type of fishing to anyone with a weak heart, because when the bass strikes, it is such a ferocious strike that your heart will jump into your throat. Jigger fishing is done by wrapping a forty-pound test line on the end of a cane fishing pole with about three feet of line hanging off the end of the pole. One may tie a treble hook to the line and put three small plastic worms to this treble hook or some pork rind or some strips of rubber balloon. You simply row about in your boat and tap your rod on the water, and this makes the hook jiggle up and down. You do this at night around boathouses, tree stumps, half-submerged bushes and treetops. This method has produced some of the largest bass I have ever seen, and in some states this is illegal.

One may take a green plastic two-hook worm and soak it with Hydron®, a fish lure scent developed by Woodstream Corporation, and dangle it in the bed of a spawning bass and entice the bass to strike. I have tried my entire life to entice a spawning bass to strike, and this fish odor added to a lure is the only method that I have found that will work.

The tackle box of my choice is a worm-proof box so that my worms will not melt.

Sometimes the fish strike a lure better if another fish has already chewed upon it. Here again I find that if one will simply coat his lure with Hydron spray, the fish will start off striking much quicker. The Hydron fish scent was developed from the glands of the inside of a fish's mouth and seems to attract another fish to strike the lure instead of swimming around and looking at it. Fish that would normally look at a lure and turn away will strike this same lure when this fish scent is added. Hydron comes in a small can and may be sprayed on any lure you have. It contains a plastic along with the fish scent and will dry up when the lure is out of the water; it holds the fish flavor until you put it back into the water. At this time your lure will turn milky-white, which shows the plastic has opened up its pores and will emit the fish odor again. Here again, I have found that once my green worms have been chewed on and take on this milky color, the bass seem to hit them better. In other words, the more the worm is chewed on, the better the bass seem to strike it, and if one simply sprays the worms with Hydron in the beginning, he is more apt to start catching fish sooner.

The addition of two small spoons to a rig is another secret I learned, to entice bass to strike. They can be added to a back hook on just about any plug or onto the top of a spoon to give the spoon a rattle.

In conclusion, I would like to say that the bass will strike a plastic worm better than any lure that I know of, and the most effective plastic worm that has been developed is one that is three or four inches long and contains ultra-small hooks. I have had letters from fishermen saying that they found the black worm better in one region while in another region they found the purple better; but as for the South, I have not run across any color more effective than the color I call "E" green. And of course, the pre-rigged two-hook is the most effective, although the lure may be made with a weedless hook.

I plan to use a larger type green worm with a small two-inch worm ahead of this with two hooks but have not found the time to leave the excellent fishing location which I enjoy. My home is located on the South Fork River, just outside of Gastonia, North Carolina, just a few hundred yards from what we call the "hot hole." The "hot hole" is simply this: the warm water that Duke Power Company distributes from its generator plants into a canal and empties into the South Fork River. The water is warm enough for a person to go swimming in the wintertime. I have just about any type of fishing I like due to this warm water outlet from the power plant. Here again the bass move in and out of this warm water and travel up and down the river, but the water stays warm enough around the "hot hole" that the green worm may be used twelve months out of the year. This area is so crowded with fishermen during the wintertime—catching boatloads of white bass with spoons, and black bass and crappie—there is hardly any room left to park. Therefore, I take my spoons into the colder water and catch my limit almost every trip.

21

THE FISHING PHYSICIAN

JOSEPH H. BELLINA

Fishing can be many things: an escape from the office, a challenge, a tax deduction, or an ancillary business. To most physicians it is a combination of escaping from the pressures of medicine and a challenge of his skill. With the mortality rate up as a result of diet, lack of exercise, smoking and tension, one should take every advantage the outdoors has to offer as a means of extending his life expectancy. Walking in the early morning to your favorite brook, in solitude or with a good friend, escaping from the world if only for a few hours, can add days to your life expectancy. Why does the doctor seem to forget his own advice to so many—"Get away for awhile and relax"?

The true fisherman is very serious about his tackle, methods, and choice fishing spots. Whether you are a weekend warrior or a vacation novice, fishing gets into your blood. As men of science we tend to analyze, perfect and concentrate on a "perfect" technique. This determination has lead many physicians to be some of today's top fishermen.

Within the following pages I have attempted to give the novice fisherman an insight into the many facets of this exciting sport. This chapter, I hope, will also stimulate others to explore the newer modes of angling, i.e. spin fishing or saltwater fly fishing. At the end of this chapter are names and addresses which may be of help.

SALT WATER FLY FISHING

The exact date on which man first landed a saltwater fish with a flyrod is unknown, and will probably remain so. In the American literature, Dr. James A. Henschall wrote of his 1878 Florida expedition, and describes tarpon, redfish and bluefish, all taken on a freshwater flyrod. Many anglers such as Bob McChristian, Holmes Allen, Red Greb and Stewart Miller, have contributed to saltwater history, but Dr. Webster Robinson of Key West, Florida, captivated the imagination of all flyrodders. In January, 1961, he landed a 74¼-pound Pacific sailfish, the world's first on fly tackle. This feat may not at first seem outstanding; however, consider that Dr. Robinson was in his late sixties and in failing health and add to this the fact that during three hundred fishing days he landed, on conventional tackle, one hundred twenty-eight black marlin—this makes him quite a *man*! Utilizing his techniques, men such as Lee Wulff have set many world records and this author has landed a 105-pound Pacific sailfish on a ten-pound tippett. A quite and noble sportsman, Dr. Robinson will remain "father of a flyrod billfish." Fly casting principles are easy to learn and after two or three sessions any man can use a flyrod effectively. As with any procedure, mental and physical, repeat performances can perfect it to a true art. In the beginning you may not be as proficient as the professional sportsman but someday you may be a professional.

Today many books on fly casting are available, and by writing any of the manufacturing companies they will be happy to send current brochures and helpful hints.

Now the matter of selecting fly tackle, a balanced rod action, line weight and reel becomes a *real* problem. Today this problem is simplified by companies attempting to produce "balanced" outfits. These outfits are priced from ten to over a hundred dollars depending on your taste and requirements. One must become keenly aware that there is no all-around fly outfit. Modern fly tackle equipment ranges from the smallest streams to the oceans. To accompany these rods there are flies that are from a few millimeters in length to over six inches in length.

The most versatile outfit is a medium action, 8½ foot rod, strung with a No. 8 or 9 line and a reel with a brake. This outfit can cast a line bug or streamers, is sensitive and yet has enough backbone to land bass or tarpon.

Beginners should learn with a level line, i.e. L8F. This line has an even weight distribution and allows the neophyte to learn the casting characteristics of his rod. Lines with an uneven distribution, i.e. weight forward taper, are more expensive and provide a greater cast distance. When an angler tackles salt-water, a torpedo taper (excessive forward weight) is used to allow casting into a stiff breeze.

Fly reels are now available for light stream fishing or heavy bill fishing. The costs are proportional to the job they are expected to perform. A simple single-action click drag may be purchased for as little as $3, while the most expensive reels cost $150. Saltwater reels are the most durable and usually have an anti-reverse to prevent the handle from injuring the fisherman. These reels have spool backing capacities of 200 to 300 yards. When an angler tackles bigger game fish he should choose a fast to medium fast rod, 9 feet with a WF10F or WF11F.

The final portion of your outfit is the leader. Much has been written on this topic but suffice it to say that it should be tailored to your fish and lure. A large fish with sharp doral fins and gill plates needs to be taken with a heavy 50-pound to 80-pound segment, followed by your weakest point in this chain—the tippit. The tippet governs the class in which you will be fishing, i.e. 15, 12, 10, 6 pound. The final segment used only in larger game fish is the shocker. This final segment should be of sufficient durability to withstand the biting and rasping effect of the fish at the strike. When tournament or world record fishing, you should obtain the complete Rules and Regulations of the Saltwater Fly Rodders of America, Post Office Box 304, Old Court House, Cape May Court House, New Jersey, 08210.

A final note of fly fishing, particularly in the big game class, is to set your adjustable drag at one-third the lightest part of your tippet and remember that the drag *increases* as the spool diameter decreases. Many a prize fish has been lost when an angler left his drag at a fixed position only to be astonished that his tippet parted when the fish had spooled off 60 to 80 percent of his line. Had he reduced the drag proportionally this may not have happened.

SPIN FISHING

A few years back a new form of reel was developed that allowed the line to spool off freely instead of being unwound from its bobbin or drum. The revolutionary concept advanced fishing techniques beyond the most skilled anglers dream. Casts of over 100 feet to 200 feet and beyond became commonplace. Today surf fisherman can be seen throwing their lures almost out of sight. Again only through the mechanical advantage of a long rod and lightning-fast spool can this be accomplished.

Beginners today can be "expert" casters in a matter of hours and avoid the infamous "backlash." The spinning reel, either closed face or open face, has the unbelievable ability to prevent a backlash. This removes one of the hazards of fishing from the angler's thoughts and permits complete concentration on casting accuracy. He now becomes truly an expert in distant and target casting.

As with all fishing tackle, outfits can be purchased to fit your location and needs. Reels can be purchased to handle light two-pound to 30-pound line depending on your needs. Whether right or left handed, a reel is available for you, either open or closed face.

The outfit which is probably the best all-around to start with is a 6 or 6½ foot light to medium action rod with a reel of 200-yard capacity topped off with 10-pound test monofilament line. This rig is versatile enough to handle six, eight or ten pound test. Today prespooled line is available and changing from one line to another requires only a few seconds.

The ultralight rods from 3½ to 5½ feet in length should be balanced with an ultralight reel and fine line. Lures should be of the light class, less than ⅛ ounce. This gear is ideal for back packing and high mountain fishing. When fighting a small rainbow or cutthroat, the angler is still put to the test.

Progressing into the medium class, the saltwater and all-around freshwater class is entered. Here a rod of 5½ to 7 feet with a reel using a 10 to 15 pound line is best. Almost all freshwater and most inland saltwater fish can be taken on the outfit, again keeping in mind the most important facts when fighting a big game fish—drag and spool capacity. If your rig has only a 100-yard capacity and you tackle a bonefish whose first run is usually 100 yards, you could be in trouble.

Reels and rods can be had to handle a multitude of assorted

lines and lures. Spinning reels are also found in the ocean class. Spool capacities of 250 plus yards with durable drags that will not freeze under the intense heat are essential for big game fishing. Rod length and backbone should match the reel. It is not uncommon to see surf anglers with 10 to 12 foot rods.

Vic Dunaway has four rules which help the novice caster become more expert:

1. Use two hands when casting, except ultralight. Two-hand casting affords much better rod control and better leverage.
2. Cast overhand at the target.
3. When you pick up the line to clear for a cast, let the line hang from your forefinger. Do not press it against the fore grip.
4. Learn to feather the line as it goes out. Cast beyond your target and slow the lure into position by applying pressure to the spooling line. This will give you the extra accuracy necessary for fishing spooky fish.

SALTWATER BIG GAME FISHING

When one jumps off here, he must be physically and financially able to cope with big game fishing stress and rising cost. If you truly want to compete in big game fishing, you must be willing to stay out for many hours, even days, spent extravagant amounts of money and accept the probability of only 10 to 20 percent success. If you feel this is acceptable, then begin by visiting your nearest tackle store and price trolling rods and reels. Of course you may rent your gear and I strongly suggest doing so unless you plan to fish regularly with professional intent.

Today the IGFA (International Game Fish Association) prescribes the rules and regulations under which an angler may compete. Manufacturing companies now produce matched outfits in 12, 20, 30, 50, 80, and 130 pound test line categories. Since the major factor again is your line, much will be said later on. Penn produces a fine trolling reel and Fenwick as well as World Wide Sportsman manufacture excellent rods with Afgo® rollers. When purchasing the rod, you need to keep in mind the tremendous frictional heat that will be applied to your guides. Afgo rollers are probably preferred. Next note that the rod separates at the butt, allowing storage of reel and butt assembly without having to disengage your reel. This is not imperative, but when you spend 30 minutes attaching your trolling reel properly, this becomes important.

Purchasing a reel is your next problem. The older stardrag models are cheaper, but remember that under a fast run, the friction may fuse the brass washers or explode your reel seat. Thus, a good reel should have a monoblock spool and shaft, disc brake and have a 3:1 retrieve at least. When 600 yards of line are out, the 3:1 retrieve is a lifesaver. I have mentioned a disc brake, as this modern modification has a marked advantage over the old stardrag. Discs of heat-resistant metals with brake shoes can give infinite increments of pressure and allow all the versatility needed for big game. The more popular reels of this type are Pen International series, Fin Nor and Garcis.

Line cost will vary as will the cost of materials. Monofilament line is excellent and has the advantage of stretch forgiveness. However, braid Dacron®-Micron is my preference. Braided Micron [squiding] has a smaller diameter, hence more line on any given reel. It has been postulated that, within reason, any line strength could land any fish regardless of size given adequate line capacity, drag system and gear ratio. This line can be purchased with an IGFA guarantee of breaking point. Please take note particularly if you are after tournament or record fish: should your line break above the class entered then all your plans and hopes will go up in smoke.

While on the subject of line, a small discussion of line testing seems necessary. Once you bring your fish in, the weighmaster will remove a segment of your line and place it in a device to test its true breaking point. The point of breakage determines your class regardless of what you purchased. Again make sure you obtain the rules and regulations of your tournament; most follow the IGFA but this is not always the rule. A final note to aid the neoplyte troller: most reels have a drag lever marked "free—strike—full." To make certain that you never lose your fish from over-applied drag, set the drag lever to almost full. Next adjust the spring tension screw to prevent your line from breaking even though almost full drag is applied. I would not recommend setting this adjustment at "full," because you may want to save some line should you suddenly realize your fish is spooling off all your line. Simply apply full drag and your line will part.

The technique of attaching baits and lures are many, and each area may vary as to type of lures, etc. In general the bait should be attached to a leader, usually of metal, to prevent cutting by the bill or teeth of the fish. The leader from six to twelve feet is attached to a swivel, usually the ball bearing type to prevent the line from twisting. Finally the line is back-spliced about 15 to 20 feet to give a double line. Most big game sporting stores will prepare your equipment at the time of purchase, but learn the techniques and modify them to fit your needs.

Teasers are very large hookless lures which attract fish to the surface. They are generally trolled close to the stern of the boat. Once the fish surfaces, he will then attack your bait. There are many ways to present the bait. Outriggers skip the bait along the surface and allow the bait to be held away from the backwash. Downriggers hold your bait at depths, by attaching a breakaway lead, to attract deep-running fish. Finally the flat line and the kite can be used to present your bait.

As to setting the hook or trolling techniques, each angler has his own. In general when a bill fish just appears at your bait he will seem to be hitting it with his bill. The "hitting" was thought by many fishermen to be a killing or stunning technique. Others speculate that probably the fish is attempting to see his prey as the visual field of a bill fish has a blind spot directly in the line of his bill. Once your fish starts this motion he will usually turn a bright color, lighting up. At this moment your fish will swallow anything. Release your drag and count to ten allowing the fish a moment to swallow the bait—gut hook technique. Apply two or three quick pulls to drive the hook into the fish and hang on.

MONOFILAMENT LINE

This section is written to aid in choosing the proper line for fishing. The newer monofilaments permit a wide range of performance. A small discussion about the physical characteristics is needed to allow you an educated choice.

Monofilament is a nylon which is pulled into threads and rated by its ability to support a given weight, i.e. 6 pounds, 10 pounds, etc. Monofilament should be analyzed by the following:

Visibility	Stretch
Strength	Limpness
Knot strength	Shock resistance
Abrasion resistance	

Visibility. The ability of a line to blend with its background is visibility. A good line should disappear in the water to give your lure a natural self-propelled appearance. This property of monofilament is probably the least important, but in extremely clear water may play a major role.

Strength. Tensile strength may be defined as the longitudinal stress per diameter. The optimum strength with the least diameter gives a low wind resistance and greater spool capacity. Many brands of monofilament are available and the same strength may vary greatly in diameter. Check clearly before purchasing and note whether the monofilament has been exposed to direct sunlight. Ultra violet light has a deteriorating effect and the fiber will loose its tensile strength after exposed.

Knot strength. Knots usually weaken a line by causing pressure points which tend to cut rather than pull the line apart. A properly tied improved clinch knot gives almost 100 percent strength, while an overhand knot reduces the strength by 50 percent. This means that even the most expensive monofilament is only as good as your ability to tie the knot.

Abrasion resistance. Monofilament is made of a core and outer shell. This outer shell is abrasive resistant and permits repeated abuse, i.e. tail cutting, coral and rocks. However should the monofilament become abraded, which is easily felt by passing through your fingertips, it should be replaced. The cheapest part of your fishing trip is the line.

Stretch. This property permits the angler to make mistakes. If you overcompensate, the line will have a slight forgiving give and may save you a fish. However too much stretch property will not allow you to set your hook properly. Thus a blend of forgiveness and resistance is necessary. The property of stretch is closely related to shock or impact resistance. The sudden strike of a fish may snap your taut line if the stretch factor is improper.

Shock resistance. Probably more fish are lost because of the initial strike causing a line to part than due to excessive studding. The line should give enough to absorb the shock and prevent a break. This property is similar to taffy. If sharply pulled it will crack cleanly; however, if the pull pressure is gradually applied, it will stretch quite a distance before parting.

Limpness. The final property of a good line is limpness or the ability of a line to be bent. Proper line should be flaccid enough to be spooled without recoiling from the reels, but still be resilient during casting.

Remember, purchase a good quality line, protect it from the sun, replace abraded portions and, above all, when in doubt, replace. Monofilament is inexpensive.

RECOMMENDED KNOTS TO USE*

When you tie a knot, which you have to do on any line, you weaken it to some degree, so you want the best retention of strength possible—the higher the better. The knot stands between you and the fish. The happiness and the success of your entire fishing trip, in the final analysis, eventually depends on the knot you tied in the line you bought. Just any knot will not do, and the proper knot must be tied with care.

The ability to tie proper fishing knots is most important. It is one of the most important factors in angling success. A fisherman needs to master only a few basic knots. None are difficult to learn.

The basic fishing knots illustrated are the ones most commonly used by anglers. Each knot answers a practical need and is easy to tie with very little practice. Each knot has been thoroughly tested in the Du Pont research laboratories and in actual use.

Monofilament must be tied carefully to be tied properly. We know certain precautions must be taken with monofilament. For

---

* From *Fishing With Du Pont Stren*® Technical Bulletin No. 3. Reprinted with permission of Du Pont.

example, in any knot where the friction is against any other material than monofilament itself, the knot has a tendency to slip. This eliminates the so-called "jam" knots. In any type of knot in which the friction is largely on the turns of the material itself there is less tendency to slip or untie.

All monofilaments are strongly affected by the type of knot used and the technique of tying. For example, with most other monofilaments, the wind or overhand knot may have as little as 40 to 50 percent of the unknotted line strength. With Stren®, you will get up to 75 percent and higher of the unknotted line strength.

The overhand knot is the weakest knot that can be tied and is therefore a good measure of the worst condition that might occur with a poorly tied knot of any type. Because of its high overhand knot strength, Stren is more forgiving for poorly tied or poorly selected knots than other lines.

As much as 100 percent of the unknotted line strength can be achieved by using the Improved Clinch or Blood Knot. However, to get ratings this high, five or more turns must be taken around the standing part of the line. The knot strength of ordinary monofilament drops off sharply as the number of turns decreases. A four-turn blood knot drops the strength of 10-pound monofilament down to 8.5 pounds. Three turns drop this to 7.5 pounds, and two turns to 6 pounds, or a loss of 40 percent.

This discovery is based on our study of high-speed motion pictures of knot failures. They showed that properly tied knots break at the very edge, where the last turn of the knot is wrapped around the center filament. Poorly tied knots tend to break in the center because the knot slips slightly and allows the total load to be carried by only one turn of the monofilament. The knot at that instant acts very much like an overhand knot and prematurely fails. Properly tied 5-turn knots distribute the load evenly over the entire length of the knot.

As a result of outside research plus years of actual fishing tests, we have come up with several different knots for specific uses. Descriptions and illustrations of these knots and the uses for which they are recommended appear on the following pages.

Improved Clinch Knot

The basic cinch knot with variations is an excellent knot for tying flies, lures and bait hooks to spinning lines or leaders. As shown in the accompanying chart, the Improved Clinch Knot retains almost all of the unknotted line strength. Using a double strand or double loop through the eye merely complicates tying without contributing to improved line strength. It is important to tie the Improved Clinch Knot to prevent slippage.

To tie this knot, stick the end of the piece of Stren through the eye of the hook or swivel and make five or more twists around the standing part of the line. Then thrust the end between the eye and the first loop, and then back through the big loop as shown in the sketch. Hold on to it and pull tight. Be sure to always cut Stren. Do not ever try to break it with your hands.

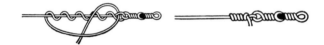

Continued research in our laboratories has proved that greater knot strength is achieved when several twists are made around the standing part of the line. So be sure you make at least five or more twists when tying the Improved Clinch Knot; and tie it up slowly and tie it up tight.

Blood Knot

This is the best knot we know of for tying Du Pont Stren to Stren when the diameters of the two strands are approximately the same. Here is the easy step-by-step way of tying it.

1. Lap the ends of the strands to be joined and twist one around the other, making at least five turns. Count the turns made. Place the end between the strands, following the arrow.

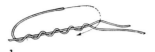

2. Hold the end against the turns already made, between the thumb and forefinger at point marked "X," to keep from unwinding. Now wind the other short end around the other strand for the same number of turns, but in the opposite direction.

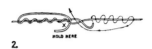

3. This shows how the knot would look if held firmly in place. Actually, as soon as released, the turns equalize.

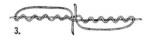

4. And the turns look like this. Now pull on both ends of the monofilaments.

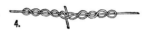

5. As pulling on the ends is continued, the turns gather as above and draw closer together (at this point the short ends may be worked backward, if desired, to avoid cutting off too much of the material).

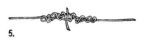

6. Appearance of the finished knot. All that remains to be done is to cut off the short ends close to the knot.

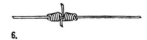

Perfection Loop Knot

If you would prefer to use the Perfection Loop Knot instead of the Improved End Loop Knot, and lose a slight amount of the un-knotted line strength, this knot is one you will find safe to use and relatively easy to tie.

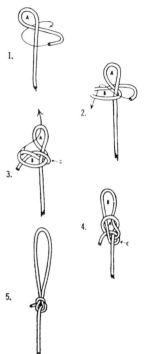

1. Take one turn around the monofilament, and hold the crossing between thumb and forefinger.

2. Take a second turn around the crossing, and bring the end around again between the turns.

3. Pass Loop B through Loop A.

4. Pull this loop up tight until jammed.

5. The finished knot.

Surgeon's Knot

This knot is also recommended for joining two strands of unequal diameter. It is particularly good for tying a heavy shock tippet to your leader point.

Lay the two strands parallel with ample overlap. Then, treating the two as a single strand, tie a simple overhand knot in the two lines. Now repeat the overhand knot, again pulling the two strands all the way through the loop. Hold both strands and both ends, pull tight and clip the ends short.

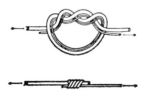

Bimini Twist
(20-times-around knot)

The Bimini Twist is one of the most useful and difficult knots a fisherman can learn to tie. Its function is to create a double line with the full strength of an unknotted line. You'll see it used for all kinds of fishing.

It requires some practice to get right, so start slowly and carefully, follow each step.

To make a long loop, it would be helpful to have two people. However, you can make a short loop by placing the loop over your knees to spread the lines apart.

In the drawings the loop has been made small and the number of twists in the line has been reduced from the necessary 20 because it would make the drawings too long.

1. Double the line to form a loop somewhat longer than what you intend to end up with. One person (B) should hold the end of the line. The other person (A) holding the loop end, proceeds to twist the loop 20 times—by keeping his index finger in the loop and making circular motions with his wrist.

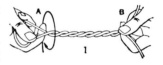

2. Once the 20 twists have been completed, separate the two strands of the loop (which will be much larger than illustrated) and work back toward the other end being held firmly by (B) to tighten the twist. Then (B) pulls the lines apart.

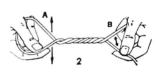

3. (B) Should place his forefinger on the twist and bring the running end of the line toward the loop. As (A) continues to open the loop, the twist begins to rotate.

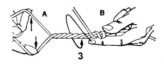

4. As the twist rotates, the running end is automatically wound around it. Care must be taken at this point not to let the running end wrap over itself. The wrap should continue until the end of the twist is reached.

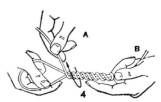

5. Now (B) must hold the wrap carefully to stop the rotation and at the same time execute a half hitch around the right base of the loop. (A) is still keeping the two lines of the loop separated.

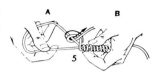

6. Then another half hitch is tied about the left base of the loop. It is now safe to let go of the wrap; it can no longer get away from you.

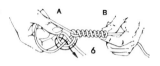

7. To finish the knot off, a little clinch knot it tied about both lines of the loop at the base. To do this (A) places the lines of the loop together while (B) takes three or four wraps around both lines and comes through as illustrated. Now the knot is pulled up tight.

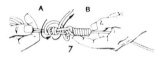

8. With the clinch knot pulled tight and clipped, the Bimini twist is completed.

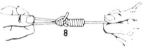

Double Turtle Knot

For use in tying your wet or dry fly to the tippet end of your leader. This knot is not as strong as the Improved Clinch Knot for this use, but if tied properly it allows the hackles of the dry fly to sit better on the water and the fly is therefore given a more life-like presentation. Here is the way we suggest you tie it.

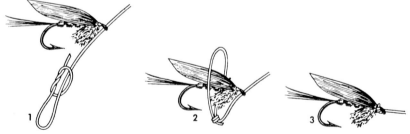

1. Run the end of the leader through the eye of the hook toward the bend. Make a slip knot in the end of the leader, bringing the end around twice (one turn would make a Single Turtle Knot), and pull the knot up tightly.
2. Open the loop large enough to permit the fly to pass through, and place the loop around the neck of the fly.
3. With the loop tight against the neck of the fly, pull on the leader until the knot is tight against the neck of the fly. All that remains to be done is to draw the slack of the Stren through the eye and pull it tight.

Improved End Loop Knot

We recommend the improved End Loop Knot for tying a loop on the end of your line or leader. To tie this knot, first bend over the strand of Stren about 4 to 6 inches from the end so that you have a "U" bend as shown in 1.

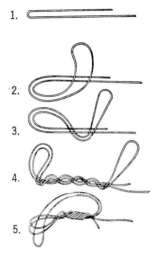

Then bend the "U" bend backwards and around itself at least 3 to 5 times depending on the thickness of the line. See 2, 3, and 4.

Now insert the end of the "U" bend through the first loop made by its backward turn and pull up tight. See 5.

Payne's End Loop Knot

This knot is tied exactly as the improved end loop knot. However, tie with a lure, fly, swivel or bait hook.

To tie this knot, first run the end of the line through the eye of the hook and slide the loop down the line about 6 inches. Next bend over the strand of Stren so that you have a "U" bend as shown in 1.

Then bend the "U" bend backwards and around itself at least three to five times depending on the thickness of the line. See 2, 3 and 4.

Now insert the end of the "U" bend through the first loop made by its backward turn and pull up tight. See 5.

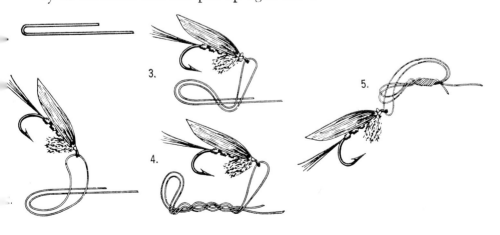

Stu Apte Improved Blood Knot

For tying a heavy Stren monofilament shock leader to a lighter Stren monofilament line or tippet. (Two greatly unequal diameters of monofilament.)

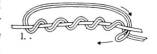

1. Double a sufficient length of the smaller diameter line so that it can be wrapped around the standing part of the larger diameter line with at least five turns. Place the doubled end down between the strands.

2. Hold the looped line between the thumb and the forefinger at the point marked "X" to keep from unwinding.

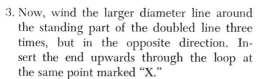

3. Now, wind the larger diameter line around the standing part of the doubled line three times, but in the opposite direction. Insert the end upwards through the loop at the same point marked "X."

4. Pull the knot up slowly and tightly to keep it from slipping.

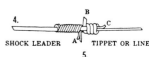

5. Now, cut off the ends of the doubled loop (A) and the end of the heavy line (B), both about a quarter-inch from the knot.

Cut off the loose end of the doubled line (C) about a quarter-inch from the knot.

Nail Knot (Tube Knot)

The Nail Knot is used to tie the butt end of your leader to the forward end of your fly line. It is also used to tie backing to a fly line. This knot gives a smooth, streamlined connection and the flat-lying knot will move freely through the guides of your rod, and if tied properly this knot cannot slip, cut, or pull out.

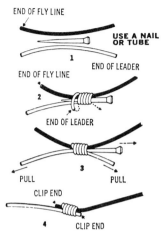

This knot is tied using either a tapered nail or piece of small tubing. Here's how to tie it.

Hold the line, leader and tapered nail or tubing alongside each other as shown in 1.

Allow ample overlap. Then wind leader downward around nail or tubing, line and itself six times and run end of leader back along nail or through tubing up under loops,

See 2. Pull both ends of leader tight. Slip knot down nail or tubing, tightening by pulling both ends of leader as it goes. Slip nail or tubing out and retighten by again pulling leader ends, See 3. Finally, pull line and leader tight and clip end of line and leader close to knot, See 4.

Recommended Uses of Knots

ADVANTAGES	RECOMMENDED KNOT	CONDITIONS	SITUATION	% OF UNKNOTTED LINE STRENGTH RETAINED	
				Ord. Mono.	Stren
LEADER TO LINE	Equal or slightly different diameter lines	Blood Knot	Dependable (basic knot)	90-95	95-100
		Surgeons' Knot	Easier to tie than Blood Knot	90-95	95-100
	Largely different diameter lines	Stu Apte Improved Blood Knot	Dependable	90-95	95-100
		Double Surgeons Knot	Easy to tie	90-95	95-100
		Bimini Twist	*	90-95	95-100
	Fly line to leader	Nail Knot	Gives a smooth flat-lying knot that will move freely through guides	90-95	95-100
LEADER TO LURE OR SWIVEL	Rigid lure or swivel	Improved Clinch	Dependable (basic knot)	90-95	95-100
		Improved End Loop	Easier and Quicker to Tie	70-75	95-100
		Turle	Quick and easy	55-60	90-95
		Perfection Loop	Quick and easy	60-65	90-95
	Free swinging lure	Payne's End Loop	Strongest of this type	70-75	95-100
LEADER TO LEADER	Equal or slightly different diameter leaders (e.g. tapered fly leader).	Blood Knot	Dependable smooth—free running in guides	90-95	95-100
	Largely different diameter leaders (e.g. shock leader or long butt section).	Stu Apte Improved Blood Knot	Dependable easier to tie than Blood Knot	90-95	95-100

*Useful to make a double strand leader on end of a line. Very difficult to tie.

HELPFUL HINTS

Line. Purchase the best and make sure it is rated by IGFA if you want a record. Prevent prolonged sunlight exposure of your monofilament line. Replace any line you suspect might have a defect. Each season respoon your reels.

Hooks. Use sharp triangular hooks. Carry a file and sharpen the edge of your hooks. Throw away old rusty hooks; a dull hook does not bite.

Rods. Always check your roller guide to see that they are free. Replace any guides that are defective—a sharp edge will quickly cut your line.

License. Always purchase the proper legal documents necessary for fishing. A red face and fine can ruin any trip.

Rules and regulations. Before going after records always check your rules and regulations.

Guides and boats. Always get a complete cost analysis before agreeing to charter. One trip recently taught me this lesson. When a price is quoted, inquire regarding what this includes— gas, food, mate, bait? You may save yourself many dollars.

Names and Addresses

I have listed below the names of three sources for equipment which I have mentioned in this chapter.

Fin and Feathers Sporting Goods, Inc.
3442 Kable Drive
New Orleans, La. 70114

World Wide Sportsman, Inc.
P.O. Box 46
Islamorada, Florida

Sevenstand Tackle Manufacturing Co.
14799 Chestnut St.
Westminister, California 92683
(makers of Fenwick rods)

MY FISH STORY

As the early morning sunrise jetted across the horizon, the Traviesa knifed her way through the green gulf waters. Our course was westward and the deep blue waters and where the linea lay. Acapulco slowly became a smear along the rugged mountain slopes as we crossed the ten-mile point. Within two hours, the linea-rip was sighted. Today the formation was poor, but still visible from the flying bridge. Captain Limones gave the orders and the crew quickly set the outriggers.

Today the outriggers carried mullets and the mates had received instructions not to attempt to hook any billfish using these rigs. If a bill was sighted, they were to use the mullets as teasers, and attract the fish within range of my flyline. Flyline,

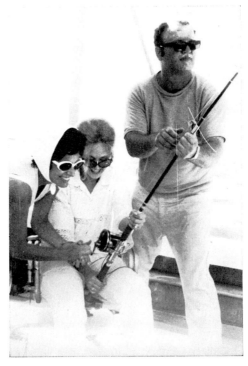

Figure 21–13. Fishing can be a family affair. This is the author, his wife, and a friend. Author's face is covered with suntan oil, a good measure for protection against excessive burning.

I thought hard as the words "flyline" and "ten pound tippet" struck me. What a way to throw away good money. One quick pass and a snap would probably be all that I would remember.

After an hour of trolling eastward, a sail was sighted. The Traviesa coursed near the area where the fish was playing near the surface of the water. The sun shimmered through the crystal waters. Like a curious child, the sailfish made a quick pass toward the stern of the boat. The silver mullet teasers struck a fiery note and his curiosity changed to rage.

Earlier in the week, while talking to A.G. Owens at Fin and Feathers in New Orleans, the idea of hooking a billfish on a fly rod seemed exciting, but now near the moment of truth, the thought "What the hell am I doing here?" seemed more appropriate.

"Strike," Victor Comancho shouted, as a lightning blue flash passed the port outrigger. Quickly the line was reeled in, and

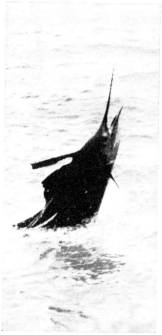

Figure 21–14. Pacific sailfish on the hook. A thrilling moment in any angler's lifetime.

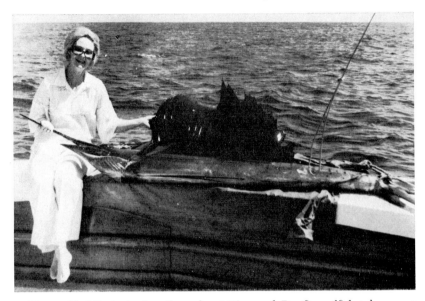

Figure 21–15. Author's wife and a 135-pound Pacific sailfish taken on a conventional tackle.

like a nautilus on the kill, the bill steamed through the Traviesa's wake. My armament consisted of a World Wide Sportsman rod, Seamaster reel, 350 yards of # 17 Trilene backing, 37 yards of #11 Scientific Flyline, a 10-pound Trilene tippet (six feet), and a 100-pound shocker of monofilament. The fly, a white streamer tied on 4/0 Pfleuger hook was instantly cast toward the oncoming bill. With lightning speed, the mullet was jerked away from the billfish and the fly presented, One pass, and down he went. Slowly, with zero drag, I counted to ten, and at this point about 200 yards out. The hairtrigger drag of the Seamaster was set, and two quick heaves set the razor sharp hook. The line went slack and quickly I backed off the drag, as I knew the great fish was racing toward the surface and the water drag alone could part my tippet. A magnificent leap, which seemed to last for an eternity, gave me the thrill of a lifetime. The drag was reset and the line quickly retrieved. The fish made a maddening pass toward the starboard, and the captain paralleled the boat to this course. During the pass, the fish surfaced and grayhounded six times.

The fight continued, and again and again the drag was set and reset to prevent the shock effect on the light monofilament line.

Slowly the Pacific bill gave way and was coaxed near the Traviesa. Here the touchy problems of boating a billfish with a #10 tippet gave me much thought. One quick lunge or slash could part the thread which held what I hoped would be a world record. The *1970 Saltwater Fly Rod World Record Catalog* had a beautiful blank for the 100-pound class Pacific sailfish.

The bill finally was airborn and the agile mate's first pass was lethal. The fish, as though given a shot of adrenalin,

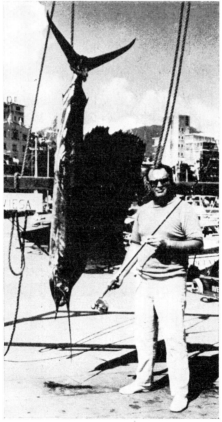

Figure 21–16. Author with his 105-pound Pacific sailfish, taken on 10-pound test tippit and a saltwater fly rod.

thrashed but was quickly sedated with a club applied to the cranium. It was done. Small bowel and stomach was present in the fish's mouth as an indictment for the effective gut hook technique. At the dock, the Pacific sailfish weighed 105 pounds and was boated thirty minutes after setting the hook.

I would sincerely like to thank Mrs. Carl Butler for her typing and Mrs. Joan Owens for her editing of my work. Also may I extend my thanks to my fishing associates Dr. Wayne Owens and Dr. Jerry Smith for their suggestions.

22

WILDWATER PADDLING

PAUL DAVIDSON

Move in your bed lovely river,
There is a new generation come to play with you;
A generation appreciative of your subtle movements,
A generation that loves you for your wrinkles and untamed ways,
A generation that only wants to help you clean and heal the
   damage left by those roughneck, greedy loggers and miners
   who used you as a depository and then abandoned you.

Wildwater paddling is maneuvering a featherweight boat over tons of surging water. It is the thrill of challenging a natural force knowing one's skill is all that stands between success and catastrophe.

Yet the challenge and catastrophe of wildwater are more apparent than real. Failure is more ego deflating than physically damaging. Flowing river water is a forgiving cushion unlike other natural forces and media used in related motion sports, e.g. soaring, skydiving, skiing, sledding, riding. The water cushion makes it far safer than involvement with the motor-driven land sports. The speed involved is actually minimal, but the sensation of great speed is present. The most apparent danger is drowning and this is virtually eliminated by life vests, helmets, and supervised graded wildwater experience.

Wildwater is interchangeably known as white water. The latter name is derived from the aeration churned in as water tumbles over an irregular rocky stream bed.

Wildwater paddling is one of the handful of sports in which man with minimal equipment allows himself to be moved by one of nature's forces and learns to control the movement to avoid potential disaster. During this controlled natural propulsion, man recaptures the moment of elation he first felt as a tossed infant. Perhaps the sensation and satisfactions of wild-water are even more primitive. It may be reenactment of the weightlessness of intrauterine life, the force of uterine contractions, the frightening stress of delivery, the elation of gasping for air and life. All these sensations are part of wildwater. Perhaps wildwater boating's appeal is the orgasm-like experience of being driven by an uncontrollable force with the confidence that the outcome will be pleasant. One can easily symbolize the boat as a phallus and the river as a frenzied mistress.

The personal requirement of the white water paddler is only that he be confident in the water. When overturned and bobbing along beside one's boat through a long rapids there is little to do but relax and let one's flotation keep him up until the river spends its energy in a pool. In the boat, finesse gained by experience is far more important than strength. The smallest girl can negotiate the biggest water if she has the appropriate skill.

HISTORY

Sports change as new equipment is developed. The change may be evolutionary, as in team sports, pole vaulting, sailing, skiing, hunting and fishing. The change may be the emergence of an entirely new sport based on a new technological development, e.g. scuba diving, skydiving, and the myriad of activities based on the internal combustion engine.

Of all the examples of change in an old sport based on technological developments, none are as dramatic as that in canoeing. This placid, utilitarian activity has been a leisurely mode of transportation since man first developed tools. Various forms of canoes serve as basic modes of transportation for every primitive society. In North America the canoe reached a pinnacle of development as the durable, lightweight birch-bark craft. Excluding tobacco, potatoes, and fictitiously syphilis, the birch-bark style canoe is the American Indian's most-adopted gift to the modern world.

The canoe was altered initially by constructing it from milled lumber covered with waterproofed canvas. A spin-off from the World War II aircraft industry was the development of the aluminum canoe. This was a hallmark breakthrough. The aluminum canoe combines much of the navigability and portability of its predecessor with tremendous durability. For the first time the canoeist had a craft that could bang into or slide over rocks without requiring elaborate repairs. A new era began. The "aluminum canoeist" could stop portaging past every turbulent stream constriction. Only the most experienced voyageur with a cavalier attitude toward his craft ran rapids in the wooden canoe. The aluminum canoe is forgiving enough to allow any paddler the thrill of pitting his skill against the seemingly hostile tumbling water. The nature of aluminum canoe construction limits the design flexibility and necessitates the construction of expensive dies. Large volume production is necessary and experimentation in design is prohibitively expensive.

The next technologic development in canoeing was from the chemical industry—the development of polymerized resin-supported fiber construction techniques, popularly referred to as fiberglass. Fiberglass products range from dune buggy bodies to bathtubs. This progress is ideal wherever large, strong, lightweight structures are to be built with simple tools, minimally skilled labor, low cost, design flexibility, and limited production.

Two North American canoes have fathered the currently used white-water boats—the Indian's birch-bark canoe known as the Canadian and the Eskimo's kayak. These craft were exported, modified by Europeans, and then in the 1960's returned to America as the currently used white-water craft.

Another related technologic development has been the development of the rubber raft. This has allowed persons without the desire or ability to learn to manage the more responsive and more challenging white-water boats to see wild rivers and experience some of the thrill of the force of moving water. It has been a stepping stone to true wildwater paddling for many.

EQUIPMENT

The specific boats used for wildwater paddling are largely dictated by the models used for competition. These boats are based on dimensions determined by the International Canoeing

Federation. The width is minimized and the length maximized for speed. The volume and rocker are varied for ultimate maneuverability.

The boats are of two basic types: the Canadian, or canoe, and the kayak. The Canadian may be designed for one (Fig. 22–1) or two paddlers (Fig. 22–2). The paddlers kneel with their butts braced against a seat, their thighs fixed against straps, and their feet braced against blocks. They paddle with a single-bladed paddle, primarily limiting all propelling and uprighting maneuvers to a single dominant side.

The kayaker in wild water uses a narrower boat, 60 cm, but a lower center of gravity (Fig. 22–3). He sits with his legs ex-

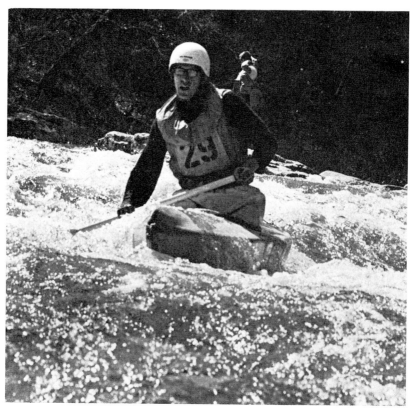

Figure 22–1. The author racing in a Czechoslovakian designed canoe. The paddle is in a low bracing position.

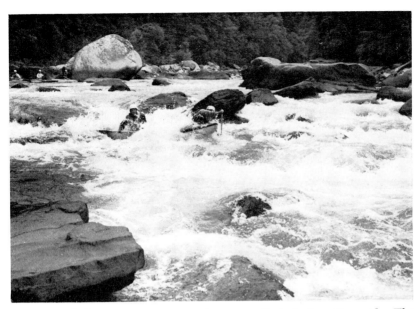

Figure 22–2. A two-man canoe in a complicated class V rapids. The bowman is driving forward as the sternman reaches for a downstream low brace. The boat is coming up out of a diagonal stopper and will momentarily be pushed sideways into another. The partially washed-over rock in the center foreground is a hazard. If the boat broaches against it, the weight of the paddles in the ends and the force of the divided current may break the canoe in two. Photo by R. Burrell.

tended and paddles with a double-bladed paddle, thus being able to exert force on both sides of the boat. The wildwater kayak is always limited to a single paddler, unlike flat-water kayaks.

In the current mode both the wildwater canoe and the kayak are decked with solid fiberglass. The paddler is in a small cockpit with the water sealed out by an elasticized skirt.

Great controversy rages between the canoer and the kayaker regarding the relative superiority of their single-man craft. Taking a stand for one or the other is comparable to a political or denominational affiliation. One must defend his chosen craft and downgrade the opposition with great emotion and without regard to reason. It is one of the jocular and harmless outlets for a paddler's latent bigotry. The real advantages of the canoe are

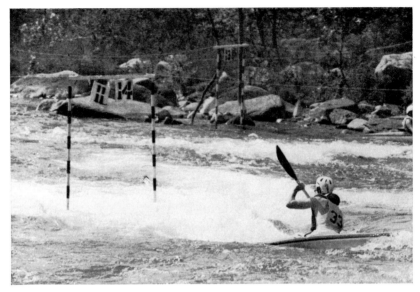

Figure 22–3. A slalom course in a class III rapids. The kayaker is approaching gate 14 after having run gate 13 upstream in the side eddy, ferried across and turned downstream on a high brace. The approach is complicated by a small roller wave forming a white eddy. The boiling water may deflect the bow of the kayak outside the gate as the stern is pushed on by the current. Photo by R. Burrell.

its greater displacement and bouyancy and the increased reach and vision of the kneeling paddler. The advantages of the basically tippier kayak are the lower center of gravity of the seated paddler and paddle-bracing stability associated with the double-bladed implement. In the western mountains, the kayak is the favorite. In the eastern mountains the paddlers are evenly split.

Both the canoe and kayak are further modified depending on the intended use. At one extreme is the boat which is maximally elongated and vee-hulled for fastest downriver racing. At the other extreme is the boat designed for slalom racing. It has minimal length and width. The hull is rounded in both directions until the waterline approaches that of a circle and the boat is the ultimate in maneuverability. The boats built for non-competitive cruising are batardizations of the two designs and are generally less satisfactory than using a slalom boat for cruising.

BUILDING

One of the many appealing facets of this sport is that the paddler can make and maintain his own equipment. Not only does this put the sport within economic reach of almost anyone but more important it adds to the more complete enjoyment of the sport. It permits a personalization of equipment like tying one's own flies, loading one's own shells, carving one's own decoys, rebuilding one's own engines, etc. A white water boat is more satisfactory if built by an experienced paddler to his specifications for his type of use than if stamped out with a cookie cutter by some disinterested factory worker. A white-water boat is an expendable item and building one's own boat is preparation for repairing the boat—an inevitable task. Building the boat as recreation and at cost of materials makes it much easier to accept its eventual destruction. By that time the paddler is enthused about building the next model with some improving modification.

Prior to 1969 there were no large manufacturers of wildwater boats in the United States. A few were imported from a German manufacturer of kayaks. No white-water canoes were available on the general market. A trickle of boats was launched from garage factories and sold by avocation builders. These builders are more often evangelists than entrepreneurs. They use their hobby time to popularize their sport. The cost of such boats is usually at bargain prices. Recently several commercial builders are offering a slicker, decidedly more expensive, but often inferior product.

Currently most paddlers build their own boat. This is a relatively simple process, thanks to the development of glass-reinforced plastics. To build one's first boat requires a mold and about $50 to $75 worth of fiberglass cloth and polyester or epoxy resin. The technique is simple and readily learned by volunteering a few evenings of labor to an experienced builder. The potential builder should contact his local affiliate of the American White Water Affiliation to locate a source of materials, molds, and instruction. It requires a weekend and two fellow workers to build one's first boat.

Other specific equipment required by the wildwater paddler is as follows:

Paddles. These are probably most satisfactorily purchased unless an expert builder's advice and mold is readily available. The usual boat store canoe paddle is not satisfactory—too narrow, too heavy, too breakable. The canoe paddler should have two paddles as insurance against breaking or loosing one in the wilderness. The paddle length is short compared to the lake canoer's paddle. This permits quick moves to counteract the effect of the turbulent currents. The best paddles are square bladed for maximum surface in shallow water and have T-grips for greatest control. They are made of fiberglass and aluminum or laminated spruce.

Skirt. This is an elasticised cover sealing the cockpit from water. It stretches tightly around the paddler's waist and extends to fit tightly around the cockpit rim. It is made of any waterproof material.

Flotation. Occasionally it is necessary for an overturned paddler to abandon his boat. A water-filled boat weighs over 1000 pounds and is certain to be crushed against boulders in a current. This is avoided by excluding water from the boat with flotation. The cheapest flotation is to fill the boat with beach balls but preferable flotation is fitted vinyl air bags.

Life jacket. This is considered an absolute must for a white-water paddler. The preferred jacket is a multiple-celled close-fitting vest which permits maximum mobility with maximum flotation.

Helmet. This is another absolute must for the wildwater paddler. While the paddler is upside-down projecting from his boat like a keel board and being swept along at over ten miles per hour, it gives a secure feeling to know that something other than one's skull will be dented by the approaching jagged boulder. The helmet must not cover the ears and shield the paddler from the road of an approaching waterfall.

Protective clothing. Since the best wildwater is in the fall, winter and spring, it is necessary for the paddler to have clothing for cold-water protection. This includes a waterproof windbreaker and sweater for more moderate weather and a roomy shorty wetsuit, wetsuit booties and mitts for near freezing weather.

Miscellaneous equipment should include a waterproof bag for lunch; sweater; duct tape for emergency repairs; fire-starting equipment; first-aid kit, etc.; and a throw line.

The cost of wildwatering is minimal relative to most sports.

To go first class with the best of equipment can cost $500, but one can get on the water with adequate used equipment for $50. A paddler-built new boat costs about $100. A boat lasts for over 500 miles of wildwater which is a good many five to ten mile per day trips. A wetsuit lasts until the stench can no longer be tolerated. Compare these costs to flying, soaring, skiing, motor boating, sailing, or belonging to a golf, tennis, or swimming club.

APPLIED HYDROLOGY

Paddling wildwater, like bikeriding, skiing, or surfing, must be learned by experience. After years of paddling there is still more to learn about the wily ways turbulent flowing water can affect a 30-pound boat. However, there are some basic facts that can be learned before getting on the water.

An understanding of simple hydrology is important. Water in an irregular, boulder-strewn, eroded, sloping river bed flows at different velocities in different parts of the stream. Shores, ledges, and boulders obstruct the free flow. As though the current were light, flow shadows form behind these obstructions. These shadows are known as eddies. Eddies are to the wildwater paddler as ledges are to the mountain climber—sites for resting and surveying the next stop. By hopping from one to another the paddler can control his descent or even ascent in a fast flowing stream.

A special eddy-forming phenomenon results in wave formation. When fast-moving water flowing over a shallow surface is stopped by deeper slow-moving water, it piles up into waves. Depending on the gradient, volume and velocity differential, the waves may be large haystacks, boiling mushrooms, undulating rooster tails, smooth ascending slopes suitable for surfing, or roller waves with aerated water rising from the bottom and rushing upstream to meet and fold in with the upcoming green water. The latter is known as a stopper, for it can form a wall of aerated water that can stop an unwary paddler coming downstream, turn him sideways, and roll the boat over and over (Fig. 22–4).

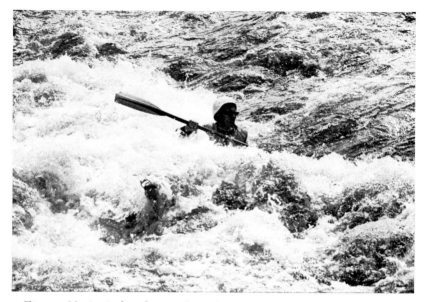

Figure 22–4. A kayak punches through the downstream wall of a
roller wave. This type of unavoidable stopper is characteristic of class IV
wildwater. Going into this sideways would be certain to upset any but the
most advanced paddler. Photo by R. Burrell.

Wildwater is classified primarily on the basis of these waves.
The classification is formalized by the American White Water
Affiliation from the first appearance of white foam and irregu-
larity, class I, to the ultimate in navigability with over six-foot
falls, greater than five-foot waves, and risk to life and boats for
even the most experienced, class VI.

DIFFERENT STROKES FOR DIFFERENT FOLKS

The techniques of wildwater paddling are not self-evident
and must be learned by wet experience. A few basic short cuts
can be outlined by instructors in non-paddling sessions, but
without immediate application their significance is lost. The
techniques of wildwater paddling differ from those of flat-water
paddling. These differences are profound enough that many
instructors would rather train a complete neophyte than try to
switch a seasoned lake paddler to the river.

The first problem is learning to paddle a wildwater boat in a straight line. Most of these boats are built with maximum fore and aft rocker and with no keel. This permits quick turning and sliding the boat sideways to avoid obstructions, but it makes the boat track erratically. The beginner will frequently spin out while trying to paddle fast. Paddling a white-water boat in a straight line requires constant attention to course correction. Each forward stroke must be individually canted to bring the boat into line. One stroke which neglects correction results in a spin-out or at least herniating straining on subsequent correcting strokes.

The kayak has an advantage for straight track paddling with its double blades stroking first on one side then the other. The canoeist paddles on one side with the consequent veering of the boat to the opposite side with each power stroke. The neophyte's inclination is to correct this by switching the paddle to the other side. This, however, is a risky maneuver in turbulent water, as the paddler must momentarily give up his stabilizing outrigger—an important secondary function of the paddle. The alternative is to terminate the forward propelling stroke with a prying motion, kicking the swinging stern back into line. The lake canoeist's smooth J-stroke is not suitable since it leaves the paddle in a poor position for boat stabilization as the driving face of the paddle is tilted upward and out. Instead of the paddle inscribing a "J" in the water, it should be a checkmark—powering backward and then turning toward the boat and kicking the nonpower face outward with a levering action against the side of the boat.

Many of the course controlling strokes in lake canoeing are rudder strokes. The boat is driven forward and the paddle is angled to act as a rudder as it rushes through the water. Rudder strokes are inadequate in a fast current, for while the boat is moving forward, in reality it is virtually standing still in relation to the moving water around it. Directing strokes must be positive power strokes if one is to avoid being pushed into rocks or over waterfalls. The basic strokes of the wildwater paddler are seldom used on a lake. They are the draw and the pry. The former is performed by leaning and reaching far out from the boat inserting the paddle perpendicularly to the water surface with the blade parallel to the boat and pulling or drawing the boat sideways toward the paddle. This keeps the alignment of the boat parallel to the current but slides it sideways to avoid an oncoming obstruction. Failure to move sideways may result in a head-on collision with an immobile object. Steering to the side without maintaining an alignment parallel to the current will messily wrap the boat around the object as the bow goes to one side and the stern to the other. Running sideways to the current is referred to as broaching and is a sure technique for locating boulders and eliminating boats.

In the kayak the draw may be performed bilaterally. The canoeist can only slide toward his paddle with this stroke. To go in the opposite direction he relies on the weaker pry stroke. The paddle is again inserted perpendicularly to the surface, with the blade parallel to the side of the boat, but this time very close to the side of the boat and slightly angled under it. The shaft of the paddle is steadied against the side of the boat and the handle is pulled toward the paddler. The short choppy pumping stroke can be repeated very rapidly by twisting the handle and recovering with a feathered blade beneath the surface. Another technique the canoeist uses to slide his boat to the off-paddle side is the crossbow draw. This is more powerful than the pry but less stable since it necessitates lifting the paddle over the front of the boat, twisting and reaching to the opposite side and drawing with the arms crossed.

Sweeping strokes are variations of the basic forward and backward propelling strokes moved in an arc to pivot the boat around a central axis.

Another family of strokes basic and unique to wildwater are the braces (Figs. 22–1 and 22–5). These are the infinitely variable, instantly adaptable outriggers of a white-water boat. The paddle stroke is directed downward against the water surface or against the current to right or stabilize the boat. Usually the brace is used at arm's length from the boat. Occasionally it is reversed and used in a hydrofoil-like manner beneath the boat. A few expert canoeists can twist across their craft and brace on the opposite side.

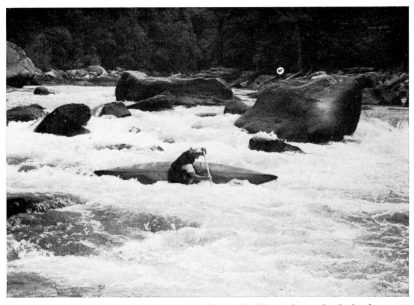

Figure 22–5. A single-man canoe being held up by a high brake as it emerges from the downstream end of a diagonal roller wave in a very complicated rapids. Photo by R. Burrell.

The ultimate application of the brace is to roll up an inverted boat. The roll is the best safety measure for the paddler and his boat. A paddler who can confidently right his boat in erratically surging waves can avoid most of the hazards of wildwater. It is a technique to be learned early and strengthened with practice. An emergency roll is seldom needed by the expert because as he practices rolling, he develops the bracing finesse to avoid unexpected flips.

The bracing strokes are not only for uprighting the boat but are also used to maneuver. Reaching a brace stroke out into slower moving eddy water will serve as a sea anchor to spin the boat out of the current and upstream into the shelter of the eddy. Leaving the eddy can be accomplished by driving the boat upstream back into the current and then leaning on a brace in the side current to swing the bow downstream. These eddy-hopping techniques are the way a paddler can rest and survey what lies ahead in the rapids.

The final basic wildwater technique is ferrying. This is a method of crossing a moving current without being swept downstream. It is a practical lesson in vectors. The summation of paddling upstream at an angle and the force of the rushing water moves the boat across the current from one side eddy to the other.

Techniques beyond these basic ones are best learned by example and with experience. Several good river-paddling technique books are available. They contain more details on these basics with helpful diagrams and illustrations. Teaching films are also available. Many canoeing clubs have white-water paddling clinics each year.

Cruising

White water paddling opportunities are available wherever there are hills and precipitation. The sport is most popular in the middle-Atlantic states. In that area there is a combination of an adequate population, adequate rainfall, mountains, and a short winter season. Good water but a shorter season is to be had in New England and New York. Excellent white water is found in the region of the Great Smoky Mountains. Northern Wisconsin and Minnesota have some white-water streams with limited gradient. Spring-fed streams flow from the Ozarks. Excellent white water which is as yet largely unused abounds in the Rocky Mountain and Pacific Coast states. Northern Ontario has a short but worthy white-water season.

There are 47 canoe clubs in the country which are associated as the American White Water Affiliation. The distribution of clubs relates to population as well as proximity of mountains. The best paddlers in the world come from central Europe. Undoubtedly there are wildwater streams within one day's travel of most of the world's population.

Wildwater seldom freezes over in most of the United States. Flood control, hydroelectric, and augmented flow dams extend adequate river levels through dry seasons. Spring thaws raise the levels in mountain rivers which are otherwise trickles. Mountains are conducive to rainfall and rapid runoff into the streams that arise in them. Thus with modern mobility and some informed planning the wildwater paddler enjoys a perennial sport.

Planning a specific trip can initially be done through wildwater clubs. These organizations generally have a series of scheduled cruises on regional rivers led by capable, instructive paddlers. A trip with such a group insures the beginner against catastrophe. He can be assured his equipment and skill are appropriate for the difficulty of the trip.

Subsequently the paddler and his associates may plan their own trips with the aid of regional guidebooks. Very good books are available for most of the Appalachians. Most paddling organizations compile files of trip reports on regional rivers.

For the advanced paddler one of the more exciting aspects of wildwater paddling is exploring unknown rivers. Obviously in the twentieth century these rivers are not unexplored. People live along them, fishermen wade them, children swim in the pools, bridges cross them, railraods parallel them, the effluent of villages is carried away and purified in them, but from the paddler's viewpoint, they are unexplored and/or unrecorded. Within a few miles of the road head, the Eastern paddler can be in wilderness comparable to that of the eighteenth century. He sees the area as it has never been seen. In a few hours he can travel forested mountains which would take days to penetrate on foot. He can travel with safety along a stream that has previously only been crossed at selected spots. Here is a last glimpse at an unspoiled world just a few hours from home.

For these exploratory trips the most valuable guides are United States Geological Survey topographic maps. These maps can be ordered through Washington, D.C., or state geologic survey offices at a very minimal cost. Since many of the more primitive and thus more interesting areas have not been remapped since the early part of this century, the maps must often be supplemented by county department of highway maps.

The logistics of a wildwater cruise involve going from point A to point B downstream 5 to 20 miles. It is then necessary to get boats and road vehicles together again. This is most readily accomplished by having all cars, boats, and paddlers meet at the start or put-in point, unload their car-top transported boats and drive to the end or take-out point. The drivers are then returned to the put-in by one car to start the trip. When the trip is completed all paddlers can head for home or camp except for the two drivers necessary to return for the car at the put-in.

With regard to camping, canoe camping in the manner of the Canadian wilderness camper is not appropriate for white-water boaters. The attrition rate on equipment is too great with occasional upsets, and the capacity of the boats is too limited. It is more satisfactory to plan trips so that camping can be done from one's vehicle each night. On some Western and Canadian rivers the roads may be too infrequent to permit this. Large volume cruising boats, elimination of flotation bags, and light weight camping equipment are then necessary or else support of a slower moving rafting party.

Cruising on wildwater has many facets. The appeal which it holds will vary with the individual and will vary for the individual on different trips. The appeal may be a desire to escape the rigidity of civilization and return to the simple solitude of the wilderness. The appeal may be the camaraderie of a group with a common mission. It may be the companionship that may arise from having together faced and subdued a common adversary—the unknown force of the river, the transient loss of the security of society, personal fear. The appeal may be a need to take a calculated risk, as society works hard to legislate away all risks. The appeal of wildwater may be a need to test oneself against a dragon. The appeal may be just the animal joy of frolicking.

The latter is an important part of wildwater cruising. One does not simply ride down the river. That soon becomes too simple unless one progressively seeks out more and more dangerous rivers. The end point of seeking progressively more dangerous waters to float is Niagara in a barrel. This is the course of the suicidal daredevil. A more reasonable avenue for the developing paddler is to test his skill against moderate streams by playing them. He may eddy hop his way up and down them. He may ferry from side to side across vigorous chutes of water. He may surf on the upstream side of a haystack wave balancing the force of gravity against the current. He may stand still in rushing water by locking his boat into a roller wave and keeping it upright. He may drive his boat end over end. All these playing techniques develop the paddler's skill while simultaneously awarding him physical and psychological pleasure for his efforts.

Racing

Most paddlers will be cruisers satisfied to challenge the river with their paddling skill. The more competitive will be attracted by racing. White-water racing is of two sorts, downriver and slalom. The former is hellbent for fiberglass for five miles, with the paddlers started at one-minute intervals and running against time over rapids which are only moderately difficult for the skill of the racers. The slalom event is run over a quarter-mile rapid of moderate difficulty with downstream, upstream and reverse gates directing the racer over the most challenging portions of the rapids (Fig. 22–3). The paddler races against time but is penalized for not running the gates precisely. Slalom racing started in the United States in 1953 and is growing rapidly until there are now races in each section of the country almost every weekend. Since 1959 the United States has sent a team to Europe biannually for international competition, and in 1972 white-water slalom is being added to the Olympics. Currently white-water racing involves a small club, and one can easily know and paddle with the champions. This is one of the appeals of this sport.

Surfing

Another locale for wildwater boats and techniques which is only beginning to be utilized is the beach. Outrigger canoe surfing developed in parallel with board surfing in Hawaii, but it was not exported to the mainland. Now with the variant of eliminating the outrigger and using single-man boats, boat surfing has been revived. The advocates of this activity cite a number of advantages which it has over board surfing. It is easier to get out through the surf and easier to catch a wave because of paddle power. Smaller waves can be utilized. This is particularly an advantage on the East coast where a lack of good surf has retarded the development of surfing. With a wipe-out, the surf-kayaker is more likely to stay with his craft eliminating the possibility that he will be clobbered.

The author has had minimal experience surfing in small to moderate Atlantic surf. The experience of sliding downhill across the leading surface of a wave is exhilarating. The experience of sliding too rapidly and pearling the bow into the water at the bottom of the wave as it breaks over the stern is initially horrifying, but it turns out to be a simple end-over-end flip with an easy roll-up after the wave moves on. The experience of having the wave collapse on the boat as it is surfing sideways is handled by leaning seaward and bracing into the foam as the boat washes sideways up the beach. This is much easier than the shallow-water wipe-out from a board. The ideal seems to be to catch the wave and surf diagonally across its face away from where it is breaking, and at the last second draw seaward over the crest letting it break beachside, then turn and paddle out for the next big wave.

Competitive kayak-surfing events and especially designed surfing kayaks are being introduced in California and New England but are unfamiliar to the author.

SAFETY

The uninitiated person has an exaggereated concept of the dangers involved in wildwater. Each year there are reports of drownings on free-flowing rivers. There is no doubt that the novice is in great danger in this sport if his ill-advised enthusiasm cannot be tempered by persons with more experience. Virtually all drownings related to whitewater can be attributed to a failure to heed at least two of four following cardinal taboos of the sport: (a) paddling in water beyond one's experience; (b) paddling in very cold water without protection; (c) failing to wear a life preserver and helmet; and (d) paddling alone. To my knowledge there have been no drownings involving experienced organized white-water paddlers.

Injuries are frequent but minor until the paddler learns to keep his boat upright or to roll it up. Injuries usually consist of bruised shins and hips from banging over rocks. Injuries are minor because the body is buoyed up to weightlessness by the water, most rocks are eroded smooth and rounded, and each is cushioned with a layer of rushing water. Almost entirely lacking are the broken bones and sprained ankles that skiers take for granted.

FUTURE

Wildwater paddling is now on the threshold of a boom. It is at a state comparable to that of skiing at the end of World War II. It is a bittersweet prospect to see the sport growing with the fear that soon the rapids will be as overrun with paddlers as the slopes are with skiers. One shudders at the thought of canoe resorts, queuing-up for lifts at the bottom of the best runs, awaiting turns to run the rapids, and dressing in an appropriately stylish manner for an aprés-canoe cocktail hour.

On the positive side, wildwater paddling is an exciting, satisfying pastime which allows persons to spread out into the unused wilderness for recreation without doing ecologic damage. No roads need to be cut, no internal combustion fumes or noises are emitted, no tire tracks tear up the forest floor, no wildlife is killed, no dams need to be built to flood the valleys, no garbage is left for lack of a way to carry it out. The wilderness is seen and enjoyed by the paddler and the only damages left behind are a few fiberglass boat scrapings on the surface rocks.

REFERENCES

1. *American White Water,* Quarterly Journal of the American White Water Affiliation, Box 1584, San Bruno, California.
2. Evans, R. J.: *Fundamentals of Kayaking.* Hanover, New Hampshire, Ledyard Canoe Club, Dartmouth College, $3.00.
3. McNair, R. E.: *Basic River Canoeing,* Martinsville, Indiana, American Camping Association Inc., 1969, $1.50.
4. Urban, J. T.: *A White Water Handbook for Canoe and Kayak,* Boston, Massachusetts, Appalachian Mountain Club, 1965, $1.50.
5. Whitney, P. D.: *White Water Sport.* New York, Ronald Press, 1960, $4.50.

23

SOARING

WYLIE H. MULLEN, JR.

Undoubtedly, even the great Aesculapius on his Wednesday afternoon off watched with fascination, as has man long before and since, the beauty of birds in soaring flight. These graceful creatures, maneuvering in the invisible ocean of air around us, have intrigued all mankind and inspired many, including legendary Icarus, to attempt to emulate their flight. Icarus undoubtedly had the answer, became so enthralled with the ecstasy of soaring that he climbed up and up, finally flying so close to the sun that his wings of wax and feathers disintegrated. It was not until the great Otto Lillienthal flew in the first glider that man actually recorded free flight. Unfortunately, intrepid birdman that he was, Lillienthal in several hundred flights, never experienced the exhilaration of soaring. He was solely a glider pilot; and although he flew, it was only earthward toward the valley from his hilltop launches. In the early part of the twentieth century, in Germany, man first sustained soaring flight and actually gained altitude above his release point. Since that time, the sport and art of soaring has become a refined and well understood diversion for thousands of avid pilots and pilot physicians.

Today's soaring pilot, like Lillienthal, is constantly gliding downward in the mass of air in which he flies. It is only with his skill and the use of sensitive instruments that he is able to seek and circle in masses of air, which are rising at a greater rate than the sink-rate of his sailplane. Most soaring flights utilize rising air created by the uneven heating of the earth's surface. The dark, dry areas absorb more heat than do the light or wet areas. This absorbed heat warms the adjacent air

290

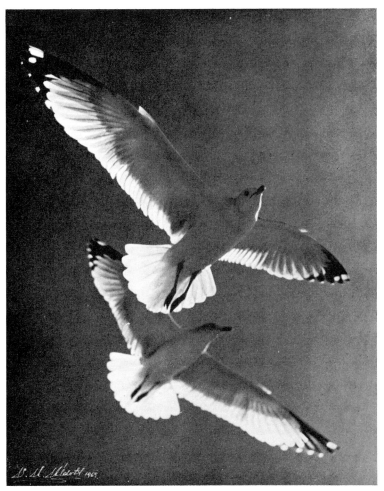

Figure 23–1. Soaring seagulls, California coast. Photo by Sandor Alcott.

to a state of expansive buoyancy, so that it rises upward in great columns and bubbles from the heated ground to form "thermals." Thermals can visually be identified by even the nonpilot as barnyard whirlwinds or as giant dust devils in the arid southwest. If conditions are right, and the air contains sufficient moisture, the top of the thermal will be marked with a beautiful white fair-weather cumulus cloud. They can be felt as the fresh, sudden, welcome breezes on a hot, summer day, as cooler air rushes in on all sides to replace the rising thermal. They are also marked by an assortment of floating debris, as well as hawks, eagles, and other species of soaring birds. A less attractice characteristic is that occasionally one produces an identifiable smell, if it truly arises from a heated barnyard.

Other types of lift are also used in soaring, both by birds and man, and include the upward movement of air over a ridge when a strong wind is blowing at right angles. This is known as ridge-lift; and as long as one has a ridge and the wind is of sufficient velocity, he can soar to his heart's content, even for several days and nights. This same type of lift is what soaring birds use along the seacoast.

The third powerful source of lift is the mountain wave. This develops on the leeside of a mountain, when the wind direction, velocity, and air mass present favorable conditions. Its presence is marked by a beautiful alto-lenticular cloud. This very high lens-shaped cloud is fascinating because even though the winds at cloud altitude are usually moving at over one hundred miles per hour, the cloud stands still! This is because it is being constantly formed on its leading edge as the wave carries the air sufficiently high for the temperature and dew point to come together and produce visible moisture, and is constantly disintegrating on the trailing edge where the wave is moving downward toward the ground, and as the temperature and dew point spread, the moisture again becomes invisible. This great source of lift has taken man to his highest soaring altitudes of over 46,000 feet. It is also one of the causes of CAT (clear air turbulence).

It's a great thrill just to be in a glider in nearly silent flight with only the whisper of air passing over its beautiful long flexing wings and graceful fuselage. But, it is even more of a thrill to find your first termal, circle tightly in steeply banked turns, and watch the altimeter show upward progress. You are soaring, soaring, above and away from the earthbound world—its problems, its cares, its telephones—and you are truly free.

I have been flying off and on for over thirty years; this experience includes flying with an airline transport rating, instructor's rating in all categories, and varied experience in

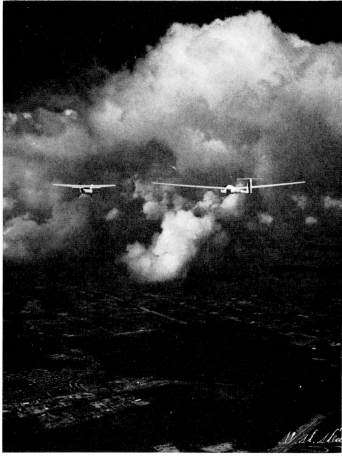

Figure 23–2. Standard Cirrus on tow, Odessa, Texas. Photo by Sandor Alcott.

multi- and single-engine seaplanes, helicopters and all varieties of land planes. This all became somewhat mundane and relatively uninteresting after my introduction to soaring some ten years ago. I became so stimulated that I avidly pursued the sport with such enthusiasm that within a month, I had a silver "C" badge; within six months, a gold "C" badge; and, in one year, became Illinois' first Diamond Soaring Pilot. This was some sort of record, and I was, of course, quite proud of these accomplishments at the time. Now, they seem insignificant af-

ter discovering the skill of others whom I have met in competitive soaring. During this period, I have met many other
physicians who have also been ensnared in this, the most interesting, challenging, and artistic type of flying. Indeed, soaring is to flying what sailing is to stinkpotting. Some of these
physicians are competitive pilots—others are content and
happy to spend three to four hours flying locally on a beautiful,
sunny day, detached and free of their medical worries.

Inevitably, as with all other types of vehicles, as soon as two
or more become available, somebody wants to find out which
is the better. Hence comes the competition with the gaggles
of beautiful white competing sailplanes and their eager, talented pilots. The contests are usually sponsored by the Soaring
Society of America and are delightful events, lasting over a
weekend, or in the case of the national and world championships, nearly two weeks. In addition to the flying, they offer a
camaraderie among the pilots and crews not found in many
other sports. The contests are never based on altitude or endurance, but instead, either on distance or speed over a prescribed course up to 300 miles in length. The distance tasks
can be one of two varieties: "free distance" in which the object is for every pilot to get as far as he can from the starting airport. It is usually called on days when the weather is
bad or uncertain, offering opportunity for great discretion and
individual choice of direction of flight. The second distance
task is within a prescribed area. There are multiple turn points,
and again the pilot has the choice of deciding between which
points he shall fly and photograph. The individual who goes
the greatest distance in either of these tasks is awarded one
thousand points, and the others are scored proportionately.
Speed tasks may be around a triangular course—an out and
return to a turnpoint, or a race to a goal. Again, the fastest
time wins one thousand points and the slower speeds are
scored proportionately. The pilots do not know the task until
the daily pilots' meeting when it is announced by the competition director. He and two or three other experienced soaring pilots have made their task selection, based on predicted
weather conditions, hoping its difficulty will permit approxi-

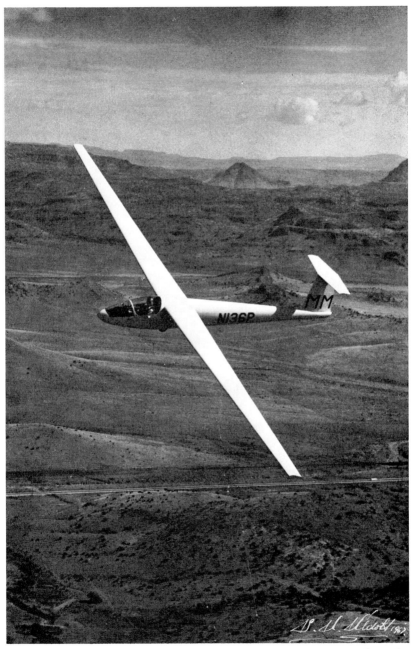

Figure 23–3. Author in PRUE UHP-1, over Marsa, Texas. Photo by
Sandor Alcott.

mately three-fourths of the pilots to complete it. In prescribed area distance, there have been many flights of over four hundred miles, even when some of the legs must be worked against cross and headwinds. On free distance days, there have been flights of over five hundred miles even though the weather was predicted to be poor. This is quite unusual since the world's distance record is only slightly over seven hundred miles. On the speed task, pilots, after their selected take-off times, soar locally until they feel conditions are right for the particular task. They are then timed through a starting gate and are off on course. If they are not making good progress, they may return for additional starts through the gate, or even reland and restart at no penalty. If an unusually short task is selected, pilots have the option of flying around the course twice and taking their best elapsed time. When the task is an out and return, or a triangle, they must make proper photographs of the turn points from a designated position over the point. These films are always processed and evaluated before the final scores are computed. The task ends with a final glide over the finish time, often with beautiful high speed dives, climbing turns, associated with white jets of trailing water vapor. The latter is the dumping of water ballast carried in many competition ships to give additional speed on strong days. This ballast may amount to more than two hundred pounds and can be jettisoned at any time. It lessens the rate of climb in thermals, but on strong days, this is more than compensated for the faster speeds one is able to fly between thermals at the same glide ratios.

The speeds accomplished are not tremendous compared to powered vehicles, and sixty miles per hour will win on all but exceptional days. These sailplanes can and do fly at time over 100 mph, but a great deal of time is spent, literally, in one spot making tight climbing circling turns in the best lift. The competitive soaring pilot is so busy that flights of eight to ten hours have been accomplished in what seems like only a few minutes. In addition to the mechanics of flying the glider, there is navigating, searching, and finding lift, evaluating its strength, centering it, and decisions, decisions, decisions, as to

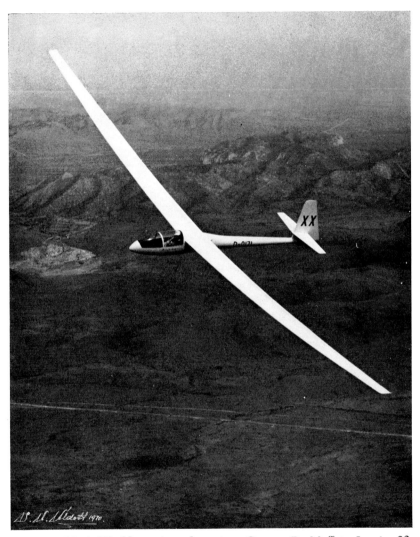

Figure 23–4. World soaring champion, George B. Moffat, Jr., in 22-meter super ship, Nimbus. Photo by Sandor Alcott.

which lift to work, how high, when, and which direction to depart, photography of turnpoints, and constant attention to the best speed to fly. One must constantly be evaluating weather conditions ahead, keeping track of the competition, and saving every possible second. The good competition pilots are learned meteorologists, and use this knowledge to good advantage in selection of takeoff and starting times, choice of course and evaluation of enroute conditions.

The sport is usually challenging and exciting, but at times it can be frustrating and disappointing. For example, you may be sitting in some farmer's soybean field or stubblefield, waiting for your crew to arrive, while above you your competitors can be seen climbing and flying onward to the finish line; the "cues" (cumulus clouds) are still popping and you pushed too hard, simply goofed, and fell out of the sky. The other challenging thing about competition is that you learn to fly on difficult days, weak days, when you must literally make hundreds of turns to gain a few hundred feet; or days when strong winds are blowing and forward progress is agonizingly slow. A cross-country flight under any conditions never ceases to be a thrill, and as soon as you cut the umbilical cord which holds you within gliding distance of your own base airport, the excitement rises—as you know you must take potluck on landing fields, and that if you should fall down and must realight, your chances of winning are slim. The availability of landing spots is, of course, variable, depending on your soaring locale. In the Midwest, adequate fields are ubiquitous and you do not need to look for a landing spot until you are below a thousand feet. In the formidable terrain of the great Southwest, other desert and mountain areas, a decision to pick out a field must be made at a greater altitude. I have landed in all sorts of fields, highways, baseball diamonds, parking lots, golf courses, and every imaginable type of cultivated field. You are usually a very welcome visitor and only occasionally does a glider pilot have to buy a few bushels of overpriced wheat, oats, or soybeans. I have been offered many a cold beer and even an occasional steak by charming farmer's daughters.

This brings us down to the most often asked question, "How safe is soaring"? This is as difficult to answer as "How safe is the kitchen knife or the medical X ray machine"? It depends upon how and by whom it is used. There have been accidents and deaths in sailplanes, almost entirely limited to the neophyte student pilot who has the same kind of accidents that beginning power pilots have, namely, too low, too slow and a stall-spin into

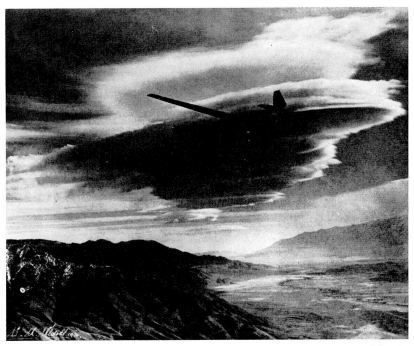

Figure 23–5. KA-7 soaring in mountain wave at Bishop, California. Note stacked altolenticular clouds in background. Photo by Sandor Alcott.

the ground. The incidence of accidents with injuries is extremely low in competent, cross-country and competitive soaring pilots who "keep it flying." In skilled hands, sailplanes are extremely safe because they continue to fly and land at very slow speeds and are designed to be easily maneuvered and stopped in extremely short distances. Competition pilots are more likely to prang their sailplane by a poor choice of fields on a delayed decision to land than they are to injure themselves. High performance single-place sailplanes usually have glide ratios in excess of forty to one. This means that at their best gliding speed, for each foot they lose in altitude, they move forward forty feet longitudinally. With a little bit of arithmetic, you can see that from an altitude of 5000 feet above the ground, the soaring pilot has a choice of landing fields anywhere within a circle of eighty miles diameter (under no wind conditions). Furthermore, his sailplane is equipped with descent controlling devices, such as flaps, spoilers, or dive brakes. With these, he can increase his rate of descent to as small a glide angle as ten to one. It is, therefore, quite simple to maneuver for a landing spot using approximately half spoilers or dive brakes. If he is still too high for the field, he pulls them out the rest of the way and descends more steeply; if he appears a little short and low, he retracts them and it is just like adding throttle—and they are always available—while the power pilot has to worry about whether one or both engines will keep running. Additionally, most sailplanes stall (and hence, land) as slow as 40 mph, and, thus, if one lands into a wind of even 10 mph, he makes ground contact at only 30 mph. All soaring pilots have and wear both seat belts and shoulder harnesses. If a mishap should occur, there is nothing to burn since no gasoline or hot engine is present to compound the accident with fire. A sailplane is equipped with a wheel brake for quick stopping, and when only extremely short or rough fields are available, can be landed on the belly with little damage. The problem is not landing; the problem is staying up! There have been fatalities related to competitive soaring, but they have occurred in the automobiles of the pilots and crews driving to and from the meets, and following the gliders around the task course, rather than in the glider.

A good crew is essential to competitive soaring for many reasons. If you fall down early and they are nearby on radio contact, they can retrieve you soon enough for a second start on the task without penalty. All sailplanes have detachable wings and usually in a matter of minutes can be disarticulated at the wing-roots, placed into a long, specially-built trailer, and back on their way for another day. Wives make excellent crew chiefs, not because they are necessarily eager, but mainly because they are readily available and inexpensive. Do not get her too interested in soaring—she might be better than you and displace the good doctor to the position of driving down the dusty road in hot pursuit of the graceful white bird.

The next most frequently asked question is, "How much does it cost"? It can be very inexpensive to the member of the fifty-man club that jointly owns a tow plane and one or more sailplanes. It can be quite expensive to the competition pilot who

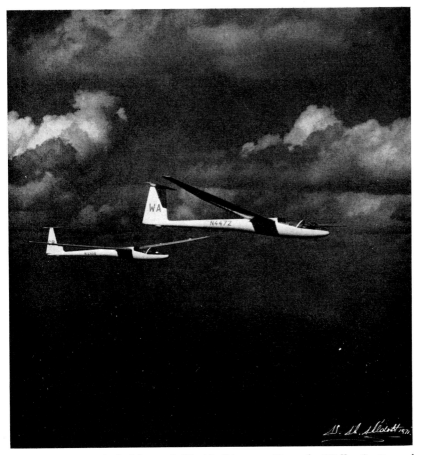

Figure 23–6. Co-holders of World Distance Record, Wally Scott and Ben Greene in ASW-12, leaving Odessa, Texas. Photo by Sandor Alcott.

owns a $15,000 well-equipped fiberglass ship and who insists on charging all over the country to enter every competition. Learning to fly will be the first expense, and this, too, is variable. There are several commerical operators in the United States who give complete instruction, including ground school and the final rating rides in sailplanes. Some of the glider clubs around the country also give instruction to new members. Names of these commercial operators and clubs can be obtained from the Soaring Society of America or from the advertisements in *Soaring Magazine*. Today, most towing is done with small aircraft and a relatively short tow rope; however, some operations use power-driven winches and, occasionally, auto tows with much longer ropes or cables. With the latter two types of tows, there often is some savings in training costs. It is usually cheaper to learn how to fly a power plane first and then make the transition into gliders, since power plane training requires only an instructor and an airplane. Sailplane instruction requires a tow plane and a tow pilot, instructor, and a two-place sailplane. A skilled power pilot can usually make this transition within a few flights because most gliders have straightforward aerodynamic characteristics, are quite easy and simple to fly, are effortless on the controls, and are unbelievably maneuverable. The problem and the challenge is not to fly it or land it, it is to stay up and to go somewhere, in incomparable soaring flight with the condors and the eagles.

24

BALLOONING

WILLIAM C. GRABB

Modern hot-air ballooning began in the early 1960's when a
nylon envelope and a propane-fueled source of heat were
combined to produce a reliable thermal balloon. During the
late 1950's, Paul E. Yost and his co-workers at Raven Industries
in Minneapolis worked on this project under a Navy contract
for the purpose of providing a rugged, reusable balloon to be
used for balloon pilot training and low altitude research. As an
offspring of this work, the hot-air sport balloon was developed,
so that there are now approximately 100 of these aerostats in
the United States.

There are two types of balloons—the hot-air and the gas
balloon. Hot-air balloons are most common in North America,
while the venerable gas balloons are most common in Europe,
there being between 70 and 80 of them, mostly in West Germany
and Switzerland. Hot-air balloons are much larger due to the
fact that hot air heated to 100 C above ambient temperature
will lift 21 pounds per 1000 cubic feet, while hydrogen will lift
70 pounds per 1000 cubic feet. Hot-air balloons typically vary
from 30,000 to 60,000 cubic feet, carrying one to three passengers
and costing four to eight dollars for propane fuel during a
typical two-hour flight. Gas balloons require about $400 of
hydrogen for a three to six hour flight, although cheaper cooking
gas which has less lift, or much more expensive but nonflam-
mable helium can also be used as the lighter-than-air gas (Fig.
24–1).

Man first conquered the air in a hot-air balloon. A wave of

Dr. Grabb is Clinical Associate Professor of Surgery (Plastic Surgery) at the
University of Michigan School of Medicine. He is currently the President of the
Balloon Federation of America.

303

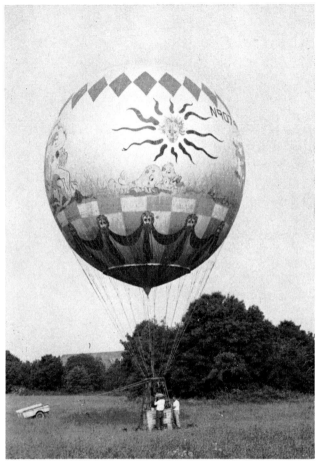

Figure 24–1. The gas balloon "La Coquette" is familiar to millions, following its appearance in the movie *Around the World in 80 Days*. The rubberized fabric of the envelope encloses 19,000 cubic feet of hydrogen. This former World War II Navy balloon is still flying in the Philadelphia area.

excitement spread throughout the world following the ascension of the Montgolfier brothers' linen-and-paper straw smoke-filled balloon from Paris on November 21, 1783. Two men flying in this aerostat for thirty minutes created a sensation throughout the world that probably surpassed the present-day rocket-powered flights to the moon. About a year later in 1784, the hydrogen gas balloon was designed by Professor J.A.C. Charles and successfully flown by him. There are many books written about the history of ballooning during the ensuing years, especially during the heyday of gas ballooning which began to wane after the invention of the airplane in 1903. But there is little written about present-day ballooning; in fact, there are no books available on the subject.

FLYING A HOT AIR BALLOON

Most hot air ballooning is done in the hour or two after sunrise or in the hour or two before sunset, when the winds are most likely to be under the maximum of 10 mph and there are no thermals. High wind and ballooning are not compatible, due to the difficulties of inflating the struggling monster when the wind wants to carry it away like a spinnaker sail.

The balloon envelope is pulled out of its bag and rolled out on the grass with the mouth of the balloon facing into the wind. The steel support cables from the envelope are attached to the gondola and the balloon is ready to inflate.

I use a gasoline motor-powered fan to force air into the mouth of the envelope which is held open, although the same thing can be done by vigorously flapping the envelope at the mouth to trap a large bubble of air inside (Fig. 24–2). With leather gloves on, the burner jet pilot light is ignited. Then pointing the cylindrical burner into the eight-foot diameter mouth of the balloon, a steady blast of burning propane rapidly heats the air, so that the baloon envelope lifts into the upright position in one or two minutes. The heat and the noise are considerable. The three-foot-long flame of my one-man balloon produces 2,400,000 BTU/h, burning propane near its maximum of 1900 degrees C. Once the balloon is aloft, the burner must continue to replace the heat lost by conduction at a rate of about 700,000 BTU/h. This is roughly the rate at which a furnace burns to heat a six-story apartment house.

With the envelope in the upright position, another two or three minutes are required to heat the air sufficiently to provide

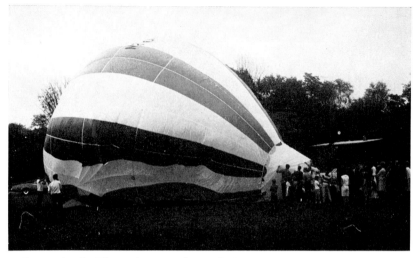

Figure 24–2. The nylon envelope of the hot air balloon is filled with air by a fan directed into the eight-foot diameter open mouth.

the life necessary to carry aloft 450 pounds of envelope, gondola, fuel, and a passenger (Fig. 24–3).

I usually fly at 1000 to 2000 feet above the ground, though I have gone to the 10,000 feet maximum allowed for pilots not using an oxygen inhalation system.

It is exhilarating to be free of the earth and float majestically through the sky propelled by the whims of the wind, then to come down to treetop level and float across the panorama of the countryside as it unfolds before you. I thought I would tire of this sport after a year or two, but just the opposite has happened. Each flight brings back the freedom and joy of my first ride in an aerostat.

The balloon can be controlled in its up and down flight by turning the burner flame up or down. A maneuvering vent on the side of the envelope can be pulled open and closed with a rope to release hot air and accelerate the descent. With a ton and a half of hot air aboard, the main skill involved is to keep the inertia of rapid up and down flight from getting out of hand. A variometer, as used on soaring planes, is of considerable help in assisting the pilot to keep ascent and descent within

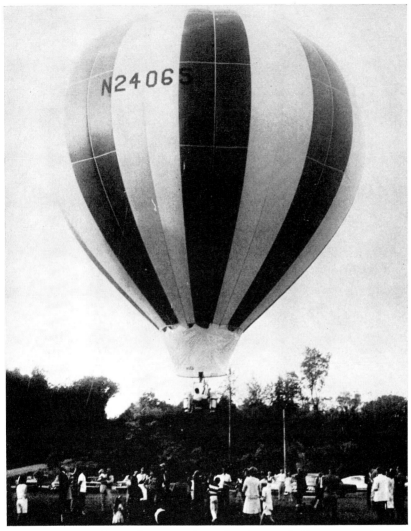

Figure 24–3. The author ascends in his Raven S-40 one-man hot air balloon. There are usually a great many volunteer ground crew members.

2 to 4 ft/sec. An altimeter, a pyrometer, and a fuel indicator complete the instrumentation.

After one and a half or two hours, when I am ready to land, I start looking ten or fifteen minutes ahead of time for an open field which does not have a farmer's cash crop growing in it or a bull grazing there. The balloon can then be gradually let down (1 to 4 ft/sec) in the same trajectory as in the landing of a fixed-wing aircraft—except that the stop is more sudden. A few feet above the ground, the burner is turned off to avoid burning the nylon. The pull out deflation port at the crown of the balloon is then peeled open by a vigorous pull on the red deflation cord. The hot air pours out of the top of the envelope and you have landed. It all happens in 30 seconds.

Returning home requires the assistance of my wife, who follows in the car. The envelope is rolled into its bag. The gondola is put on the trailer and we are on our way.

BALLOON PILOT'S LICENSE

The Federal Aeronautic Association requires that persons who operate lighter-than-air free balloons be certified by the association. To obtain a balloon pilot's license, the basic requirements are to make eight training flights, each of one hour's duration (6 flights with an instructor, one solo flight, and one flight to 5000 feet), pass a written examination, and obtain a second-class medical certificate.

Four detailed manuals on hot-air ballooning (*Introduction to Club Ballooning, Commercial Pilot Training Manual, Commercial Balloon Pilot Flight Curriculum,* and *Commercial Balloon Pilot Examination Guide*) can be obtained for $10 each from the LERC Wind Drifters Balloon Club, 2814 Empire Avenue, Burbank, California 91503.

BALLOON MANUFACTURERS

The two largest manufacturers of these $3000 to $6000 hot-air balloons are Raven Industries, P.O. Box 916, Sioux Falls, South Dakota 57101, and Don Piccard Balloons, 427 Fullerton Avenue, Newport Beach, California 92660.

FURTHER INFORMATION

The Balloon Federation of America, a division of the National Aeronautics Association, was formed to promote, develop, and

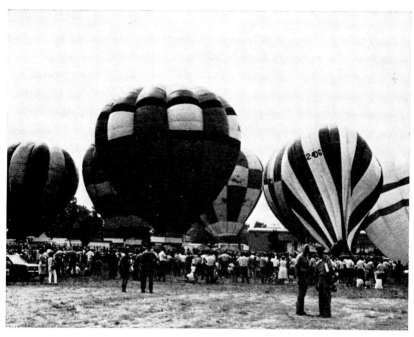

Figure 24–4. Several hot-air aerostats prepare to take off in the 1970 Columbus International Hot Air Balloon Race.

aid the art and science of ballooning in the United States. A quarterly journal, *Ballooning*, is published by the Balloon Federation, which is the best up-to-date source on hot-air balloon races, rallies, and other information of value to the balloonist (Fig. 24–4. The $10 dues for annual membership in the BFA include a subscription to *Ballooning*. Application for membership (both pilots and nonpilots) should be directed to The Balloon Federation of America, Suite 610, 806 15th Street, N.W., Washington, D.C. 20005.

25

PHYSICIAN, FLY THYSELF

DONALD B. FRANKEL

A pilot has his recompense
For who in the world but such as we,
May climb the sky to God's own knee
And ponder his wondrous artistry.

Gill Robb Wilson

The trouble with the first man who tried to fly was that he did not have enough information. His name was Icarus and when the wax and feathers melted, down he went.

My purpose in this chapter is to give you enough information to tempt you into your first lesson, to show you that any doctor with average mental and physical equipment, no matter how shopworn, can learn to fly.

Richard Collins, the editor of the magazine *Air Facts*, named the private plane the "time machine." No matter where you live, within a few hours you can be hundreds of miles away with a minimum of effort and more safety than if you used a car.

The first question anyone asks is "Is it safe?" Figure 25-1 lists 1968 and 1969 fatalities in transportation accidents. Statistics show that private and business aviation is safer than walking. Mile for mile, hour for hour, flying is safer than being in a car or boat as driver or passenger.

Year after year general aviation carries more people more hours than do domestic airlines. Federal government statistics show that in 1969 only 2 percent of the total airplane fleet was airline and commercial aviation. The other 98 percent (more than 133,000 planes) were owned and flown by general aviation. Of the 10 busiest airports in the United States (and in the world), moreover, six made the list because more than 90

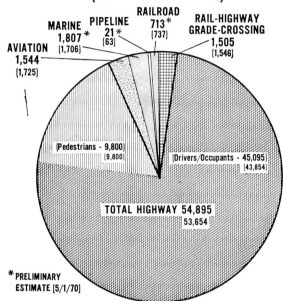

60,485 FATALITIES
IN
TRANSPORTATION ACCIDENTS
1969
(1968 IN PARENTHESES)

MARINE PIPELINE   RAILROAD   RAIL-HIGHWAY
1,807*   21*   713*   GRADE-CROSSING
         (63)   (737)   1,505
AVIATION (1,706)   (1,546)
1,544
(1,725)

(Pedestrians - 9,800)
(9,800)
(Drivers/Occupants - 45,095)
(43,854)

TOTAL HIGHWAY 54,895
53,654

*PRELIMINARY
ESTIMATE (5/1/70)

NATIONAL TRANSPORTATION SAFETY BOARD

Figure 25–1.

percent of the takeoffs and landings were made by general aviation.

OPERATIONS AT TEN BUSIEST AIRPORTS WITH TOWERS

Airport	Total	Airline	General Aviation	
Chicago O'Hare	676,473	632,030	41,111	(6 %)
Los Angeles	613,938	443,236	161,083	(26%)
Long Beach (California)	550,867	13,019	524,555	(95%)
Santa Ana (California)	545,299	18,443	525,727	(94%)
Ft. Lauderdale (Florida)	532,416	51,666	475,965	(89%)
Opa Locka (Florida)	526,402	46	516,009	(99%)
Van Nuys (California)	526,230	2,123	519,563	(98%)
Tamiami (Florida)	502,716	0	499,899	(99%)
J.F. Kennedy (New York)	436,298	376,404	59,452	(13%)
Atlanta	432,110	361,287	69,361	(16%)

Difference between airline and general aviation and total is military.

There are two aspects in learning to fly. First, the actual mechanical handling of the airplane and second, the theory. To learn to fly an airplane, you must learn with an instructor; learn to take off, land, fly straight and level, make turns, handle yourself in forced landings and in other emergencies. In short, you learn every procedure for the actual mechanical handling of the airplane itself.

The theory covers flight planning, navigation, a study of weather and meteorology, flight rules, federal aviation regulations, the use of a circular hand computer and many other things. The basic knowledge and skills necessary for safe flying are easy to learn and are fascinating to play with. For a doctor to become more knowledgable about meteorology and the air we live in, to know how mountains, trees, paved roads and the like affect the environment which we breathe and walk through, is a thrill that adds zest and facts to his storehouse of knowledge. To be able to chart a course, like the sea captain of old, through a medium where there are no roads, stop signs, stop lights or policemen, and arrive safely at your destination, is satisfaction as far from the humdrum as one can go.

Step one is to take a physical. There are many physicians in every specialty and general medicine who are licensed aviation medical examiners. All of these men are interested in flying and their findings will determine your ability to fly. The physical is neither difficult nor time-consuming. It is necessary to know that you can hear the radios or an instructor, that you are able to see the ground and distinguish colors, and that you have no diseases which might impair your ability to fly. Our country would be a safer place if everyone took the same physical before they were allowed to drive. The doctor who does the physical for the prospective pilot issues him not only his medical certificate but his student's pilot license as well. With this in hand, you can fly for two years, at which time you must take another physical.

Step two would be to contact the organization known as the Flying Physicians Association. This organization is comprised of 2500 flying M.D.'s from every corner of the Union and from every specialty. They will be of inestimable value. Any member

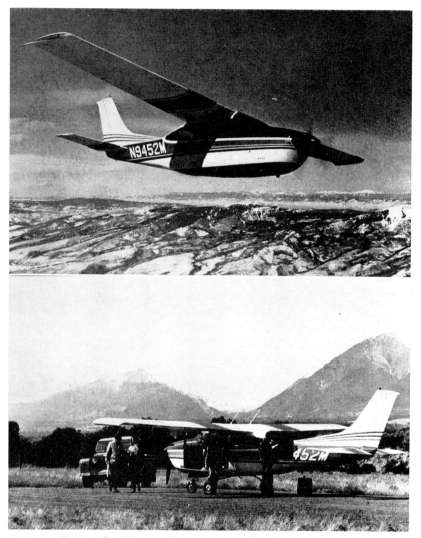

Figure 25–2. The doctor who learns to fly adds a new dimension to his life . . . one which the entire family can enjoy.

would be pleased to help another physician who wants to fly.

Next step is the airport. Here a flight school will take you in hand. You will be assigned an instructor, who will teach you the mechanics of flying a plane. During your first lesson, you will sit in the airplane, while the instructor patiently explains the use of rudders, ailerons, throttle, mixture controls and so forth. Your Boy Scout memories will be evoked, as you once again learn the compass and how to tell not only North from South but your right hand from your left. Levity not withstanding, physicians learn more quickly than the average person and retain it better, therefore making better pilots.

There are many connotations for the simple word "airport." In the Chicago area, more pilots think of O'Hare or Midway, or perhaps a military field like Glenview Naval Air Station. It would surprise many to know that the greater Chicago area has over 38 public airports plus about 35 private airports. Add the big ones and you can find a total over 75. A small airport like Sky Harbor in a near north suburb of Chicago has had as many as 1200 plane movements on a busy day, and this is a very small airport. Therefore, you can see there is no need to worry about competing with jets or large prop planes. You will learn at a place suited to your level of flying.

When you are somewhat familiar with the cockpit, you will taxi to the end of the runway. You will then take off (while the instructor's hands and feet follow you on the controls). He will not allow you to get into any difficulty or trouble, since any bad situation that you may become involved in would also involve him and he is certainly not anxious for that to occur. As the plane climbs out of the traffic pattern, the instructor will direct you to the practice area where you will learn to make turns, then a long slow lazy turn back to the airport, reenter the pattern and land. The main thing the instructor will teach you is to have control of the airplane at all times. You must also have control of yourself, always; thus, if you learn all the mechanical and theoretical aspects you will be an excellent and safe pilot.

The main thing you learn when you fly is discipline. You must be a precise pilot and live by the rules. In other words, a mature approach to flying will make you a good pilot as well as a safe one.

Practice, practice and more practice. While all this mechanical learning is progressing by the day—or week—you are learning theory at night. Why does a plane fly? What are thrust and drag? Why does it climb or descend? Why must elevators and ailerons be coordinated, and why throttle changes are made? The theory of flight is a fascinating journey through old and newly acquired facts that will entrance you as each new concept is grasped.

One day, as you come in and land for the umpteenth time, the instructor opens the door and gets out. You know—yes, as your autonomic system goes wild, you know—today you solo! "But am I ready?" is the usual cry, or "But I'm not ready!" But you are, and have been for the past two flying hours. No instructor believes in rushing the student into solo flight. He holds off until he is confident that the student can handle the plane in any emergency and especially in conditions prevailing that day.

And so you taxi out *alone*, and do all the things you were trained to do, *alone*, and suddenly you are airborne—*alone*. There is no comparable sensation to that of your first solo flight. You are master of your ship, master of the sky, master of yourself, and the immense satisfaction is exceeded only by the fantastic thrill of flying alone.

I do not think there is a thrill in the world, including the memorable words of your wedding, or the words of the Dean bestowing upon you your medical degree, that can compare to the feeling of the plane leaping skyward with you at the controls and in the airplane for the first time—alone.

> The fun of it! Oh, the fun of it!
> The soul-cleansing, mind-clearing fun of it!
> You have broken away from the spider web below
> The river is naught but a silver thread
> Caught in the needle eye of a moonbeam
> The winking lights of earth
> Are as the flittering of fireflies.
> In the meadows of your youth.
> You are free, free, free!
>
> Gill Robb Wilson

After solo, you go back for more practice. You learn how to use various radios to navigate and communicate, to file flight plans, to read air maps and a host of other things. It will become second nature to call "radar," when you want to keep free of other traffic in a congested area. But how anyone can complain

316 Games Doctors Play

of a "crowded sky" after driving home on a city expressway is beyond my comprehension.

There is still much to learn. One learns radio procedures and how to talk to a tower, how to call Center or Air Traffic Control. You will become familiar with all the cockpit instruments, which appear complicated and complex, but in reality, are very simple.

There are really only four fundamentals. All other maneuvers and procedures are variations of these. They are in turn, the normal climb, the normal glide, and flying straight and level. Once you master these and are able to correlate them with the various procedures, you have mastered the art of flying.

The next big step is cross-country flying. This is the *raison d'etre* of flying, the travelling from place to place. Map reading and flight planning are reviewed and the flight is planned. Weather is checked with all possible sources. Then off on a dual cross-country flight with the instructor. If you are successful, the next step is a solo cross-country trip. These are repeated for longer and longer distances until your proficiency becomes a matter of course.

The ability to leave a point, perhaps a pencil dot on a map and then travel 600 to 900 miles without road signs to arrive at another pencil dot can cause emotions only the explorer or traveler of old experienced. To do this as a captain of your ship, responsible for all aboard, avoiding bad weather, chatting with the voices of more than helpful flight service stations or tower controllers will make you feel truly a man among men. When the Tower says, "Cleared to land," you guide your plane in with as much aplomb and a great deal more pride than an airline captain.

More practice and finally—the check ride. You preflight the plane, plan your flight cross country, execute your trip and run the whole gamut of maneuvers and emergency procedures. The only drawback is the presence at your side of the FAA inspector. This doughty representative of the Federal Aviation Administration just wants to make sure you really know the rules, the theory, and the mechanical processes of flight. He must be positive that you are a safe and sane pilot—if you are, you will get your private license and become a full-fledged pilot.

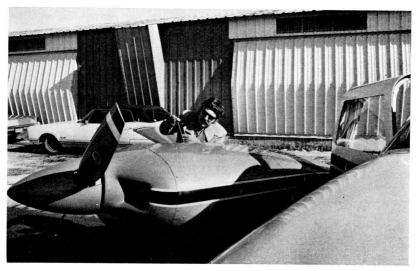

Figure 25–3. Checking the oil of each engine on twin Comanche 8788Y preparatory for the luncheon flight to northern Wisconsin.

But the inspector is really on your side and wants you to succeed. Since he will be in the air with you, he insists that you know what you are doing.

It is a balmy May morning when you awaken. As you lie in bed you review in your mind what has been done and is to be done. Your patients have all been arranged for: emergencies, chronics, etc. Grandma is ensconced in the guest bedroom to act as the weekend babysitter for your children. You earlier talked to the flight service station and aviation weather bureau and have been assured of a beautiful storm-free trip. You checked to see that the airport that you are using is open and in good order. The plane you have rented (or own) has been checked and is functioning perfectly. Tanks are topped and it is waiting on the flight line for your pleasure.

You and your wife drive to the airport and put your baggage in the back. This may include fishing gear, golf equipment, hunting equipment, any type of vacation equipment that you like. While your wife settles herself for the flight with the coffee thermos at hand, you carefully preflight the aircraft, checking propellor, wings, engines, wheels, gas tanks, controls etc. Around the plane you go, slowly checking each thing as you have been taught to do before any flight. The preflight check is in order; you climb into the plane, and you are a king.

The propellor is clear, the engine is turned over. The propellor starts to spin, you check your gauges professionally, turn on your radios and make a thorough check of the cockpit. You then call Ground Control on 121.9, and in your professional voice, impressing your wife with your calmness and ability, say "This is Cessna six-nine-one-zero Romeo ready for taxi and takeoff." Ground control directs you to the end of the active runway and while you are taxiing, keeping a lookout for planes and personnel, your wife (newly appointed navigator) is arranging the maps, computers, and pencils in proper order for the lord of the realm, the pilot. On arriving at the end of the runway the plane is checked; the engine is runup, both magnetos check, propellor check, carb heat check, final radio check, and again a complete cockpit check. The radio is then tuned to the tower frequency and you say, "Cessna one-zero Romeo ready for takeoff."

The Tower answers a United Airline pilot advising him which runway to use for landing and in the next breath says to you, "One-zero Romeo, taxi into position and hold." You obey this order and the plane sits poised and ready for your weekend adventure. Tower's calm voice says "one-zero Romeo cleared for takeoff." Feed the power in gradually and the plane accelerates down the runway and suddenly you are free. You have lifted off the ground and the plane begins to climb into the sparkling sunrise and the quiet air of the atmosphere which so few of us know.

You leave the airport pattern, turn your frequency to the flight service station, and notify them as to exact time you were off the ground. The station activates your flight plan. You next turn the aircraft to the proper heading and climb until the flight level of your plane has been reached. The plane is then trimmed, the mixture is leaned and the plane hums along toward your destination.

The maps are now put to use. Each checkpoint is marked off as you pass it. Between checkpoint 2 and 3 you have determined your speed over the ground; you can now much more accurately estimate the time of arrival. Straight as an arrow you follow the line of flight across the unmarked earth. Periodically, you check each flight service station within your range, identify your plane, tell them where you are and at what time, and request weather ahead. Other information such as turbulence, fast-moving cloud cover, storms, or unusual events will be reported to you far in advance so you can avoid trouble.

It is now three hours since you left and you are close to the six hundred mile destination, so you prepare for your descent. Check the map, check the cockpit and switch to approach control.

"Approach control this is Cessna six-nine-one-zero Romeo twenty-five miles out, estimate landing your airport in fifteen minutes."

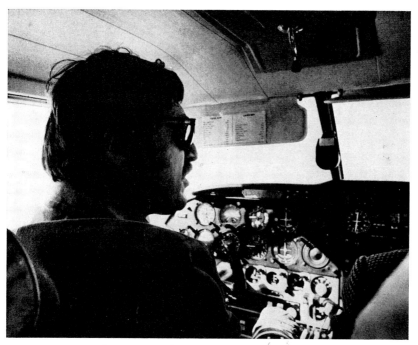

Figure 25–4. Flying over Chicago at 3500 feet at controls of twin Comanche 8788Y. Full instrument panel, ultrasophisticated navigation and communication avionics, autopilot, etc. This plane is equipped for all weather flying up to 24,000 feet.

"Continue present heading and descend to 2000 feet," replies Approach Control. "When you are ten miles out, call the Tower on 118.3"

You throttle back to descend gradually to the 2000 foot level. When you are ten miles out, you switch to the Tower and you say, "Tower, this is one-zero Romeo landing your airport." The Tower gives you the runway, the direction and strength of the winds, and the number of planes in the traffic pattern. The towers directs you to make a right or a left pattern or a straight-in approach. On a given day, the Tower will tell you to make a right base leg for runway 22, which means that as you come down the final approach to land on the runway your heading will be 220 degrees (or southwest).

When the airport is in sight, you make the turn into the right base leg, at a right angle to the runway on which you are going to land. You notify the Tower you are there, and Tower says, "One-zero Romeo cleared to land." You execute a right turn for the final approach, make a final cockpit check, all systems are in working order and you are prepared for your landing. As you come in over the airport boundary, the throttle is fully retarded, the plane is flared out and it settles to the earth as gently as a butterfly landing on a summer rose. You taxi to the gas pump at the transient area and shut down your engine.

It is not yet time for lunch and you have a full weekend of pleasure ahead of you and the most pleasant part of the weekend is still in the offing: the flight back.

This may sound like oversimplification, but it is not. As one becomes more and more familiar with the airplane, the navigation planning, the weather planning, the handling of the plane, the use of the radio and other facilities that are available, one does not become complacent. You become knowledgable and able to handle yourself in the air with a great deal of efficiency and aplomb. No matter how many years you fly or how many hours a year at least you will never be bored, because it is never the same.

There is no reason why you cannot learn to fly at night or day, to fly in bad weather or good weather, or to fly single engine or multi-engine. There is no limit to what you can learn or how high you can go. Some doctors who fly so-called "puddle-jumpers" make total trips away from the airport no more than one hundred miles. There are other doctors such as the two who flew the Lindbergh Trail in a single-engine Bonanza all the way around the world.

You may remain a private pilot or go all the way up to air transport and jet ratings if you like. Some even race planes such as the P-51. There are no limits other than those you set yourself. In flying there are always more goals if you wish to aspire to them.

You can even find out if you are going to like it before you get in too deeply. Both Cessna and Piper, manufacturers of general aviation airplanes for private use, offer a five-dollar demonstration ride. Any dealer at any airport will give you a ride with an instructor who will give you your first lesson for five dollars to determine if you are at all oriented to fly.

But, beware! Once you get up in the air and look around at a sky of blazing blue, not obscured with smoke and fumes that form the sullen opaque lid that seals us in most of the time, your whole way of life may change. You will begin to live for those hours when you are free of the bonds of the earth and in the air. As a pilot named McGee once said:

> I've topped the windswept heights with easy grace
> Where never lark, or even eagle flew;
> And while with silent lifting mind I've trod
> The high untrespassed sanctity of space,
> Put out my hand and touched the face of God.

There are almost as many variations in flying as there are reasons for flying. Some people love to build and fly antique airplanes, some restore World War II and even World War I planes and fly them. Other people fly for the peace and solitude, others fly because of the sense of accomplishment. With all of this there is one salient fact: the man that flys is responsible for his own destiny. The accident that could not have been avoided is just about nonexistent. Almost without exception accidents are due to a pilot who has made a bad judgment. There is no place in flying for an excuser, the second guesser, or the second-hander—this is the one place where *you* are master of your fate and king of all you survey.

It will be the most memorable, the most honest and the most thrilling, the most all-consuming thing that you have ever done and it can only be compared to other great accomplishments such as the ability to practice medicine.

To get started, write, call for, request or buy the following:

Invitation to Flying, H. Davis Publishing Company, One Park Avenue, New York, N.Y.   10016, 1969.

AOPA Washington, D.C.   20014   (Aircraft Owners and Pilots Assn)

Flying Physicians Association, 801 Green Bay Road Lake Bluff, Illinois   60044.

Federal Aviation Agency, Washington, D.C. and almost any other city.

Cessna Aircraft Company, Wichita, Kansas   67201.

Anyone Can Fly by Jules Bergman, Doubleday and Company.

Flights of Fancy and *I'd Rather by Flying* by Frank K. Smith, Random House.

Let's Go Flying by Martin Caidin, E.T. Dutton and Co.

Who, Me Fly? by Robert Schraff, Power Publications (paperback).

Student's Pilot Flight Manual by William K. Kersher, Iowa State University Press.

There are dozens of books on where to fly. Some tell of flying around Florida or island-hopping the Bahamas and the Caribbean. Books on where to fly and fish from Canada to Baja, California. Books by AOPA such as *Let's Fly,* and/or vacation and fly-in directories are also available. There are innumerable books on how to fly, where to fly, when to fly, and when not to fly. The important thing is first of all to try to fly.

People seem to think that flying is an expensive sport and only for the rich. If you are a moderately avid golfer, your expenses for less than one season would be more than adequate to cover the cost of obtaining a complete private license. Once this occurs, you may go as far as you like.

You could own a plane with one, two, three or four other people or, if you are able, own one by yourself. Planes do not depreciate like cars. I once owned an airplane called "Stinson Station Wagon," which was old when I bought it in 1949. I flew it for two years and then sold it for the $3000 that I paid for it. Today in 1971 you can still buy that same airplane with somewhat slightly better equipment for the grand total of $3800 to $3900.

You can start flying at any age. There are doctor friends of mine who started their first lessons at the age of forty-eight, and now at fifty-two are multiengine rated, instrument-rated and accomplished pilots. They would not think of taking a trip anywhere by any means of transportation other than a private plane.

There is for each pilot an immense sense of pride because it is a special skill, a special accomplishment. The sailor can heave-to, the driver can pull over, the golfer can sit and rest. The pilot can never forget, backdown or give up his responsibility. Nor is there anything as convenient as flying for "going and doing," but beyond this convenience is the physical, mental and emotional sense of completion that flying gives to the man who lives by the strength of his mind, the physician.

FOR FURTHER READING

The Airman's World. Gill Robb Wilson, Random House.

Around the World on the Lindbergh Trail. Francis X. (Cy) Sommer.

Invitation to Flying. Ziff Davis Publishing Company 1969.

Cessna Aircraft Company, Wichita, Kansas 67201.

Piper Aircraft Corporation, Lock Haven, Pa. 17745.

Federal Aviation Agency, Washington, D.C. 20553.

Superintendent of Documents, U.S. Government Printing Office, Washington, D.C. 20402.

Places to Fly. Volumes I, II, III, AOPA.

Lets Fly. AOPA (Aircraft Owners and Pilots Assn.).

Flying Magazine

AOPA Pilot   All available at Newsstands or

Plane and Pilot   by subscription

Private Pilot

26

EQUINUS MEDICORUM

ROBERT J. SPENCER AND JACK BRAINARD

Horsemanship is still growing in the United States; there are now more saddle horses in the United States than there were prior to the introduction of automobiles. Obviously, there are a lot more people in the country States than there were prior to Henry Ford's invention; still there is an increasing utilization of horses for pleasure.

The sport of kings is still very appealing and probably will continue to be for it offers something for everyone who has the slightest inclination toward becoming involved. The sport of horsemanship can become appealing because there are various aspects, each of which has its own particular appeal. Some will be primarily interested in the riding, whereas others can get pleasure from raising, training, showing, or merely keeping horses. Still other individuals will find an outlet for their energies by owning race horses or perhaps participating in the social events of riding to the hounds.

Our endeavor here is to present various hints and suggestions to those who wish to become involved in this sport. Although this is the sport of kings, we feel that a royal treasury is not an absolute prerequisite to partaking in the sport; still, it would be very helpful. The other and most sage advice we wish to deliver is that an amateur can get a lot of pleasure out of the sport if he or she is willing to recognize his lack of real knowledge, and therefore obtain truly expert advice as needed. As with many sports, almost everyone who becomes interested feels that he is an expert in the area, but this is far from true. The unjustifiably self-proclaimed experts should be avoided, or at least their advice should not be taken, for this can cause considerable trouble in the handling, management or riding of horses.

What are the advantages of this sport? Sports generally do not need to have their advantages defined. There is, of course, the pleasure of getting involved in something that does not need a practical commercial advantage or rationale for existence; but obviously there are many benefits that can be derived from horsemanship. It is an endeavor which an entire family can enjoy and which can be a unifying family activity, frequently initiated by a preteen or young teenage girl in the family. As the activity is examined, we see that there are certain benefits which can be easily obtained from this endeavor. Obviously, physical activity is a significant dividend for it is virtually impossible to become involved in any part of this sport without reaping the benefits of physical exercise. Unfortunately, sometimes most of the exercise is obtained just chasing the horse around the pasture in an attempt to catch it for a short ride. There are social advantages of riding, for it is a sport that is enjoyed in groups of people and obviously this is the greatest advantage and benefit from any hobby, the advantage of being with humans who also enjoy the activity. Many physicians have farms or acreage, and this is a sport that can truly be worked in with land and the proper utilization of it. The advantage of babysitting is an obvious one, for it is an activity which the younger members of the family can enjoy with assurance that it is a relatively safe and wholesome activity, one that will give them a feeling of achievement and which they can enjoy as they progress to the various levels of competence. Children with supervision can progress rapidly, developing a great deal of confidence, skill and ability to overcome frustrations while partaking in the sport, particularly when ponies or small horses are available to them. We feel that children really are never too young to start in the sport for there are ways and activities in this leisure activity that are appealing even to three and four year olds. There is a great advantage for little children to be around horses, for the horses sense that this is a small person and will be particularly gentle with children. A little child with a newborn colt is a joyous, thrilling sight to behold.

Probably the most significant benefit obtained from equitation is that it is a family project, one that even the youngest members can enjoy because they are included; thus, this becomes partially a babysitting service. Of course, supervision of small children is needed. After one considers the benefits of this sport and its obligations, if he still feels an overwhelming urge to become involved, then he should set out to define his objectives in the sport. The objectives can be raising, training, riding, showing or having harness horses or race horses. One of the easiest ways to succumb to this disease is to use the pony route. Ponies are relatively easier animals to keep than horses, for they require considerably less care than horses. Ponies by their own nature are extremely rugged animals. The ruggedness probably is an expression of their meanness but, of course, ponies have their own particular appeal, especially to children, because their small size makes them less overwhelming for a tot. No matter what route an individual takes in becoming involved in this sport, he should anticipate that through the years he will try to increase the quality of the animals he maintains and uses. I am addressing most of my comments to those who plan to own their own animal, for many of these comments or suggestions really would be unnecessary for persons or families who plan to use commercial riding stable horses. When one becomes involved in the ownership of horses, he tends to lose some degree of cold judgment in that he feels an emotional attachment, and it is not uncommon for a person to become quite sentimental about an old horse that has been in the family for 20 years. I, unfortunately, am one who does not have a great personal love for a particular horse, for I feel that as long as the horse is useful, I will maintain it. Once the horse becomes useless from age or injuries, I feel that he should be relegated to a more practical use, even if that use is merely a nutritional adjunct to the care of dogs or foxes. When one decides that he is going to keep his own horse, it means that he is making a considerable commitment to the sport, a commitment that will require planning, a commitment from which one is not easily released, but one that really is most enjoyable.

We started with two ponies and a horse. Through the years we have developed a herd that now numbers 12 animals, half of which are ponies. As our children are maturing, the ponies are becoming less significant and used less. We anticipate that we will be totally free of the pony activities except for the pony horses—half-pony, half-horse—that we are using for breeding I have found it a considerable advantage to have horses of various types. Currently we maintain a Tennessee walker, a hunter-jumper and a three-gaited saddle horse. This gives all of us an opportunity to enjoy a different type of ride, depending upon our whims. Also it gives the children the opportunity to practice various skills in equitation, skills that really only can be obtained when a special type of animal is used. In addition to the previously mentioned animals, we maintain two western-trained horses, and we use these horses to learn the English style of riding or the Western style of riding. Once one has thrown caution to the wind and decided to become involved, he should consider the equipment that will be needed for this sport. The equipment for riding on the local trails would be quite minimal, whereas equipment needed for riding in horse shows, hunts, extensive trail rides, or rodeos obviously would be special. Probably the most reasonable way to approach this problem is to ask what attire is used in the particular event locally. Obviously, for just hacking about on a casual basis, extremely casual riding attire is perfectly appropriate. This can consist of any type of jeans or britches and a comfortable boot of appropriate style. The boots can be leather or rubber, can be polished or unpolished for casual riding. For safety's sake, we have a rather strict family rule that a protective hard-hat must be worn by everyone when any serious or extensive riding is in the offing. There are various colors and styles of hard-hats for riding that are not overly expensive.

When one becomes involved in a more formalized type of riding such as horse shows, fox hunts and rodeos, special attire is needed. The traditional attire required for these sports is of great significance, and one should not try to engage in these activities without the appropriate attire. The discipline of this proper dress is extremely good training for youngsters, and it is a thrill for more mature people to see a group of youngsters turned out in the proper attire with well cared-for and well-groomed horses with clean, well-oiled tack. We have found by attending shows that it is the best way to get all our equipment in proper order with the least amount of nagging.

When the horse is maintained by some commercial stable, the owner of the horse should recognize that he shares the responsibility with the operator who is providing the care. I feel the owner is responsible to see that the horse gets some type of exercise at a regular and fairly frequent interval. The owner is also responsible to report any physical change he notes in the horse such as cough, foot damage or injury, and should recognize that although someone else is responsible for most of the care for the horse, the horse will be subject to the usual diseases and infections. As a matter of fact, in most commercial stables there is a high incidence of infectious problems with the stock, for there is a more rapid turnover in the herd introducing contagious diseases at frequent intervals. The ideal stable would offer a reasonably large indoor riding ring and several outdoor rings for riding and training of horses. It should also have easy access to bridle paths and trails. Above all, one should try to keep his horse in the stable where there is a minimal turnover in the herd so that the horses are not exposed to too many infectious diseases. The barn should be clean, above all should be safe; that is, they should have the horses in tie stalls or box stalls that are constructed of strong enough materials to prevent the horses from injuring themselves on broken equipment. Ideally, box stalls should be of minimum size, 8 feet $\times$ 10 feet with good ventilation and the floors of the stalls should be of sand. There should be adequate, clean, straw bedding. There should be an area in the barn for grooming horses and a secure place for storage of owner's tack.

For family participation in the sport, one should try to find commercial stables for maintenance of his horse where lessons can be obtained for the younger members of the family. The lessons should be of various levels so that a young rider can progress as his skills develop.

KEEPING YOUR OWN HORSES

Physicians with the land and inclination may succumb to advanced stages of this hobby. He will undoubtedly endeavor to keep his own herd either at home or some relatively convenient location so that he can watch progress of his horses and can enjoy them more. There is a definite pleasure to be obtained by just keeping horses. The grooming and also managing the barn need not be overwhelming tasks, and with some thought and planning an environment can be developed in which horses can be maintained without excess of work. Horses being grazing animals, the most important necessity for their keep is an adequate pasture; in most parts of the United States an acre or two per head is sufficient for the maintenance of an adult horse. Lesser amounts are needed for the maintenance of ponies and young stock. This would give the animals sufficient room for exercise and summer grazing. In the less watered parts of the United States, an additional space would be necessary for summer grazing. Ideally the pasture should be what the farmers call a permanent pasture; that is, a good stand of grass that is developed on the land where secure fencing of the area is maintained. Ideally there should be ample water available either by means of a stream going through the pasture or by a watering tank. If a watering tank is used, it should be installed so that a muddy patch about the tank is nonexistent or minimal. The pasture should be clipped at regular intervals to prevent overgrowth of undesirable weeds, and the pasture should be inspected so that dangerous objects which could injure the horse can be removed. Some area of shade in the pasture would be of great comfort to the horses in the hot summer days. The pasture may have to be sprayed occasionally to remove noxious weeds and also to minimize insects. Ideally one should consider cultivating the pasture every two to three years so that the ova of the intestinal parasites of the horses will be removed from the surface, thereby terminating their life cycle.

Some type of barn is necessary, and this can vary from an extremely elaborate paneled structure with numerous amenities including showers and fancy tack room with fireplace to a simply corrugated pole-shed closed on three sides. The barn should be in keeping with the challenge to which the horse is placed; that is, five gaited hot-blooded horses in intense training cannot be kept sound in a very basic type environment. This horse would require a relatively air-tight box stall with fresh bedding once or twice a day, with ample water supply furnished in the stalls. An idle horse or a relatively idle horse can be maintained adequately in grazing type of environment. The real critical feature is the challenge to which the horse is placed; that is, the amount of exercise and training required from the horse per day. Obviously, even Whirlaway could have survived the rough and tumble environment of a Montana ranch.

Horse Nutrition

Horses can only be as good as the food that is available to them and only as good as the exercise and care that they receive. The most significant item in their entire nutrition is the roughage in the form of grazing or in the form of hay. Horses who have time for sufficient grazing can do considerable work, but a horse who is exercised optimally very likely does not have sufficient grazing. Therefore, horses that are expected to perform should have supplement to their grazing. Obviously, the supplement is essential when grazing is not available, such as in extremely arid parts of the United States or in the winter. Under these conditions, hay of good quality must be provided at a rate of approximately 40 pounds per horse per day. If alfalfa hay is available to the horse, this should be used for the weight of the daily hay portion. Alfalfa hay is an excellent hay for horses, but the traditional hay for horses has been timothy. The idea that timothy has been the only proper hay for horses should be exposed as a myth. Timothy is relatively deficient in both protein and vitamin A. If the animal has ample protein in the form of grain and vitamin A, the form of feed supplements, timothy could be acceptable, but alfalfa generally is a much more reasonable source of both these nutritional requirements for horses both in an ideal state and in conditions of stress. One must be cognizant of the fact that a horse on a fairly rich protein feed requires an abundant supply of drinking water, particularly when that animal is being brought from idle condition to a fit condition. Horses are subjected to myoglobulinuria under stress, and this demands appropriate diuresis to prevent renal shutdown. Caution must be taken when situations of excessive exercise is demanded suddenly of the horse. This can easily be prevented by scheduling three to five days of gradually increasing exercise for animals that were previously idle. Grain offers a horse a ready source of protein, minerals, and calories. It is essential particularly for young stock and for animals who are being brought to and maintained in a fit condition. A great deal of variation in the grain formulas can be found, but one can, with some expert assistance, develop his own grain formula for his particular situation. I use a formula that amounts to approximately 40 percent oats, 20 percent corn, 10 percent soybean meal, and 10 percent bran. The remaining portion consists of vitamin A supplement, calcium supplement, trace mineral supplement, molasses, and alfalfa pellets. There are numerous commercial feeds for horses, which are variations on the previous theme. Unfortunately, some of the popular horse feeds have excessively high molasses which the horses enjoy, but so do many insects.

The saying, "healthy as a horse," is probably one of the world's most confusing statements. Horses generally are not noted for being healthy animals. Horses are subjected to numerous infectious diseases, some of which are brought on by cold rain, insignificant cuts, and even a very casual contact with an infected carrier. Horses are also extremely prone to muscle soreness and joint disorders of mysterious origins. Probably the most dangerous problems in the general maintenance of horses' health is control of parasitic diseases, which plague the equine family. Horses, being grazing animals, are prone to graze near contaminated grass; fleas and other insects use the horses as a convenient host in their life cycle. Therefore, to properly maintain the health of these animals, a schedule of routine prophylactic worming is necessary. Also special measures should be directed at interfering with the life cycle of the parasites. A convenient technique is to worm the animals twice a year, once in early fall after the first frost so that the discharged worm will freeze. The second attack on the parasitic organisms should be made in early spring to destroy the parasites which migrate to the intestine of the horse at this time of year.

The care of horses' feet is truly a task that requires a great deal of expert management. This is not something that should be attempted by amateurs nor is it a task that can be carried out by a local handyman. There is a great deal of precise care needed to properly trim the horse's hoof, especially if one hopes to achieve any unique action of the horse's gait. In addition to the precise technique of trimming the horse's hoof, there is a real but subtle art to properly fitting the shoe to the individual horse and accomplishing the goals which the owner hopes to achieve.

EQUITATION

Generally speaking, light horse breeds are divided into two divisions primarily on the basis of their usage. We call one division Western and the other English. In the English division the foaling breeds are used principally. They are the standardbreds, Tennessee walker, thoroughbred, the saddlebred and sometimes the Arabian and Morgan. The Western division has adopted these breeds primarily because they are the most adept for the job the Western horse must do. These breeds are composed of the quarter horse, the Appaloosa, the thoroughbred and the Arab. You will note that some breeds can be dual-purpose because they are used in both divisions. These are the Arabs, Morgans, and the thoroughbreds. Each of the breeds of light horses has an interesting background, and certainly no *one* breed can claim superiority. Each of the breeds must be trained for the job he has to do, and the training process, in the advanced stages at least, is widely different. First we will discuss the Western horse and the job he has to perform.

All Western horses are schooled for one of the following uses: first, the Western pleasure; second, a cutting horse; third, roping; fourth, reining; fifth, barrel racing and other games.

The Western pleasure horse is exactly what his name implies, a Western horse that is a pleasure to ride. The Western pleasure horse, as far as performance horses are concerned, is the backbone of the horse industry. There are more Western pleasure horses than all the other kinds combined. A nice Western pleasure horse has a relaxed and easy manner. He must be a horse

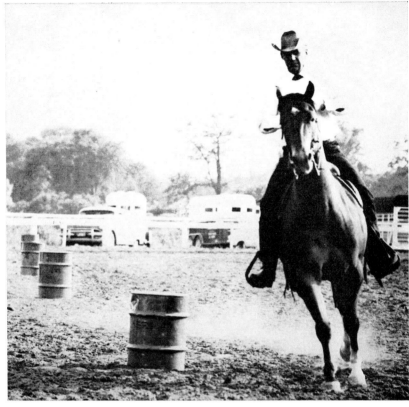

Figure 26–1. The games of a western riding contest bring out subtle skills which some observers miss. This is Jack Brainard on Blue Heather in a Western Riding Contest which requires a change of leads while weaving through a series of obstacles.

that moves fluently over the ground, a horse that has a nice even temperament and a nice disposition, and a horse that is a pleasure to ride. The gaits that he is asked to perform are basically three: the walk, the jog and the lope. Another of our Western performance horses is the cutting horse. This is probably the most highly trained of all our horses.

This horse is used primarily for cutting or sorting cattle and is a horse that was developed into a modern-day contest horse mainly because of the romance and the legend of the cow business on the great ranches years ago. At this time the favorite or best horse on each of the ranches was the cutting horse or the horse that was used to sort or cut our beef during the fall round-ups. Our present day cowboys found that it was fun to train a horse to cut cattle, and a great working event has grown out of this. Our modern-day cutting horses are judged on the manner in which they perform. A horse must enter the herd of cattle quietly, he must sort out an individual and bring him to the outside of the herd; the cow is then hazed or driven back into the herd by turnback men. The horse must perform and hold the cow out of the herd while the other horses try to drive her back into the herd. The horse must work on his own. He must work on a loose rein and must not be cued by the rider. Faults are reining the horse, jerking or spurring, or in anyway cueing or helping the horse to hold the cow out of the herd.

The roping horse is a horse primarily used for rodeo work. Cowboys depend on him for their living. He is also a horse used basically on the ranches in the West. Roping has developed into a sport and is now practiced and enjoyed by many across the United States. You will find many roping clubs and arenas everywhere. Many roping enthusiasts are boys who can definitely do a good job of roping, but do not have a ranch back-

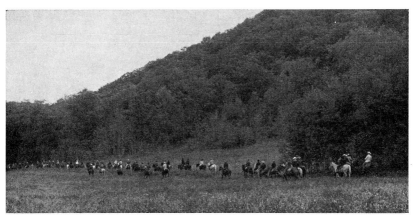

Figure 26–2. Riding itself is enjoyable, but the pleasure multiplies as the crowd increases. Organized trail rides of 50 to 150 riders are becoming a modern way to use horses and enjoy nature while having good fellowship and good food.

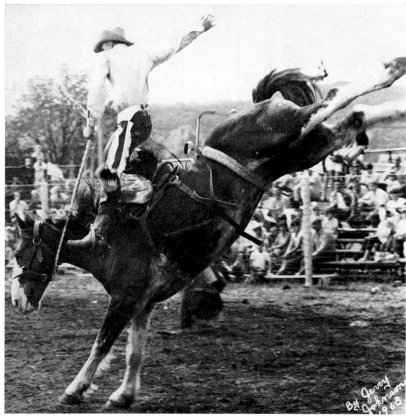

Figure 26–3. If this is your thing, remember balance and timing of rider and horse are still essential. Here is Chip Whitaker staying on Rodeo Incorporated's horse Sheep Mountain. This horse won 1967 National Finals Bucking Horse Contest.

ground. From this sport we have developed our modern-day roping horse. Primarily he is of the quarter-horse breed because he does have a burst of early speed. The roping horse must back into a barrier or box and chase the calf across the arena. As soon as the calf is roped, he must come to a sudden stop. He must then back up on the rope, keeping the rope tight until the calf is tied down. Many roping horses command high prices primarily because the cowboys can win large sums of money with them at roping contests during the year.

Another Western use is, of course, the reining horse. The reining horse is a highly trained horse. It is a horse designed for a specific job and must perform in a certain manner. He is judged on the manner in which he executes his sliding stop, how he changes leads by which he changes directions abruptly in what we call roll backs. Actually the reining horse is the ballet dancer of all the performing horses. Our modern-day pole horses are reining horses, so to speak, but not as highly trained as our present reining quarter horse which we see in horse shows and contests across the country nowadays. Reining horses are truly beautiful horses to watch as they execute movements and patterns in the horse show arena.

We have barrel-racing horses and other game horses; these are horses used in barrel-racing contests in which a horse must run a prescribed or a cloverleaf pattern around three barrels which are set up in the arena. These horses are not judged on the manner or the style in which they work. The stopwatch is the sole judge. Whichever horse can get around the course the fastest is declared the winner. Barrel-racing horses are extremely popular, especially among the younger set.

The English horse, like his Western counterpart, has been bred for a specific purpose. The English horse generally falls into one of these classifications: (a) the English pleasure, (b) the three and five gait horses, (c) hunters and jumpers, (d) the park horses, (e) Tennessee walkers, and (f) the harness horses. The English pleasure horse is also what its name implies: a horse tacked up in English equipment and a pleasure to ride. It can be one of many breeds. We find many English pleasure horses in all the breeds which we have mentioned in the English division. The English pleasure horse should be a well-mannered horse that is fun to ride and travels easily. The basic difference between the English pleasure horse and the Western pleasure horse is that the Western horse travels in a little freer and more relaxed manner. A nice English pleasure horse shows more spirit and animation than does the Western Pleasure horse. Here again the English pleasure horse is judged up to three gaits; the walk, the trot and the canter.

Three- and five-gaited horses are almost exclusively sad-

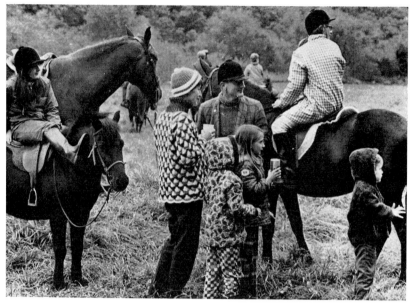

Figure 26–4. There is proper attire for every riding event; some are rather stylized. It is important for the rider to turn out neatly without overdressing. Hard hats are a must for jumping events and should be worn for protection when just riding. Pictured here is the Spencer family in conference during a trail ride.

dle breeds. The saddle bred make an excellent English pleasure horse, but most of the time they are trained for show ring competition and when in the show ring they generally fall into two classifications, the three-gaited and the five-gaited horses, the difference being that the three-gaited horse performs at the walk, trot and canter, and the five-gaited horse performs at two additional gaits which are the rack and slow gait. In other words, a five-gaited horse would perform at the walk, the trot, the canter, the slow gait and the rack. In the show ring, animation is of prime importance. These horses have been described as the most beautiful of all the light horse breeds.

Hunters and jumpers also constitute a large division in our English horse field. The hunters and jumpers are mainly thoroughbred horses. Fox hunting has been a sport for hundreds of years both in this country and in Europe, and a horse has evolved for this sport which we find to be very important today. Hunters, as the name implies, are horses used in fox hunting, and when we say field hunting, we mean horses that travel across the country and go over jumps, obstacles, and hurdles, or anything they might find in their way. The jumpers we think of as show ring jumpers. Here these horses are pitted one against the other over a series of obstacles, and the horse which jumps the highest is the winner. When we are thinking about hunting horses in terms of show ring hunters, this type of horse is judged differently than the jumper. He is judged in the manner in which he approaches the jump and the safety with which he goes over it; he is judged on pace and the manner in which he covers the ground and gets over his jumps. Height of the jumps in these classes are varied, and the hunters are not asked to jump as high as an open jumper.

Park horses are horses much like English pleasure horses. They can be of any of the four mentioned breeds. The main difference between a nice park horse and an English pleasure horse is that the park horse possibly shows a little more animation and a little more carriage than does the English Pleasure horse.

Tennessee walkers, of course, are an American breed of horse. They are developed in the southern part of the United States on the large plantations where the overseers rode this horse to look over and manage the field operations. Of course, as the name implies, they are extremely fast walking horses and here again they are an easy horse to ride which makes them popular in this area. We do have the contest Tennessee walking horse. This horse, when shown in the show ring, is shown at a flat walk, at the extended or running walk and, of course, at the canter. These horses do not trot.

Harness horses are horses which we use to pull a vehicle of some type. They are standard bred horses which we call road horses and are hitched to an appropriate two-wheel vehicle. Other horses which we call fine harness horses can be hitched to a four-wheeled vehicle as shown in this category. Harness horses are popular in the show ring, and we find that primarily they are the standard bred.

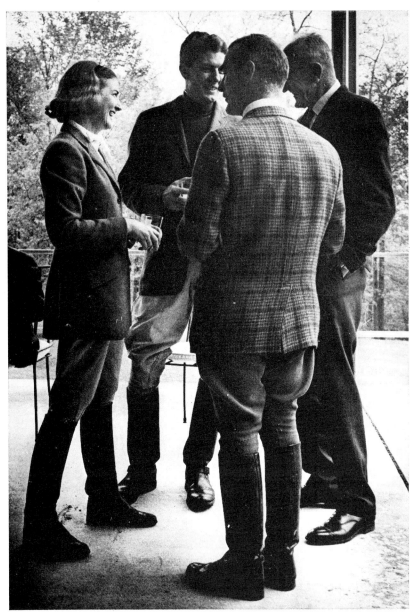

Figure 26–5. Riding horses can be a social function and this aspect should not be overlooked. This picture was taken after a hunt ride at the home of Dr. and Mrs. F. E. Donoghue. (*Left to right,* Mrs. F. E. Donoghue, Dr. Mark B. Coventry, Mr. Cutter and Dr. R. J. Spencer with his back to the camera.

Training

Although the advanced training techniques vary widely in the different breeds, the basic training methods are essentially the same. The primary object in schooling the young horse is, of course, control. A horse with basic training is one who will respond to the cues or "aids," and one who will walk, trot, canter, stop and back up in a willing manner. All horses are trained by the use of aids. Aids are the means by which we teach the horse to respond. Aids are of two kinds, the natural and the artificial. The natural aids are the hands, the legs and the seat, and the artificial aids are the whip, spur and the bit. After having ridden the young horse or colt a few times, the first order of training, of course, is to teach him to walk. We cue the horse to walk by a squeeze with our legs. We also relax on the reins at this time, and we dive the horse off. Sometimes it is called impulsing the horse off, since we squeeze the horse with our legs and relax the reins. The horse should walk off in a business-like manner. He should walk relaxed and also in a straight line. Simple as it may seem, it is sometimes hard to teach a colt to walk properly and correctly. After we have started the horse walking, we can usually increase his speed at the walk by continually squeezing him with our legs and driving him into the bit or forward with our legs. If the horse tries to break out of the walk and into a trot or attempts to break into a canter, we immediately pull him back to the walk by use of the reins. We want the horse to carry his head in a natural manner. By this we mean it should neither be too high nor too low, and the horse must be willing to accept the bit and go forward without twisting his head, mouthing the bit or any of the other habits that an untrained horse has. We must teach the horse to walk and perform in an area where he will not be distracted by other horses or objects which might take his mind off the trainer. We must remember that the walk is the basic gait. This is the gait we use the most, and a horse should perform it well. We should be extremely careful not to canter or trot the horse away from the training area or back to the training area at the end of the training period. Remember that our object at this gait is to teach our horse to walk in a straight line, to walk in a relaxed and easy manner and to walk at a business-like speed.

In teaching a horse to trot, we merely urge the horse into a trot which is the faster gait after the walk. We want the horse here again to trot in a straight line. We want the horse to trot as easily and smoothly as possible. At this gait most horses are a little inclined to lower their heads, especially if they are trotting at the extended trot which is the fastest speed of the trot. Here again head position is important. Through all of the gaits, at the walk, trot and the canter, we want the horse to carry his head in a natural position. We should be extremely careful not to be pulling on the reins, or the horse might mouth or chew on the bit which is definitely a fault for which the horse would be severely penalized if he were in a show ring.

The canter is the third gait with which we are concerned in the horse's basic training. It is, of course, nothing more than a controlled gallop or run. It is of prime importance that if a horse is cantering he is not merely running away. Speed is extremely important in the canter, and we do not want a fast canter. Actually, it should be a relaxed gallop without the horses trying to charge or run away at full speed. We teach the canter by urging him out of the trot and into this gait by the use of our legs. If the horse tries to run away or to extend his canter, then we immediately pull him back with the bit until he is cantering at the gait which we desire. Once the horse is into the gait or traveling at the proper speed in a relaxed easy canter, we immediately relax the reins as a reward, telling him that this is the speed at which we would like him to travel.

After the horse is cantering in a relaxed manner, we begin to teach the horse leads, and leads are extremely important. When a horse canters to the left, then his left foreleg and his left rear leg are extended farthest in the stride. In other words, they reach out farther on the left side than they do on the right if the horse is cantering in a circle to the left. By the same token, if the horse is cantering in a circle to the right, then his right foreleg and his right rear leg are extended in the stride. This is known as a lead, and a horse must canter in the correct lead while he is traveling around the show ring. We find that if a show horse does canter to the right in the opposite or left lead, then he is awkward and clumsy and he is not at all efficient on his feet.*

In teaching the horse leads, we depend primarily on leg aids. For instance, if we are to ask a horse to canter on the left lead, our cues would be to squeeze him hard with our outside or the right leg. We press our right leg firmly into the horse's side behind the cinch and impulse him out of the trot into the canter. If the horse takes the wrong lead, then we immediately stop him with the reins, present a new set of cues and try him again. It is very important not to let the horse canter in the wrong lead for any time. If we immediately stop him, this is punishment for taking it wrong and soon he will respond to the cues by taking the lead correctly. After we have taught the horse to canter correctly in the lead, we immediately reverse our cues and start on the other lead, remembering, of course, if we are to move the horse in the left lead we squeeze him with the right leg, pull his head slightly to the right and lean over his left shoulder as we impulse him or drive him into the canter with the leg. To teach the horse to stop we squeeze him with our legs, manipulate our bridal reins and pull back on them until he slows down. We are careful not to ask this horse for a complete stop by a hard steady pull on the reins. The primary role of all great horsemen is never to dwell on the reins, never to give a horse a hard steady pull but only a tug and a relax, and a tug and a relax, and so forth. After the horse breaks or slows up his speed, we continually manipulate the reins until the horse drops to a walk and then stops. Soon he will associate the manipulation of a reins and the squeezing of a leg with a stop, and he will drop to a stop immediately, which is what we want. We must be very careful not to pull hard on the reins, which would tend to deaden the horse's mouth or to lose the sensitivity or the feel which he has there. To teach a horse to back up, use much the same technique or aids which we have described in teaching a horse to stop. We squeeze him with our legs, manipulate the reins from a standing position until the horse takes one step backwards. As soon as he does, we immediately relax the reins

---

* In dressage riding, the counter lead is required for certain maneuvers.

and reward him by patting him on the neck or shoulder. Again we pick up the reins and ask him for one more step back. If he takes it, we again relax. Soon we can give him a series of pulls, and he will take a series of steps backward. It is extremely simple to teach a horse to back up provided we remember the cardinal rule which is, "Never pull hard on a horse's mouth."

Shoeing and Foot Care

There is an old horseman's adage about a horse being no better than his feet. This is certainly true. Many horsemen neglect the care of their horse's feet, which is certainly a mistake. In dealing with a horse's foot and the foot problems which our modern-day stable facilities provide, we must remember that in the wild or natural state, a horse did not need his feet trimmed because he was on the move continually and there was natural wear enough to take care of his feet. With our modern facilities, with our barnyards where the horse is confined and he is not allowed to run and to roam as was the wild horse, his feet naturally grow longer. Also today's modern roads are sometimes rocky and are of a surface which wears on the horse's feet. A horse soon becomes sore, and we must shoe him. Under normal circumstances we are riding horses on this type of terrain and on footing where there is considerable wear, and it is reasonable to assume that we should shoe or reshoe our horse at six-week intervals depending on the usage we give him. We must remember in shoeing a horse we should keep his foot in as near natural a position as we can. All horse's feet are different. They strike the ground at different angles. Due to the confirmation of the horse's foot, it can also be trimmed at different angles on different horses. Most horse shoers will agree, however, it is best to shoe the horse at his natural angle. If we do shoe the horse at an unnatural angle, we can cause a strain on the tendons and the horse will immediately become tendon sore rather than foot sore. A horse's foot needs moisture. If the horse does not have access to mud holes, to stream crossings, to grassy areas where the grass will become wet, then his foot becomes dry, and he can develop a problem. We must get moisture to the horse's foot either through natural or artificial means. Routine care for the horse's feet should be daily cleaning or "picking the horse's foot," as it is termed in horse language. We should be careful that we scratch all the dirt, manure and so forth out of the frog of the foot so that it is clean and there is no evidence of thrush. Foot care is extremely important in the young colt or foal. A competent farrier can work wonders with a colt's foot. By routine trimming he can form and shape the foot and even change the carriage of the colt. I cannot overemphasize the fact that we must routinely take care of our horse's feet. Nothing can be truer than the old adage than an ounce of prevention is worth a pound of cure, especially around the horse's foot.

BIBLIOGRAPHY

1. Ensminser, M.E.: *Horses and Horsemanship*, 4th ed. Danville, Ill., The Interstate Printers and Publishers, 1969.
2. Goodall, D.M. and Millan, Mae: *Horses of the World.* New York, 1965.
3. Ricci, J.A.: *Understanding and Training Horses.* Philadelphia, J.B. Lippincott, 1964.
4. Wright, Gordon: *Learning to Ride, Hunt and Show.* Sandem City Books, 1960.

27

SAILING

H. W. VIRGIN, JR.

O f all sports, sailing is probably the most comforting to the busy physician. It is a sport in which the physician can become buried in his entirety, and it can thereby prevent him from thinking about his busy practice, the ringing telephone and the social engagements. I have been a sailor since age nine and owned boats from the famous 12-ft X-class dinghy designed by John Alden up to an 85-footer. I have sailed for pleasure, for family cruising, for individual class-boat competition and ocean racing. I am presently the proud owner of the famed *Touche,* and have been fortunate in amassing a houseful of trophies.

Sailing can start at any level in terms of the size of the boat, the size of the body of water available, and the number of persons you wish to have participate with you. You may sail a small dinghy for solitude and the comfortable feeling of being in command of your ship, or you may sail as the skipper of an ocean racer, driving your ship through all manner of weather and commanding a crew of four to fourteen people. You may extend your interest in sailing to joining a sailing club, or a yacht club, and you may become involved in the organized side of sailing.

Ask me, "How shall I start?" and I must answer, "First tell me where you will sail." If you are on an inland lake, five miles in diameter, then you should start with a small one- two- or three-person boat. My preference would be a glass hull with an aluminum mast and boom and with Dacron® sails and rigging. Everything should be as simple as possible so that you can spend your time sailing and not caring for the boat. The desire to care for the boat can come later, when you know the fundamentals and some of the fine points of sailing, and will be interested in "tun-

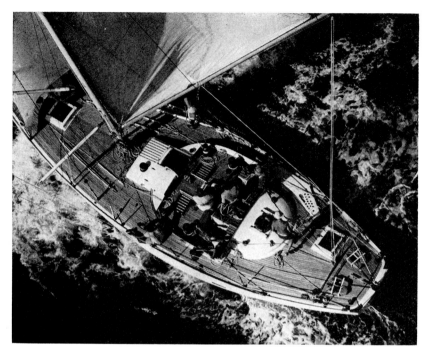

ing your boat" (arranging the mast and rigging) so that you can get the most out of it in terms of speed and performance.

Now that you have decided that you will sail on a certain size lake, a bay or an ocean and that you will fit a boat to this certain body of water, you will want to know something about how to make the boat actually sail. Of course, you may get in the boat, hoist the sails and have the wind blow you back and forth until it dawns on you that the boat will go in a given direction, depending on how your sails are trimmed, i.e. how your sails are brought in close to the boat or allowed to swing far away from the boat. We describe beating into the wind, or "tacking" into the wind, as that maneuver which enables one to actually sail at approximately 45° into the direction of the wind. You move from where your boat is to a point upwind by changing the direction of the boat, shifting the sail from one side of the boat to the other as you "tack" against the wind toward your destination. If you make a series of these, 45° to the wind tacks (from one tack to the other is actually 90°), you will eventually arrive at your destination. This is the finest art of sailing. If you wish to sail toward a point which is across the wind, or at 90° to the direction of the wind instead of 45° as in tacking, you are then "reaching." "Reaching" is that maneuver in which the wind is from the side of your boat and your sail is allowed to swing away from the boat, perhaps 30° to 40°. This maneuver will enable you to sail with the wind coming toward the side of the boat at right angles. Now if you wish to get away from the wind, or as sailors express it, "downwind," or even more technically, "running," you will turn the stern of the boat toward the wind and run away from the direction of the wind. Allow your sails to swing away from the boat so that the boom, which is attached to the mast, is now approximately 90° to the side of the boat. Thus, you may sail or tack into the wind, reach across the wind, or sail running in a downwind direction.

Better still, purchase a book which will explain the action of the boat in relation to the wind and the function of the sails in relation to the wind. Subscribe to several sailing magazines. Read them!

I like to think of sailing as a continuation of a formerly useful commercial venture into the form of sport. Probably the first modern racing was done in fairly large yachts that belonged to wealthy people in Europe and England. In this country, the oldest yacht club is in the Carolinas and has become a little-known club, due to the prominence acquired by such prestigious clubs as the Chicago Yacht Club, the New York Yacht Club, the New Orleans Southern Yacht Club, Miami's Coral Reef and Biscayne Bay yacht clubs, the San Francisco St. Francis Yacht Club, and others. Yacht clubs have banded themselves together for mutual service into an organization called NAYRU, which controls the racing rules and the governing of racing of boats.

Other than buying a book, finding a professional who will teach you to sail, or bungling along yourself until you ultimately discover the method of making your boat go, the best form of teaching is found in the brotherhood of yachtsmen who have formed yacht clubs. There are yacht clubs in almost every size-able community on the waterfront and many yacht clubs are inland where bodies of water have attracted people and have formed pleasant arenas for sailing. Many yacht clubs do not have clubhouses, but function out of the homes of members, and have their meetings in hotels or public buildings. One of these with which I am familiar is the Gulfstream Yacht Club in Fort Lauderdale, Florida, which runs among the finest children's teaching program, adult teaching program, and competitive sailing programs that exist in the United States. Boats of all kinds and variety are found in this club, and the club membership runs from blue-collar workers to professional people. It seems to make no difference in the sailing fraternity what your economic status is.

Another excellent club is the Coconut Grove Sailing Club in Miami, which is made up of blue-collar workers, bankers, lawyers, letter-carriers, school teachers, filling-station attendants, etc. It is one of the finest clubs, and can boast of a truly healthy atmosphere of friendship and helpfulness. These clubs may have very small fee schedules, such as $25 initiation fees and $25 to $40 a year membership fees. Most of the dinners and parties are dutch-treat, and there are frequent club events that do not involve racing at all, but are events in which the whole club fleet might sail to a pleasant cove and rendevous, or "raft-up" for an overnight dinner and bash.

Those doctors who find themselves circumscribed in time by their specialty, especially the obstetrician, the young surgeon who cannot afford to miss a case by being away very long, the orthopaedic surgeon who must cover the emergency room properly, can find sailing a real possibility. With the modern VHF line-of-sight inexpensive ship-to-shore radios, they can keep in communication constantly and inexpensively with their offices. I have in mind my daughter-in-law's obstetrician who has a 30-ft sloop which he and his brother-in-law designed and constructed themselves. He sails up and down the shore close enough so that if at anytime he is called, it is only a matter of a few minutes for him to dock his boat, get in his car and proceed to the hospital. An engine helps him.

As an orthopaedic surgeon, I have found that bay sailing, or close-ashore sailing is quite compatible with an honest coverage of the emergency room, except for dire emergencies that require instant care to save life. After all, most of us would require fifteen to twenty minutes, if we were asleep, to dress, get in the car and get to the hospital. We are not far away from that kind of time schedule when it would require ten or fifteen minutes to sail to the dock, get in the car and get to the emergency at hand. Those of us who are able to ask a colleague to cover for us for several hours can extend the sail, take a party out for entertainment, take our families out for a lovely ride on a brilliant, sparkling day and enjoy relaxation without any feeling of tension or compulsiveness to be "available." It is this sailing that I like to think of as the most worthwhile of all. It is known as "day sailing."

There are actually a host of boats in the range of 25 to 30 ft which are less expensive than a good car, are made of glass, are sturdy in construction, have stalwart mast and rigging, contain a small gasoline or diesel engine, and can tolerate the most rigorous type of storm. These are the boats that will enable you to take a family, even babies and young children, safely offshore for short distances and bring them back in the event of bad weather.

I would like to point out that there is at this time a national organization called MORC (Midget Ocean Racing Conference) which accepts for membership boats 23 to 30 ft. These boats, in my part of the world, sail across the Gulf Stream and back on cruises and races without any hesitation. They have encountered sharp storms (not just squalls), and to my knowledge have never had any serious accident occur—other than perhaps losing a mast. These boats are all strongly constructed, have radios, lifelines, motor power, and have the ability, through their fine naval architectural designing and construction, to bring their captains and crews home safely.

These boats are available and can be seen at boat shows throughout the country; they can be just as easily handled by husband and wife as can a much smaller boat. As a matter of fact, they are safer in that they do not turn over, are watertight, and can be handled in rough storms. Small boats, which are called "class-boats" (Stars, Lightnings, Comets, Solings, 505's, X-class dinghys, Snipes, etc.) do turn over, do swamp, and with

TABLE 27–I
ONE-DESIGN RACING/DAYSAILING BOATS

Name	Class Material	Boat Length	Crew	Average Cost
Soling	Glass	26	3	5,000
Star	Wood	22.5	2	4,500
Lightning	Glass	19	3	3,500
Snipe	Glass	15	2	3,000
Bullseye	Glass	15	2	5,000
505	Glass	14	2	3,000
420	Glass	12	2	1,500
Frostbite Dinghy	Glass	11	1	1,200
Finn Dinghy	Glass	11	1	1,500

heavy keels such as those of Stars, do sink. There is no question in my mind that for peace of mind, love of the water, noncompetitive as well as competitive sailing, these MORC boats are the finest.

The man who has "come up through the ranks" in sailing—started out with a dinghy, learned the trim of the sails and the way to tack, how to handle his boat in choppy water, and has then moved up to a larger class-boat such as the Lightning, the Star, the Soling or the Snipe—and has sailed competitively or for pleasure can, of course, more properly go into the MORC class. These "small boat" sailors make the greatest crews and the greatest skippers, I have learned in my experience.

My own sons and my daughter, all of whom are great sailors, and my wife, who has sailed small boats and big boats for years, have won far more cups than I have, and are considered in the sailing world highly competitive and competent sailors. They all started in X-class dinghys and graduated through Lightnings and Stars into their father's ocean racers. Two of my sons have sailed as helmsmen on *Gypsy,* the great boat of the Great Lakes, named "Boat of the Year" many times over. These boys have sailed their father's ocean racers when he was away at medical meetings, when they were as young as fifteen years of age, in such races as the Lipton Cup, the Nassau, the Lucuyan, etc. This gives you some idea of the value of starting young and learning in the small boat.

I think you can understand that when racing in class-boats, you may race three "heats" or three races each Saturday and Sunday for several years; making multiple starts and multiple

stops, you make multiple tacks, multiple sail-changes and altera-
tions, and experience hundreds of times the situations which
will later confront you in the bigger boats. It is simply a matter
of exposure to many situations many times over that makes the
small-boat sailor such a great big-boat sailor later in life.

Now in regard to some of the larger boats, you should know
that you are not allowed in most ocean NAYRU races to sail
anything over 72 ft overall-length. Actually, there are very few
of these large boats. They are quite expensive and require large
crews, and are designed primarily for long, arduous ocean racing. Someday most of us would like to have one. I like to see the
smaller of the ocean racers become dominant because it gives
sailing a great base of operation, rather than a small base as it
would be if we all had to have big boats. Some of the ocean
races require a minimum 35-ft overall-length. Such a race would
be the Bermuda race, one of the great blue-water classics. In the
Southern Ocean Racing Circuit, we are allowed to have boats
30 ft or larger in overall length.

What does it cost to maintain a boat of this sort during a year?
You will need a change of ropes, known as "sheets," and in order
to remain competitive you should get a new mainsail and Genoa
jib every third or fourth year. You will need certain painting,
varnishing, and repairs which you may either do yourself or
have done at a boat yard. Unfortunately at this time, most boat
yards charge $10 to $12 an hour for any sort of work that is
done. It is much more fun to do your own work, except for the
painting of the bottom of the boat, which has to be done (on
racing boats) with the boat hauled out at a boat yard. The
family cruising boat, on short budget, can be beached at high
tide, then scrubbed and painted at low tide. In the North, you
will have the boat stored for the winter, usually out of the water,
and you may be able to find a yard where you will be permitted
to do your own bottom work. Down here in our area, we are not
allowed to do bottom painting in most yards.

Your engine will require overhaul and maintenance, and there
is no way of knowing how much this will run. Sometimes owners
are unfortunate in having engine trouble. Other sailors of my
acquaintance do not know what the word "trouble" means. Most

MORC sailors not only do their own work, but many of them are experienced enough to design their own sails, and some of them even *make* their own sails. These are the rare, deeply committed souls who buy a zigzag sewing machine and do this as night work, or weekend work.

When you move up into the ocean racers, you should have a reasonably good income to support your sport. My wife and I rationalize as follows:

1. This is good anti-coronary insurance.
2. It is an excellent way to keep in physical condition.
3. We entertain, to a large extent, by taking out important guests on our boat for an afternoon sail, or occasionally, an overnight party. We have them actively sail the boat, and they enjoy it. Some guests ocean race with us.
4. Taking your vacation on a boat is an enormous saving, and we translate this saving into the expense money, and thus rationalize a great deal of the maintenance and care of the boat in terms of dollars saved on a boating vacation as against the typical resort vacation, or air flight to a foreign country.

Now, cruising is different. No matter where you live, no matter the thickness of your purse, no matter your age, weight or experience, cruising can become the *all* in life. Planned or unplanned, spontaneous or designed for one, two or four couples, a cruise becomes the memory to cherish through the winter, and plan for and anticipate all spring.

Take a 36-ft yawl, drawing 5 ft of water, with a small diesel engine driving her 6 knots an hour. Put on board 75 lbs of cake ice, a 10 lb roast, vegetables, fruit, beer and snacks. A few clothes to suit the temperature, foul-weather gear, tow a dinghy, and start out with small sails. Ask the wife, or a guest, to take the wheel while you go below to make sure all is stowed and things are shipshape against heeling in a sudden squall, and you are master of your own world; happiness may be thirty miles down the coast in a snug harbor. Cruising can be easy or hard, short or long. The destination can be planned or come-as-may.

Mrs. Virgin and our family of three children have made over fifty trips into the Bahamas, Jamaica, Cuba, around into the Gulf of Mexico, Bermuda, around the Great Lakes and up the Atlantic coast to New England.

Our happiest cruises would find us selecting a safe harbor at night where children and guests could swim, fish, shell, skin-dive and explore old ruins of centuries ago. Meeting the cruising crowd becomes an ever expanding delight, and part of the fun is never knowing who might pull in and drop an anchor next to you in a remote island harbor, perhaps a family not seen for years.

SMALL CRUISING BOATS

Name	Length	Sleeps		Crew	Approx. Base Cost
Columbia	26	gas	5	3	7,500
Erickson	27	gas	4	3	unknown
Ranger	23		4	2	5,450
Seacraft	22		5	2	2,400
Irwin	28	gas	6	3	12,000
Venture	24	gas	5	2	3,000
C and C	24		4	2	unknown
Seafarer	29		4 or 5	2	8,800
Huntley	27		5	2	8,000 sails
Ranger	29	Diesel	6	3	12,500
Chance	30	gas	5	3	17,000
Yankee	24		4	2	6,000 sails

One summer, a member of my crew and I took six teenage boys for two weeks from Miami to Cat Cay, to Andros, to Nassau, to Frazier's Hog Key, up the Berry Islands and home. Later it was college friends in large numbers, and then our married children and their families. Now it is our children in their boats, cruising with their children and their children's friends.

Food is a problem. Read the books on cruising and find that good bread can be canned; unfertilized eggs last a month; can bacon as your grandmother did fruit—in a Mason jar—by steam-sterilizing it. Make up single-pot dishes like canned tuna, canned peas and rice—nickname it "pea wiggle." Do not forget the bottom-fish, lobsters, crabs, and such. Be sure you have enough! We were anchored in the lee of Cat Cay one summer morning, when a sloop crewed by four boys from our club sailed past us. They had been out for a month and were headed home.

Mrs. Virgin observed that they were sailing back and forth near us while we were eating breakfast, and it dawned on us that they wanted an invitation. Out went the fenders, and she came alongside. They had had only raw fish for two days—and just about depleted our larder of ham and eggs.

How does your wife become interested? Well, if you are lucky, she may be a yacht club companion you sailed with while growing up; or she may be the daughter of a boat owner; or you two may come head-on into the boating world after marriage. My best advice is to give her a boat. If this fails, after deciding you want sailing as your sport, recreation, and hobby, ask her to help pick a yacht club you can afford, and then join it as a family investment. Mingling with sailing wives usually "softens her up" when buying-time comes. One thing is sure; do not point her in the direction of the galley immediately. Let her believe she is a guest until she has to eat the food you cook, and the rest comes easy.

Why should a doctor boat? To get away from the office. It is great family sport for all. You can boat until you are 80. At what age can you start? Youngsters can begin at six, and older. Mrs. Virgin's father learned to sail and cruise at 68 and won many cups. Where can you sail? Sail on inland lakes, dams, big rivers, coastal waters. How should you start? Go where boats are. Ask people questions. Read boating books and magazines. Go to boat shows, wander around and see all kinds of boats. Find a professional sailing school. Join the U.S. Power Squadron. Some cities have boating schools as part of their recreational departments. Some colleges have yacht clubs and schools. Join a family yacht club. Ask other members to let you crew. Sign up for men's classes. Or start bungling yourself.

Chapman's book is the Bible of boating. It tells you the rules of the road, ordinary piloting, coastal piloting, small boat handling, how to tie knots, and all the other essential things one must understand in order to sail safely. Other excellent references are the following:

Rufus G. Smith: *Sailing Made Easy* (Told in Pictures). New York, Dodd Mead & Co, 1959.

H. A. Callahan: *Learning to Sail*. New York, Macmillan.

Robert N. Bairer, Jr.: *Sailing to Win*. New York, Dodd, Mead & Co.

George O'Day: *Learning to Sail is Fun*. New York, Grosset & Dunlap, 1961.

Cuthbert Mason: *Ocean Sailing and Racing*. New York, Macmillan, 1954.

28

THE SOCIAL USES OF ATHLETICS FOR INDIVIDUAL DEVELOPMENT

ARNOLD R. BEISSER°

A considerable part of the disability of contemporary man has been related to his sense of estrangement and alienation. The activities and institutions which heretofore have sustained him have largely become obsolete or meaningless. Freed from the servitude of material necessity, he is paralyzed in the face of his new-found opportunity to choose his way of life. A disturbing relativism has replaced the absolutes in morality and religion which guided previous generations. Now he feels swept inexorably and involuntarily by a faceless crowd into mass leisure and mass culture where he finds little sense of life or involvement. In an effort to avoid the press of mass conformity and its accompanying sense of estrangement, many young people have "dropped out" of conventional life and its organizations and institutions. Many have felt that it is hopeless to try to find self-fulfillment in a society filled with contradictory values which demand conformity. Others, similarly motivated, have taken an activist position and seek to overthrow the existing order aspiring to replace it with an incompletely defined concept of a new free society. Understandably, older generations committed to the existing order, in spite of limited opportunity for satisfactions, react stiffly against the revolutionary activism.

The social activist position does provide a sense of personal aliveness and stimulation to those involved in "the cause," making that position appealing. The reactive position of conservatism, when militant, provides an equal sense of involvement for

° Director, Center for Training in Community Psychiatry, Los Angeles, California; Associate Clinical Professor Department of Psychiatry, School of Medicine and Lecturer School of Public Health, University of California at Los Angeles.

individuals committed to enforcing the existing order. However, the large mass of the population, while acknowledging the need for change, is less willing to accept either alternative, fearing the potential destructiveness and chaos which would inevitably grow out of an all-out revolution, or the militaristic repression. Instead, they look for opportunities for personal development *within* existing institutions while supporting more incremental changes.

Yet there are few institutions which do provide this sense of aliveness to those who either support the existing order or who support a gradualism in social change. Javanovich observed that only in sex, crime and sports can contemporary man find an elemental experience.[1] The social destructiveness of crime and the biosocial limitations on sex make sports the most available communal opportunity.

Many Americans awake from the monotony of living when they arrive at the ball park or turn the television set to the sports event of the week. A sense of excitement and involvement pervades the atmosphere of the game. The peak of national interest is reached at the time of the World Series, the Rose Bowl or the Olympics. All else seems to pale in significance. The American male arises from his bed in the morning, seats himself at the breakfast table and immediately becomes more involved in the sports page than in the food before him or his wife who serves it.

Moreover, so great is our national dedication to sport that it is built into our educational institutions to mold future generations of sports fans and athletes. Throughout the educational career of an American schoolboy, more time will be devoted to physical education than to any other single subject, and physical education usually means sports. This is justified by the belief that bodies need education as well as minds.

Certainly no one can disagree, but there is unfortunately little correlation between sports activity and physical fitness. The Kraus-Weber studies have revealed that European schoolboys who ordinarily do not have sports as a prominent part of the school curriculum are stronger and more agile on standardized physical fitness tests than their American counterparts. Besides, after the school career, athletes become fans, and the man in the bleachers with the hot dog and bottle of beer is doing very little for his physical powers.

Nevertheless, there is a certain wisdom in this emphasis on sports, for it satisfies a national need and does provide a means for maturation and growth to the individual. This potential is more for the integration of the whole organism than for physical fitness, however. Sports offer a unique opportunity in our society of alienation and estrangement. The author has had an opportunity to examine the psychological uses of sports over the past fifteen years. The sources of data have been individual patients who have come to him in his role as a practicing psychiatrist— individuals for whom sports and athletics were significant influences. In addition, he has been consultant to a number of coaches and athletic teams. Now let us examine some of the features of athletics which make them an important social vehicle for individual development.

1. *Sports are an intense psychophysical activity available to everyone in some form.* The active play of youth can blend smoothy into the spectatorship of adult life. One can participate with vigor or vicariously as a fan, achieving a similar sense of expression and discharge as the players, without having their skills or taking their risks. Sports activities are thus available to all in some form: the weak, the strong, the timid, the brave, the frightened and the courageous. The structure of team sports provides a reciprocal relationship between fans and players. Each group needs the other and each is vital in its participation.

Because of the flexibility of role participation, one may have a continuity of involvement. There are few such opportunities for continuity in modern life to sustain the individual, to give him a continued place in a central activity.

The 19th century prototype of such continuity was the blacksmith occupation. The blacksmith's son first observed his father at work; as he grew, he began to help in little ways consistent with his capacity. The son gradually assumed more and more responsibility until in his father's declining years he became the "smithie"; the father's participation gradually diminished consistent with his declining capabilities. There was a perfect continuity without interruption, affording a role in the central activity for each person in childhood, adulthood and senescence.

How different from modern life. Boys rarely see their fathers at work, and because of the fragmented and specialized nature of jobs in technical industries, it is very difficult for a father to tell his son what he does. The family has also become conjugated so that elders are separated from others in senior citizens' villages; and as soon as they are able, children move away from their parents. For each generation the mainstream of activities are separated and discontinuous. Relationships and problems are fractured rather than solved.

In sports one can find continuity not unlike that in the blacksmith's family. He can visualize a place for himself, and he can continue to encounter the life problems he brings to the situation, offering the possibility of changing adjustment to them. More will be said about these problems later·

2. *In sports, there is an opportunity for the physical expression of certain impulses forbidden elsewhere.* As people live closer together and social regulations increase, the possibilities of settling differences by physical means diminish. Yet everything about us stimulates competition. Diabolically man's competitive strivings are stimulated, while the physical expression of them is blocked. In fact, in order to win in most of life's competition—economic, political or social—direct expression of anger or aggression disqualifies the participant and he loses. Many people move about their lives in some form of chronic restraint of the physical concomitants of aggressive expression, contributing materially to the prevalence of certain psychosomatic medical disorders. Elevation of blood pressure and chronic muscular tension as found in headaches and certain forms of arthritis are some somatic expressions of repressed aggression.

On the athletic field, like a Saturnalian holiday, there is liberation. The players receive their rewards for knocking an opponent down or out of the play. They are stimulated in this by the fans who shout excitedly "kill him" or "murder him." While not literally obeyed, the hardest contact has highest favor with the crowd. When the mandate to win is carried through, the fans feel a satisfaction akin to the players!

In other walks of life, aggressive physical behavior would

result in ostracism or perhaps even arrest for assault. But the context of sports preserves an element of the primal relationship between the wish and the act. The rules of the game are strictly enforced but offer considerable latitude for the physical as well as the symbolic expression of aggression. So long as the aggression occurs within the rules, no matter how devastating its results, the players and the fans' relationships with one another are facilitated. They are not ostracized but included because of aggressive display.

It is not only aggression which is restrained in contemporary society; so, too, are many affectionate expressions. This is especially true for men. Physical expression of affection between men, in most contexts, has a distinctly nonmasculine connotation. The great "fear of being queer" was so pervasive as to be the primary concern of college men a decade ago.[2] While the social pressures against male display of affection have lessened in recent times, sports offer an acceptable opportunity for young men to express such feelings.

American males grow up in an atmosphere which insists on an anachronistic model of maleness taken from the 19th century pioneer: rugged, hard working, aggressive, self-reliant, with a role entirely distinct from the woman's role. Yet in the house in which he grows up, it may be difficult to distinguish between the man and the woman on the basis of division of labor. Women frequently work outside the home so that the household chores are shared by man and wife. This even includes the physical care of infants. Since the definition of masculinity does not fit the reality, many men are in a chronic state of anxiety lest they be considered feminine. At the same time their wives are also concerned that the husbands are not aggressive or masculine enough.

For young people who reject convention it is small wonder that sexual roles have become blurred. But many still try to adhere to the old expectations. In the sports stadium the problem is solved, for this most masculine of settings allows scantily clad men to congregate together without "queer" implications. A linebacker pats his squatted linemen on their buttocks, and in moments of success the players embrace. All this is viewed and cheered by thousands of fans, male and female, who in other settings would be horrified by such displays.

Thus, a continuity of maleness with physical contact is retained without odious connotation in sports. The infant male who was diapered and fed by his father as well as his mother can continue to feel masculine in the context of sports while having close physical contact with other men or boys.

3. *Beyond the simple opportunity for expression of impulses in sports, they may be the vehicle for working through certain conflictual personal situations in an active way.* Half a century ago in Vienna, Sigmund Freud took note of the play of a certain little boy. With his great intuitive psychological mind he came to understand that the boy's play was a symbolic reenactment of the major issue in his life: that his mother would leave him during the day. In his play he chose to use a spool over and over again. He would throw it away and then retrieve it with its string. Freud surmised that this play symbolized the separation from and reuniting with the mother. Playing out the conflict allowed the boy to repeat it again and again, but in contrast to the real situation he could do so on his own terms. He thus was able to turn his helpless passivity to the real situation into a controlled symbolic activity. In the game he was not only the helpless victim, but the one who pulled the strings (sic). Followers of Freud made further elaborations on the functional significance of play and games in children. They noted that the player can take both offensive and defensive roles in a particular game and enhance the possibilities of solution by experiencing a variety of outcomes.

Sports and athletics, whether for men or boys, women or girls, afford a similar potential for achieving mastery over symbolic situations. This psychological work can continue whether as player or spectator. One has the chance of experiencing the nuclear problems of life in high intensity in a relatively therapeutic atmosphere. There are joys of victory balanced by the guild for vanquishing opponents, the despair of defeat, the anxiety of the crisis, the sadness of separation, the fear of injury. Athletes experience their competition as repetitions of life conflicts and symbolically struggle against them.[3] In sports, a person may actively seek solution. He does so, not in isolation, but with the enthusiastic support of other players and fans. Eventually he may achieve mastery.

4. *In athletics many people find a balance in the work-play dilemma.* Traditionally, work was an activity which was productive and usually dominated by a spirit of necessity. Play, at the opposite pole, was unproductive, free, with a sense of pleasure and lightheartedness. Today these definitions are at least partially obsolete.

In our technological society there is an increasingly insufficient amount of work to go around. Productivity has improved to the point that necessities are provided for everyone whether they work or not. Work thus becomes, for many people, separated from its products. At the same time, many jobs are so technical that the period of education and preparation for them must be prolonged. Coupled with early retirement and the obsolescence of many jobs, there seems only a fleeting moment of productivity for many others. Most of the focus in "work contracts" has to do with fringe benefits which are closer to play than work—break time, vacation time, improving surroundings, etc.

The major problem becomes what to do with the free time available. The spirit of work is like the spirit of dedication and does not flourish at leisure or rest. With the contemporary structure it is difficult for many people to feel dedicated to their work; and it is even more difficult for them to feel dedicated to free time. Thus there is a sense of aimlessness in people, both at work and leisure.

Just as work is being transformed, so is play. Play has largely become modern team sports. As such, the spirit of freedom seems to have left, and games are dominated by the spirit of work. The organization of sports, from team to league, are authoritarian with limited rights for "players." Discipline is severe; and practice sessions are more arduous, physically harder with longer hours, than in most "work" activities. Players have frequent injuries, runners reach the point of exhaustion, the game continues in cold or snow. Even among fans, the dedication to losers, as with the New York Met's baseball team during its early years smacks of dedication and duty rather than play. Both players and fans are eager and willing to suffer for their teams.*

The Puritans despised play and eulogized work. As Macauley opined, "The Puritan hated bearbaiting, not because it gave pain to the bear, but because it gave pleasure to the spectators." Gradually sports became acceptable as a part of religious life, and churches even built their own gymnasiums and supported their own teams. The smiling face of Bob Richards is to most Americans familiar, as he shuttles between his two callings, the pulpit and the Wheaties Sports Foundation. The Sunday sermon is as likely to deal with the virtues of play and sport as work.

In fact, for a vast secularized group of Americans, the Sunday sermon has been replaced by the Sunday double-header or "game of the week." They feel compelled to watch "the game" just as their ancestors felt compelled to attend prayer meetings. A tragic dilemma overtakes the truly dedicated sports fan when two major athletic events occur simultaneously. The result is the harried fan who attends one game while listening to the other on his transistor radio. The spirit of the dedicated worker has been transformed into the spirit of the dedicated sportsman.

5. *The players and fans are like members of a tribal society.* Goals and purposes have been supplied for individuals in the past by the traditional groups—family, clan or tribe. Modern mobile society, both geographical and social, has seen the dissolution of these traditional groups, leaving the individual without support in his choice of goals and purpose. In this state there are no absolutes, and the individual often flounders in the quest for identity.

When one becomes identified with a team, he enters a world like the tribal society. The goal is absolute—to win. The "good guys" are clearly separated from the "bad guys"—the other team. They wear different costumes to prove it, and the fans may purchase banners or caps to demonstrate their allegiance.

---

* One of the peculiar paradoxes is that those games which began as play, for example, ball games, have become dominated by the spirit of work, while the only sports which seem now to continue to be playful are those which formerly were essential work activities, i.e., hunting and fishing.

Although they may not have prior personal acquaintance with one another, by sitting in specified sections of the stadium, spectators can be certain of being among fellow tribesmen who share the same beliefs. Each member of the tribe knows the intimate biographies of their representatives, the team members, and heroic stories are exchanged about them. The rules, too, are absolute and unchanging, and the tribesmen learn them in detail.

All of this certainty has a refreshing quality for so many who live in an ambiguous state. There is a sense of membership, of purpose, and of method. There are the badges of distinction and the shared familiarity of information. All of these advantages can be had simply for the price of admission.

What does this have to do with individual development? Each person needs some island of certainty from which to grow. One must be able to stand in one place before he can run or walk. He must start from somewhere that is dependable and consistent and that he can return to in times of stress. There are a diminishing number of such institutions available to most Americans and those which are available have been reduced in their effectiveness. The family which has traditionally transmitted social values to children and sustained them for adults seems no longer able to do its job effectively in the face of social mobility and pluralism.

By contrast, sports have a consistency and a sense of certainty which stand out. The rules and the values associated with sports and athletics are relatively unchanging as compared with other aspects of society. Sports thus can serve as a secure and reliable activity to which a man can return from time to time with full knowledge that he will know what to expect.

Every opportunity for growth carries with it a risk; so obvious was this to Orientals that the Chinese character for danger is also the one for opportunity. The danger with sports is fixation: that rather than serving as a base of operations for further growth and experimentation, they may become the final answer for some individuals. If this becomes so, the game becomes not a game at all but the ultimate, if myopic, solution. The dynamic potential becomes prematurely crystallized in form. The positive characteristics of sports outlined here make such an outcome understandable although undesirable. Of course the same danger exists in any activity to which one commits himself. The qualities of sport are such that they have dominated large numbers of people.

Whatever the dangers, the potentials for growth through athletics are very strongly present. Of particular importance is their availability. For a variety of reasons, some of which have been described, sports are among the most available opportunities for expression open to Americans. Not so easily recognized is their potential for psychological experimentation and manipulation by spectators as well as players.

A segment of the school-age population now seeks alternative solutions to integrating the individual with society; the revolutionary activist is at one pole, the dropout at the other. Perhaps, as there is further change in our society and as new life styles develop, the importance of sports and athletics will become less, but today they still represent an important place where men and women attempt to find personal meaning within societal contradictions. Moreover, individual maturity can be sought by working through symbolic life problems on the athletic field whether as spectator or active player.

This actualization takes place within the context of a group which accepts and supports the individual—so long as he is on the same side. Fans and players move together in a group effort towards the common goal, but with distinctive and individual styles. Sports thereby serve as a suitable vehicle for growth for countless Americans.

REFERENCES

1. Javanovich, W.: Sex, crime and, to a lesser extent, sports. *Saturday Review of Literature,* July 18, 1964.
2. Wedge, B. M.: *Psychological Problems of College Men.* New Haven, Conn., Yale University Press, 1958.
3. Beisser, A. R.: *The Madness in Sports: Psychosocial Observations on Sports.* New York, Appleton-Century-Crofts, 1967.

29

A FAT CHANCE

JAMES P. HARNSBERGER

Weight reduction on a permanent basis is probably one of the least successful treatments in medicine. These patients are usually poorly motivated, somewhat depressed and very discouraged with the whole idea, having tried to lose weight many times. They usually come in because their husband has nagged them to "do something about that weight!" They are usually in very poor shape from lack of exercise and dislike most forms of exercise. Many of these obese people are under-exercised rather than overfed. A woman will come to the doctor with the remark, "I need to lose 10 pounds or so," when actually from an ideal weight chart she needs to lose 30 to 50 pounds.

Usually the physician gives a brief physical, a prescription for an amphetamine, 800 to 1000 calorie diet sheet, and a jovial injunction to "push away from the table." There is rarely any discussion of physical conditioning, how to do it, and its relationship to calories eaten.

I believe that weight reduction without physical conditioning is rarely successful and is almost certainly temporary. Exercise must contain some measure of pleasure or satisfaction. Boring calisthenics for 30 to 60 minutes daily or jogging alone probably will not last long. In groups these exercises last much longer.

Here at The Homestead in Hot Springs, Virginia, we have developed a program utilizing the skills of our Swiss chef and our various sports professionals. Located in the mountains of Virginia, there are 200 miles of walking and bridle paths in the area. Golf courses, tennis courts, swimming pools, horseback riding, skiing and ice skating offer great variety to anyone's taste in exercising and conditioning.

Prior to coming into our program, the patient is asked to have a general physical examination to include CBC, EKG, blood sugar, BUN, PBI, T3, cholesterol, blood lipids and urinalysis.

The results are to be brought with the patient along with any recommendations by the family physician.

On arrival all findings are reviewed with the patient and an evaluation of the patient is performed using the Obesity, Etiological and Physiological Evaluation Form by Strasenburg Pharmaceutical Company. Diet, conditioning and associated physical problems are discussed. We discuss giving bodily physical fitness a higher priority in life's schedule, the needs for it and benefits to be derived. Adjustments for back troubles, orthopedic problems, cardiovascular problems are made as needed. We use Dr. Kenneth Cooper's *Aerobics* as a guide for this phase.

A bulletin board shows the relative calories utilized in playing golf, dancing, swimming, skating, hiking, tennis, horseback riding, skiing and bowling. Finally, sunbathing is illustrated to demonstrate how long it takes to burn up foods if no exercise is performed. Six foods are compared as to number of minutes required to be consumed.

MINUTES USED TO EXPEND CALORIES EATEN

Food	Calories	Sunbathing (1.3 cal/min)	Tennis (10.2 cal/min)	Golf (5 cal/min)
Bread and butter, 1 slice	78	60	7	15
Fried chicken, ½ breast	232	178	22	46
Hamburger, large	350	269	34	70
Chocolate milk shake	502	386	49	100
Strawberry shortcake	400	308	39	80
T-Bone steak	235	180	23	47

The table below illustrates various exercises, moderate to strenuous, and the number of calories expended per minute and per hour in the performance of these activities.

We also discuss the importance of recreation (re-creation), which the dictionary describes as revive, cheer, amuse, enliven (especially after anxiety or labor), reanimate and refresh mentally and physically. Too often among business and professional people recreation is something children do after school. It is something they do not have time for in their schedule. As a result many are obese and in very poor physical condition.

We impress upon them that the two or three weeks here is only a beginning to change habits of eating and exercise.

A 900-calorie diet is prescribed and attractively served. An

CALORIES EXPENDED PER MINUTE AND PER HOUR*

	Minute	Hour
Walking—normal	3.6	216
Walking—fast	5.6	336
Jogging	7.1	426
Running—racing	15.0	900
Cycling—normal	4.5	270
Cycling—racing	11.0	660
Skating	6.0	360
Skiing—snow	9.9	594
Skiing—water	8.0	480
Horseback riding—walk	3.0	180
Horseback riding—trot	8.0	489
Swimming—slow	5.0	300
Swimming—fast	10.0	600
Golfing—walking course	5.0	300
Tennis—singles	10.2	612
Table tennis—Ping Pong	6.0	360
Rowing	5.0	300
Rowing—racing	14.0	840
Bowling	4.5	270
Volley ball	3.5	210
Canoeing	3.0	180

* From *Today's Health*, June, 1965.

hour of calisthenics each morning as a group participation—particularly for the ladies. This is designed for spot reducing—hips, thighs, legs arms and face. Following this, lunch and a rest period. In the afternoon two to three hours of a sport are prescribed. If they do not know how to play, an appointment is made for them with the pro. He also arranges games for groups of equal ability so as not to discourage beginners. Then a rest period and hot bath followed by massage. Dinner and dancing finish out the day.

The patient is checked at three-day intervals. We discuss diet or any problems that may arise. Especially, we point out the need for gradual increase in conditioning so as not to over exert. Above all, we encourage them to persevere.

On this routine many lose 15 to 20 pounds in a two- or three-week period. They show great interest in the direct relationship of exercise to food intake. They begin to understand the excess number of minutes or hours of exercise required to pay for an indiscretion in diet.

The reward to the physician is to see the patients going home leaner, more energetic and more cheerful. Many state, "I feel better than I have since I was in high school."

30

IMMEDIATE CARE OF ATHLETIC INJURIES

H. ROYER COLLINS

More than ever, the physician of today needs to keep himself fit in order to be able to respond to the tremendous demands which his profession places upon him. This has led to increasing participation in sports such as those described elsewhere in this book. The physical activity and relaxation afforded by these are certainly worthwhile. Injuries which do occur are mostly musculoskeletal and not life threatening. However, proper immediate treatment is necessary to avoid chronicity and the possible need to discontinue athletic activity.

As in other fields of medicine, the best treatment is always prevention. Too often, the busy physician is a "weekend athlete," or worse still, a once-a-year participant. He would never think of allowing an unconditioned patient to participate in a football game without going through the usual preparation. Neither would he allow a middle-aged, obese, obviously poorly conditioned man to go out and run in a marathon without previous physical examination and gradual conditioning. The same must hold true for him, although we all recognize that this does not happen.

The musculotendinous unit is only as strong as its weakest link, and if one analyzes the tremendous stresses and forces involved over small areas of the body during physical exertion, he would realize the necessity for preparticipation preparation. It is these forces that contribute to the strains, sprains, dislocations, and other injuries.

To keep fit so that the demands of sports can be met requires year-round exercise. There is no one form of exercise which can produce true fitness, so his program should include

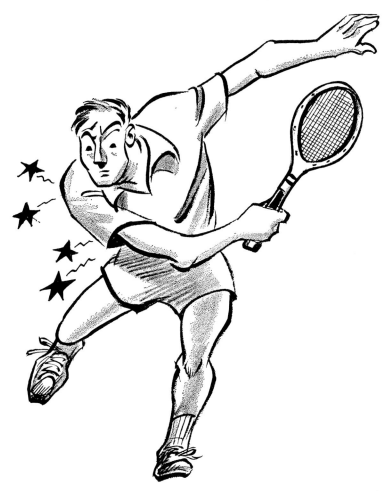

strengthening exercises as well as those which stress flexibility, agility, and endurance. These should be done at least three times per week, but preferably on a daily basis in order to be truly effective. Before participating in an activity, an adequate warm-up period is advisable to avoid pulls and strains.

Shoulder

Problems secondary to attritional changes such as rotator cuff degeneration, bursitis and bicipital tendinitis are common in all sports involving repetitive motion of the shoulder. Treatment involves resting the part to prevent the chronic friction and injection of anti-inflammatory compounds, such as the steroid derivatives, into the involved area. Heat and analgesics may help. Immobilization should not be too prolonged in order to prevent the development of adhesive capsulitis. If calcification is noted in these tissues, this may be aspirated by using two large bore needles, instilling local anesthetic and attempting to flush the liquid calcium out. If the calcium is no longer liquid, this will not work, but usually symptoms will subside with injection alone. If symptoms continue to recur, surgical removal of the calcium deposit may become necessary. The player may have to make some adjustments in his style of play, changing from an overhand to a more sidearm motion to protect a degenerative rotator cuff.

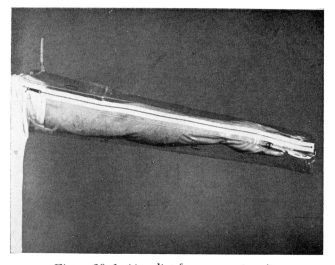

Figure 30–1. Air splint for upper extremity.

Elbow

Lateral epicondylitis or "tennis elbow" is also a common ailment. The number of forms of treatment advocated attest to the difficulty of treatment and indicate that that is no sure cure in all these cases. The pathology is not well understood, with some feeling it is a tendinitis, others a radial humeral bursitis and others something else. The usual initial treatment is ice and rest with avoidance of the activity until the pain has completely subsided. If this does not work, steroid injections into the site of pain and including the radial humeral bursa may be effective. Sometimes several injections may be necessary. If the condition is aggravated when serving or hitting an overhead shot in tennis, which produces maximum extension at the elbow and flexion of the wrist with stretch on the origin of the extensors at the elbow, an Ilfeld brace to prevent full elbow extension may be effective. Changing grip size to larger or smaller and even changing from wood to metal rackets all have helped in some instances. Changing the type of stroking may also be necessary. As a last resort, surgical release of the extensors at the elbow with or without section of the annular ligament may be necessary. A similar condition occurs on the medial side of the elbow and is called "golfer's elbow." The pathology is essentially the same and the treatment is similar to that of lateral epicondylitis.

Wrist

Strains may be placed on the wrist by sudden unexpected twists in tennis or golf or repetitive motions such as casting while fishing. De Quervain's tenosynovitis involving the short extensor and abductors of the thumb may also occur. Heat and rest may be all that is necessary, but occasionally Butazolidin® or injection with steroids as well as cast immobilization may be necessary. In de Quervain's tenosynovitis, surgical release of the extensor retinaculum may be necessary to prevent the repetitive friction which tends to produce it.

If the symptoms are the result of a fall, fracture of the navicular should be ruled out, particularly if there is pain in the anatomical snuff box. Initial x-rays may not show the fracture even on navicular views and x-rays should be obtained ten days to two weeks later if the initial films are negative and symptoms persist. If the navicular is fractured, a cast extending to the interphalangeal joint of the thumb must be applied and maintained until healing occurs.

Spine

In most movement sports, the spine plays an important role. Muscle strains are common and painful. If there is spasm, bed rest is essential, with heat, muscle relaxants and analgesics helpful. The mattress should be firm and a bed board of ¼-inch plywood between the mattress and box springs helps. Any position of comfort is acceptable. Occasionally injections of Xylocaine® and steroid into the trigger area may completely alleviate the symptoms. If symptoms do not subside or signs of a herniated nucleus pulposus develop, traction and physical therapy may help. If not, surgery may be indicated.

As soon as severe symptoms have subsided, Williams' flexion exercises should be started slowly with the numbers of repetitions increased gradually. Muscles around the abdomen and lumbar region must be kept in good condition subsequently, in order to prevent recurrence.

Occasionally jogging to the middle-aged man who has some degeneration and narrowing of the intervertebral disks of the lumbar spine may produce low back pain and one must have to consider changing to an activity which does not require the repetitive pounding which jogging does. This can often be prevented or helped by jogging on soft surfaces and wearing ripple-sole jogging shoes which absorb some of the shock.

Thigh

Strains of the musculotendinous unit are common in this are and they involve any portion of the unit from its tendinous origin to its tendinous insertion. The injury usually occurs at the weakest area and usually at the site of attritional change.

Inadequate warm-up may result in a tearing loose of the attachments to the pelvis (the so-called groin or hamstring pulls) because the muscle is too tight and is unable to either elongate sufficiently or unable to withstand the strain of a sudden muscular contraction. Rest, ice for the first 36 hours, and compression with an ace bandage wrapped in a hip spica fashion should help. Crutches may be necessary. Before returning to further activity, stretching exercises should be performed to prevent recurrence.

If the muscle fibers are weakest, they may rupture with varying degrees of damage and hemorrhage. Ice, compression and
rest using crutches if necessary, should be instituted immediately to prevent disabling hemorrhage and subsequent development of myositis ossificans. Massage is contraindicated. Motions of the leg which are not painful are permitted, and activity may be resumed as soon as this does not produce pain.
If the injury has been relatively severe, motion of the knee
may be limited. No attempt should be made to forcibly regain
motion, as this may produce further hemorrhage. With time
and active exercise just short of pain, the range of motion will
improve. Quadriceps-setting exercises should be started immediately to prevent atrophy. We have not used oral enzymes
routinely, but have injected the area with hyaluronidase 48
hours after injury in some cases. If the muscle has been completely ruptured or the musculotendinous unit at the knee is
disrupted, surgery should be carried out.

Knee

Injuries involving the knee are common. Twisting the partially flexed knee may tear the cartilage or ligaments or produce a traumatic synovitis. The disability may be immediate,
with locking of the joint, instability, and swelling, or may
come on after the activity is completed. The time honored
trio of ice, compression, and elevation are useful along with
the use of crutches. Of course, the knee should be thoroughly
examined as soon as possible to determine the integrity of the
ligaments, and an x-ray is helpful in ruling out possible fracture or osteochondral fracture. A modified cotton cast consisting of strips of mole skin covered by webril, and then plaster
splints laterally placed, followed by conforming-type bandage,
serves to limit motion as well as prevent effusion. If the swelling is severe or the diagnosis is questionable, aspiration of the
knee is done, but this is not done as a routine measure. Occas-
sionally diagnosis may be difficult initially, and repeated examinations may be indicated to make the proper diagnosis.

In a Grade I sprain, treatment is symptomatic as mentioned.
However, in Grade II sprains where there is partial tear of the

ligamentous structures, cast immobilization is carried out until the ligaments have healed. This may require three to six weeks. If the ligament is completely disrupted, indicating a Grade III tear, surgery is the treatment of choice.

Pain after activity without any known injury may be the only symptom, and one must consider the possibility of bursitis involving Voshell's bursa under the medial collateral ligament or pes anserine bursitis under the insertion of the sartorius, gracilis and semitendinosis tendons. The infrapatellar bursa may be involved as may any of the fourteen or so bursae around the knee. Injection with local anesthetic and steroid is usually effective with care to avoid repetitive stress until symptoms subside.

Pain and effusion in the knee without twist or any outside force may indicate chondromalacia patella, early degenerative arthritis, internal derangements, synovitis, or inadequate quadriceps strength or even gout. The diagnosis should be made first with rest, aspiration of fluid if necessary and injection of the joint with steroid if indicated. The underlying pathology should be corrected before returning to activity, or if this is not possible, a new form of recreation may have to be chosen.

Leg

Fractures of the lower extremity occur particularly in skiing. Usually the ski area has a well-equipped team for handling these emergencies with splints, stretchers and procedures for removing the injured skier from the slopes to the emergency room. Of course, care must be taken to prevent further damage; this must be done by splinting with the boots and clothing in place, which can be accomplished very easily with the new air-splints.

Tendo Achillis ruptures are also more common with the new rigid boots used in skiing, but may also occur in running sports due to sudden stress caused by over-elongation or sudden contracture, which is too strong for a tendon which has undergone attritional change. This must be distinguished from the less disabling although painful plantaris or medial gastrocnemius rupture. In tendo Achillis rupture, there is complete loss of integrity, which may only be detected by Thompson's gastrocnemius squeeze test. One must remember that the toe flexors can also plantar flex the foot and even permit standing on tiptoes despite rupture of the Achilles tendon, so these must be relaxed when testing. Treatment of tendo Achillis rupture is usually surgical in order to get adequate reapproximation of fibers, with cast immobilization until healing. Plantaris or medial gastrocnemius rupture can be treated by ice, ace bandate compression, elevation and crutches for a period of approximately three weeks, when ambulation may be possible.

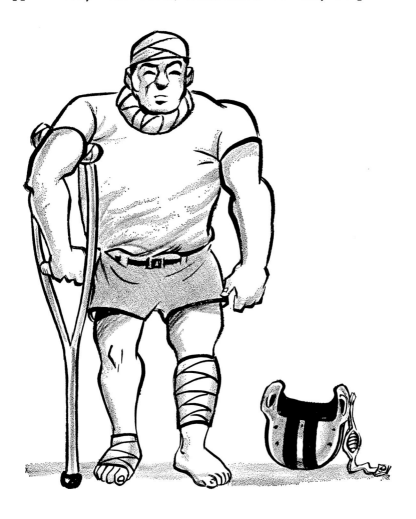

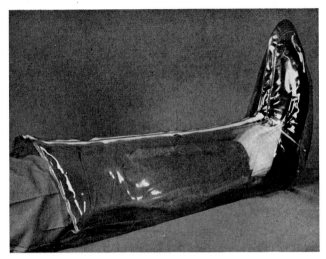

Figure 30–2. Air splint for lower extremity. Note that this can be put on without removing shoes or clothing.

The current enthuiasm for jogging has produced many cases of "shin splints" from running on hard surfaces. This term includes several conditions and is not specific but is commonly used in athletic circles despite the AMA's attempt to change it. There may be involvement of the origin of the posterior fibial or of the anterior tibial muscles. In most instances, a tight gastrocnemius contributes to the problem due to the necessity for the foot to go into valgus with dorsiflexion, producing a stress on the posterior tibial tendon. This painful condition may be prevented by proper stretching of the heel cord prior to running or by wearing ripple-sole track shoes which give some cushioning while running. Once the condition develops, rest and anti-inflammatory agents such as Butazolidin and heat may help. Before resuming activity, the underlying pathology should be corrected and ripple-sole shoes worn with avoidance of hard surfaces. We have been stress fractures of the tibia in joggers with similar symptoms, so this should be kept in mind.

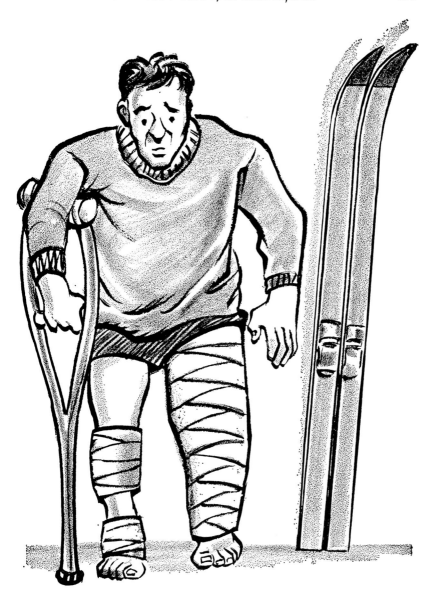

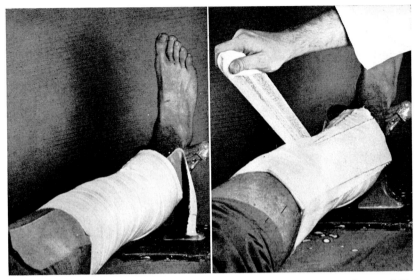

Figure 30–3 *A*, Modified cotton cast for knee compression and immobilization. Moleskin and Webril have been applied; *B*, Completion of knee dressing showing plaster splints along medial and lateral side of knee with moleskin overlapped and application of final layer of conforming gauze.

Ankle

Sprains of the ankle usually occur from an inversion stress with the foot in varying degrees of plantar flexion. The anterior talofibular ligament is most commonly involved but occasionally the anterior tibiofibular ligament and/or the fibulocalcaneal ligament may be.

Immediate application of ice, compression and elevation are necessary to prevent swelling, which prolongs the disability. I prefer to tape these ankles but a gelo-cast may be used. Crutches are also helpful for a couple of days until weight-bearing is possible. If the injury is not too severe, walking with the ankle taped is allowed. Our athletes are treated with ice and early motion after taping during the entire convalescence. If the fibulocalcaneal ligament is torn as well, with instability to inversion stress, a cast should be applied for three to six weeks depending upon the symptoms when the cast is removed. Some form of immobilization should be continued until the injured ligament is no longer tender.

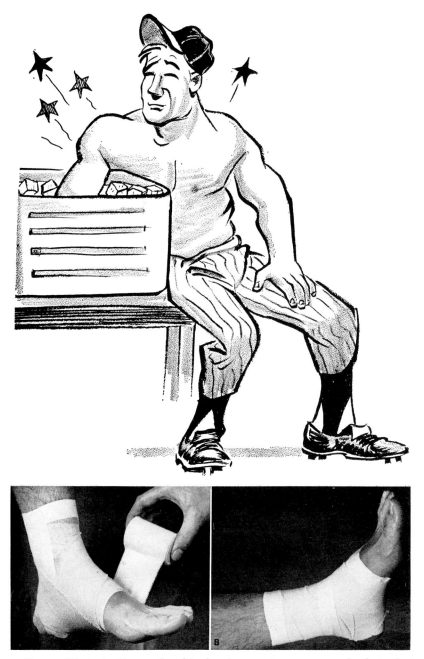

Figure 30–4 *A*, Type of ankle bandage using gauze and elastoplast immediately after sprain to prevent swelling; *B*, Completed ankle dressing.

Dislocation of the peroneal tendon or posterior tibial ten- dinitis must be considered in the differential diagnosis of ankle injuries. In the former, the tendon must be replaced and held by strapping or cast. Posterior tibial tendinitis may be treated by rest, heat, and anti-inflammatory agents such as Butazolidin. If symptoms still persist, steroid injections into the synovial sheath and/or immobilization in a cast may help. Surgery is rarely necessary as the physician usually changes to some other form of activity which will avoid aggravation long before the necessity to operate.

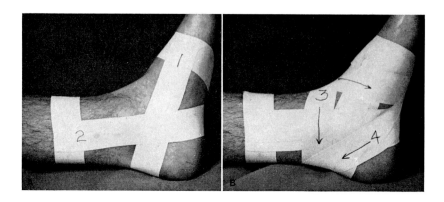

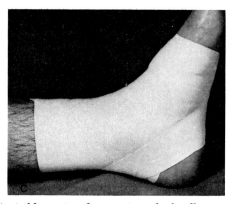

Figure 30–5 *A,* Ankle taping for sprains which allows immediate weight bearing. Note initial stirrup and anchoring pieces; *B,* Note anterior figure of eight strip (#3) and posterior heel lock (#4); *C,* Completion of ankle taping by filling in all spaces.

Foot

"Jogger's heel" is another term used to indicate irritation of the cushion under the calcaneous secondary to the repetitive blows of the heel against a hard surface. Rest, hot baths, foam-rubber heel cushions, plastic heel cups, and ripple-sole jogging shoes have all been used with varying degrees of success. Steroid injections may also help. However, when returning to jogging, ripple-sole shoes and heel pads should be worn and running should be on grass or other soft surfaces. Changing the running gait from heel-toe to flat-foot or sprinters gait may be necessary. Caution should be exercised in running too far forward on the toes, as one may substitute a stress fracture of the metatarsals for a sore heel.

Summary

Sports offer a tremendous change of pace for the busy physician and should help to prolong his life. However, activity should not be sporadic but regular. The physician will not only have more fun and prevent injuries by year-round conditioning, but will also feel the benefits of being fit.

INDEX

385

rods, ultralight, 249
rules for novice caster, 250
Sports
  dangers, 365
  emotional stress, antidote for, 176–180
  exercise
    distinguished from, 167
    fulfillment of biologic need, 167
  fun and enjoyment, 178–179
  growth potentials, 366
  opportunities, 359
  participation in, 168
  psychological aspects, 359–365
Sprinting, 157
  conditioning, 167
  expense, 166
  exercise, 167
    relationship, 169
  facilities, 166
  fun and enjoyment, 178–179
  skills, 166
  time, 166
Stance, in golf, 60
Strategy, in handball, 93
Strokes (*see* Golf; strokes)
Sugarloaf World Cup Races, 209
Swimming (*see* Long distance swimming)
Swing, in golf, 60, 61

T

Tables, for table tennis, 34–35
Table tennis, 27–36
  advantages, 28–29
  balls, 32
  clubs, 31, 33
  equipment, 30
    availability, 30–31, 35
  how to play, 33
  lack of romance, 28–29
  Ping-Ping®, 29, 36
  rackets, 28, 34
    inverted, 34
    requirements, 34
    rubber, 34

    sandpaper, 34
    sandwich, 28, 34
  scoring, 32
  tables, 34–35
  tournaments, 30, 33
    popularity, 30
    United States Open, 33
  training machine, 28
"Take-out" (*see* Curling; armamentarium)
Targets
  skeet shooting, 134
  trapshooting, 134
Target shooting, 129–141
  other facets, 140
Team games
  curling, 81
  lawn bowling, 70, 75
"Tee" 81
Tendinitis (*see* Athletic injuries)
Tennis, 3–26
  advantages, 9–11
  ball, 6
    development, 6
  clinics, 8
  commandments, 24, 25
  courts, 6
    backcourt, 21
    carpet or canvas, 13
    clay or composition surface, 13
    development, 6
    hardtop surfaces, 13
    Lay-kold® surface, 13
    maintenance, 13
    "slow," 16
  doubles (*see* Doubles)
  field tennis, 26
  footwork, 7
  formations, 18
  history, 6–7, 26
  lawn tennis, 13
  learning, 7–9
    concentration, 7
  matches, 17
    "set," 9
  mutual interest, as, 10
  physical conditioning for, 14
  plays